T5-BBX-764

HOSPITAL ACCOUNTING PRACTICE

Volume I

Financial Accounting

Robert W. Broyles, Ph.D.
University of Ottawa

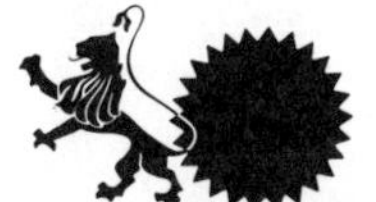

AN ASPEN PUBLICATION®
Aspen Systems Corporation
Rockville, Maryland
London
1982

Library of Congress Cataloging in Publication Data

Broyles, Robert W.
Hospital accounting practice.

Includes index.
Contents: v. 1. Financial accounting—v. 2. Managerial accounting.
1. Hospitals—Accounting. I. Title.
HF5686.H7B76 657'.8322 81-12784
ISBN: 0-89443-340-7 (v. 1) AACR2
ISBN: 0-89443-376-8 (v. 2)

Library of Congress Catalog Card Number: 81-12784
ISBN: 0-89443-340-7

Printed in the United States of America

1 2 3 4 5

Table of Contents

Preface

The purpose of this text is to familiarize practicing administrators and students of health administration with the fundamentals of accounting for health care facilities. Accordingly, the focus of discussion is on the accumulation, presentation and interpretation of information that depicts the financial position and changes in the financial position of these institutions.

The book assumes that readers are unfamiliar with the use of fund accounting and functional accounting in health care facilities. As a result, the material here is of use in health administration programs and by practicing administrators who require an understanding of accounting in the industry.

In this work, financial accounting is developed in essentially four parts. Part I is devoted to a discussion of the fundamental principles of accounting and to an examination of the accounting process. It also looks at accounting issues that are peculiar to health facilities. Part II analyzes the problem of recording and accumulating information depicting the revenues earned and expenses incurred by these institutions. Part III covers the accounting procedures that pertain to the facilities' assets, liabilities, and restricted funds. Part IV concludes with a presentation and interpretation of the institutions' financial statements.

In developing this material, the author has attempted to maintain a balance between accounting theory and practice. In addition, it is hoped that the discussion provides an understanding of the concepts required to use financial information effectively as well as the basis for further study in accounting and financial management.

Robert W. Broyles
December 1981

Acknowledgments

To acknowledge everyone who contributed to this work is an impossible task. However, a special word of gratitude must be expressed to the reviewers of the text whose suggestions were incorporated in the final manuscript and resulted in a far better product than would have been possible otherwise. The contribution of the many students who used early drafts and whose suggestions resulted in an improved presentation are gratefully acknowledged.

Further, the contribution of Mike Brown, Margot Raphael, Eileen Higgins, Jane Coyle, and Samuel M. Sharkey, Jr., are gratefully acknowledged. To Micheline Leblanc who typed many drafts and deciphered my handwriting, I wish to extend my sincere gratitude. The efforts of Johanne Bruyère, who assumed the responsibility of typing the final draft, are gratefully acknowledged.

I also wish to express my appreciation to my family, Rita and Erin, for their patience, understanding, and encouragement.

Recognizing the contribution of all others who made this work possible, the author must, of course, accept the responsibility for any errors.

Part I

Introduction

Chapter 1

Accounting Concepts and Principles

1.1 INTRODUCTION

In general, the basic concepts and principles used in accounting for non-profit organizations—and health care facilities specifically—are similar to those for commercial firms. Accounting may be defined as the accumulation and communication, in conformity with generally accepted principles, of historical and projected economic data that relate to the financial position and the operating results of any enterprise engaging in economic activity. Accounting, then, is a service function that provides information to decision-making bodies that may be internal or external to the institution. If the accounting function is to provide a set of meaningful and understandable data to widely disparate groups of decision makers, the process by which information is accumulated and communicated must adhere to commonly accepted concepts and principles.

The basic principles or conventions of accounting cannot be regarded as absolutely permanent. Rather, they emanate from a continuing evolutionary process in which changes in social, political, and economic activity, data requirements, and technology may result in modifications to basic conventions. Consequently, accounting should be regarded as an art rather than a science. It is in such a spirit that this book is presented.

1.2 FINANCIAL STATEMENTS

The financial statements of an enterprise are the vehicles by which the information accumulated during the accounting process is communicated to individuals or groups who make decisions that influence the institution's economic activity. Financial statements are of two basic types: (1) of financial position and (2) of change in financial position.

1.2.1 Statements of Financial Position

Statements of financial position, known as balance sheets, provide an indication of the financial status of the facility at a moment in time. The balance sheet may be thought of as a photograph of an enterprise's assets or resources, its economic liabilities or obligations, and the owner's equity. The basic elements of the balance sheet are depicted in Table 1-1.

This consolidated balance sheet indicates that the basic elements in the statement of financial position are assets, liabilities, and owner's equity. A discussion of each component follows.

1.2.1.1 Assets

Assets refer to the economic resources owned by the institution. Examples of assets usually found in the balance sheet are cash, inventories, accounts receivable, notes receivable, land, buildings, equipment, and the institution's investment in interest-earning securities. Resources are selected for inclusion in the balance sheet if their value may be quantified objectively and measured in monetary units. As a consequence, even though intangibles such as good community relations and employee morale are valuable resources, they are not included in the statement of financial position. As is discussed in Chapter 3, the assets of the health care facility frequently are segregated and reported in accordance with the principles of fund accounting.

To anticipate this discussion, it is important to note that the health facility frequently receives resources that must be used in accordance with restrictions imposed by donors. Fund accounting is simply a mechanism of segregating assets, liabilities, and owner's equity into essentially two sets of self-balancing accounts. One set pertains to unrestricted resources while the other reflects those resources that must be used for donor-specified purposes.

1.2.1.2 Liabilities

Liabilities may be defined as the economic obligations of the enterprise. Examples of liabilities found in the balance sheet are payables such as accounts, notes, salary and wages, mortgage, and interest. As in the case of assets, liabilities also are segregated and reported in accordance with the principles of fund accounting.

Table 1-1 Consolidated Balance Sheet

Assets	$1,000
Liabilities	800
Owner's Equity	200
	1,000

1.2.1.3 Owner's Equity

In a commercial enterprise, the owner's equity is the residual interest or equity of the company's owners. Similarly, owner's equity in the hospital is the residual equity that is the excess of assets over liabilities. As in the case of liabilities and assets, owner's equity frequently is segregated in accordance with the principles of fund accounting. The reason for this segregation and other difficulties encountered in consideration of owner's equity are discussed in Chapter 3.

1.2.1.4 The Accounting Equation

The relationship between assets (A), liabilities (L), and owner's equity (E) is expressed by

$$A = L + E \tag{1.1}$$

which is called the accounting equation. This equation, which is simply an identity, expresses the equality between total assets and the total claims on those assets. This equality is maintained in accounting and is the basis for the construction of the balance sheet.

A rearrangement of the arguments in Equation 1.1 highlights the residual nature of owner's equity. If L is subtracted from both sides of the equation, we obtain

$$A - L = E \tag{1.2}$$

which indicates that total assets less the claims of creditors yield the residual ownership in the enterprise.

1.2.2 Income or Operating Statements

Just as the balance sheet represents a photograph of the financial position of the enterprise at a point in time, the operating or income statement may be thought of as a motion picture that portrays changes during the period. The income statement provides a summary of revenues earned and expenses incurred during the period. Hence, the income statement produces information that is germane to the analysis of the extent to which the institution achieved its objective of obtaining revenues at least equal to, or in excess of, expenses during the period.

The basic elements of the income statement are: (1) the revenues earned during the period, (2) the expenses incurred in earning the income of the period, and (3) the net gain or loss of the period. Table 1-2 is a condensed income statement that expresses the relation among the three elements.

As suggested by this statement, the net income of period t (NI_t) is simply the excess of the revenues earned (R_t) over the expenses incurred (Ex_t). This relation is summarized by

$$NI_t = R_t - Ex_t \tag{1.3}$$

Similarly, a net loss (NL_t) is incurred during periods in which expenses exceed revenues; this relation is summarized by

$$NL_t = R_t - Ex_t \tag{1.4}$$

where $Ex_t > R_t$. The following analysis considers the definitions of revenues and expenses in more detail.

1.2.2.1 Revenues

The discussion of the accounting equation notes that the equity of the enterprise is simply the excess of assets over liabilities. Revenues may be defined as gross increases in assets or gross decreases in liabilities resulting from an activity that changes owner's equity. Examples of activities that earn income are the provision of inpatient and outpatient care, the receipt of investment income, and the sale of laundry or dietary services to another hospital.

It must be emphasized that not all activities that result in a gross increase in assets or a gross decrease in liabilities generate revenue. For example, an increase in cash resulting from a bank loan is not revenue, nor is the repayment of the loan and the reduction of the associated liability. It is convenient to think of revenue as resulting from a transaction in which an increase in a given asset account, such as cash, is unaccompanied by either an equal decrease in another asset, such as an account receivable, or by an equal increase in a liability account such as a note payable.

Table 1-2 Condensed Income Statement

	Year Ended December 197-
Revenues	$1,000.00
Less Expenses	750.00
Net Income	250.00

1.2.2.2 Expenses

Where revenue is defined as gross increases in assets or gross decreases in liabilities resulting from activities that change owner's equity, expenses are defined as gross decreases in assets or gross increases in liabilities resulting from activities that change that equity. Obvious examples of expenses are wages and salaries, supplies, rent, utilities, minor repairs, and depreciation. Expenses, like revenues, usually are classified by department or function.

Not all decreases in assets or increases in liabilities are regarded as expenses. For example, the decrease in cash associated with the repayment of a loan and the issuance of a liability to acquire a piece of capital equipment are not normally regarded as expenses. Consequently, it is convenient to think of an expense as a decrease in an asset, such as cash, that is not accompanied by either an equal increase in another asset or by an equal increase in a liability account.

1.2.2.3 Net Income and Net Losses

This discussion demonstrates that revenues increase owner's equity and expenses decrease it. As a result, during periods in which revenues exceed expenses, the net increase in owner's equity is equal to the net income earned during that time. Similarly, during periods in which expenses exceed revenues, the net reduction in owner's equity is equal to the net loss of the period.

1.3 ACCOUNTING PRINCIPLES AND CONCEPTS

To ensure that the information conveyed by the financial statements is relevant, understandable, consistent, and verifiable, the process of accumulating and communicating economic data must adhere to a number of basic accounting concepts and principles. This provides the basis for examining the performance of an institution during different time periods as well as comparing two or more facilities. This also tends to ensure that a given transaction will yield similar effects on the financial position of one or more facilities. The more important principles and concepts that are germane to accounting for profit and nonprofit enterprises are studied next. Accounting concepts that are peculiar to health facilities are discussed in Chapter 3.

1.3.1 Entity Concept

The health facility or any other business enterprise is viewed as an entity that is capable of taking action and engaging in economic activity. It is regarded as an independent entity whose economic activities are accounted for in a manner that is separate and distinct from those of individuals who may be associated with the institution. Further, if the facility is but one element of a larger organization such as a governmental unit or church, the accounting procedures should be designed to permit the determination of the entity's operating results and financial position as distinct from the parent organization's income statement and balance sheet.

1.3.2 Continuity Concept

A related assumption is that the institution will continue with an almost infinite life. The continuity concept is reflected in several accounting practices such as the valuation of plant and equipment at cost rather than at market value and the allocation of certain costs into future periods.

1.3.3 Transaction Concept

Given that the institution is viewed as having a relatively permanent life, the result of each transaction it enters into should be recorded and reported by the accounting system. Clearly, if the accounting system is to provide results that are valid and dependable, all transactions must be recorded. If all transactions that materially influence the financial position (and changes in it) are not included in the institution's records and reports, an element of arbitrariness is introduced and the accounting system is likely to fail in its major role of reflecting the financial situation accurately.

1.3.4 Cost Valuation Concept

The transaction concept implies that all activities that materially affect the entity must be included in its accounting records and reflected in its financial reports. Since such transactions must be given formal accounting recognition, it is necessary to consider the method of determining the value attributed to their elements. For example, retail prices, wholesale prices, replacement prices, and purchase costs can be used to record transactions in which the institution acquires needed resources.

The most useful method of recording transactions is to employ the cost to the institution or the price paid in acquiring the items. The major advantage of cost evaluation is that the price paid is verifiable as well as definite in both time and place. The major disadvantage involves the likelihood that, over time, prices probably will change in response to new technologies and general economic conditions. Under the cost valuation approach, the value of each transaction is linked to the cost of acquisition at the time the purchase is made. The disadvantage, however, may be overcome by presenting financial statements in terms of current market value so as to account for price changes.

1.3.5 Cash and Accrual Concepts

At this point, it is desirable to emphasize the difference between cash and accrual accounting systems. In a cash accounting system, transactions are recorded at the time cash is received or disbursed. For example, suppose that the institution earns revenue by providing a service in March and that the corresponding cash receipt is realized in May. Under a cash accounting system, the revenue is recognized in May rather than March. Consequently, if the institution engages in no other transactions, the reported income for March is understated while that for May is overstated. Similarly, suppose the institution incurs an expense in January that results in a cash disbursement in February. Under the cash accounting system the expense is recognized in February rather than January. Thus, assuming the institution engages in no other transactions, the reported expenses for January are understated while those for February are overstated.

These illustrations suggest that the cash accounting system does not accurately portray the financial activity or financial position of an institution that acquires assets such as accounts receivable, inventories, and notes receivable or incurs liabilities such as accounts payable and notes payable. Consequently, a cash accounting system is appropriate only when an organization has no major assets other than cash and incurs few or no liabilities.

By contrast, under the accrual concept, revenue is recognized in the period in which it is earned irrespective of when, if ever, the associated cash inflow occurs. The *realization rule* states that income should be recorded in the period in which it is earned or captured. In general, revenue is recognized when a sale is consummated or when service is provided.

Similarly, the accrual concept dictates that expenses are recognized and recorded in the time period in which they are incurred. Thus, the recognition of expenses depends on the consumption of resources in the production of revenue. The *contribution rule* states that expenses should be recorded in periods during which resources contribute to operations regardless of when, if ever, the cash outflow occurs.

In summary, under a cash accounting system, revenue is recorded only when cash is received and an expense only when cash is disbursed. As a result, a cash accounting system fails to recognize all of the revenues and expenses of a given period. Under the accrual concept, revenue and expenses are recorded in accordance with both the realization and contribution rules. All revenues and expenses thus are included in the financial records and reports of the period in which they are earned or contribute to operations. The consideration of size and volume of activity therefore suggests that accrual accounting should be used in most health care facilities.

1.3.6 Matching Concept

Closely related to the accrual concept is the matching of related revenues and expenses. The derivation of net income discussed earlier assumes that the revenues recognized under the accrual concept are matched with the expenses of the period in which the revenue is earned. Thus, in computing the net income of a period, the revenues and expenses in the calculation must pertain to the same accounting period.

1.3.7 Double Entry Accounting

The point that transactions that materially influence an institution's financial position (and changes in it) should be recorded has been discussed. Transactions that materially influence the health facility are recorded in accordance with the double entry accounting system.

The double entry system and the rules of debit and credit are based on the accounting equation introduced earlier:

$$A = L + E$$

Arguments on the left side of the equation are termed debit accounts; those on the right are called credit accounts. To increase an asset that appears on the left side of the equation, a debit entry is recorded; to reduce an asset, a credit entry is recorded. Conversely, to increase a liability or equity, which also is called the fund balance, a credit entry is required and to reduce a liability or the fund balance, a debit entry is made. These rules can be summarized as follows:

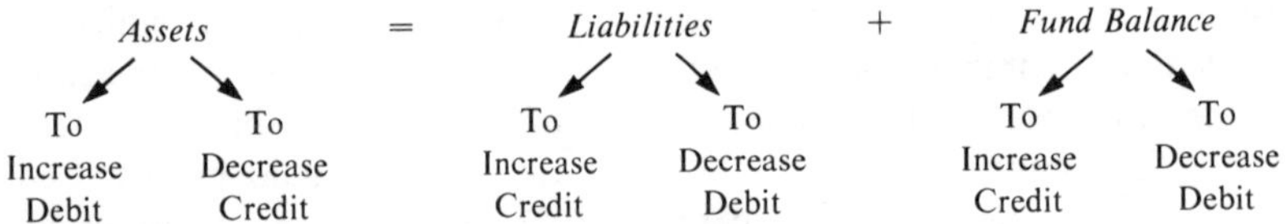

If the accounting has been performed correctly, the sum of the debit entries must equal the sum of credit entries.

To preserve the balance between debits and credits, each transaction must be analyzed and recorded from two aspects. A transaction can be analyzed as representing a direct increase or decrease in an asset, liability, or equity (fund balance) account. For example, assume the institution purchases $6,000 worth of inventory on credit. Obviously, inventory (an asset) has been increased by $6,000 and, in accordance with the accounting equation, the asset account titled Inventories must be debited by $6,000. On the other hand, a

$6,000 liability has been incurred in the inventory acquisition. Thus, in accordance with the rules of debit and credit derived from the accounting equation, the liability account Accounts Payable must be credited for $6,000. The entry required to record the transaction is:

	Debit	*Credit*
Inventory	$6,000	
Accounts Payable		$6,000

which serves to increase inventory (an asset) by the $6,000 debit entry and to increase accounts payable (a liability) by the $6,000 credit entry.

Clearly, not all transactions are analyzed easily in terms of asset, liability, or equity accounts. For example, consider the payment of cash for labor. Obviously, an asset has been reduced by the payment and the transaction results in a credit to the cash account so as to reflect the decrease. The corresponding debit entry, however, raises a serious problem. A wage cost clearly is not an asset, although some benefit presumably has been obtained from the services of labor. A similar problem is encountered when, for example, a hospital sells dietary services to another health care facility. In recording the sale, the hospital should debit an asset account such as cash or accounts receivable and credit the equity account or the fund balance. Recall, however, that the fund balance represents the *excess* of assets over liabilities. Therefore, a credit entry to the equity account in the amount of the sale, without a proper reduction reflecting resources consumed in providing the service, results in an overstatement of the hospital's equity or fund balance.

The solution to these problems is to introduce nominal or temporary accounts, which are subdivisions of the equity account, into the system. The nominal accounts are revenues earned and expenses incurred during the period. Unlike the balances appearing in the permanent accounts that are presented in the balance sheet and are retained from one period to the next, the balances associated with temporary accounts are presented in the income statement, eliminated at the end of the accounting period, and employed to determine the net income or loss of the period. Accordingly, the advantage of the nominal or temporary accounts is that they permit an analysis of net changes in equity.

As has been pointed out, revenues increase, and expenses reduce, owner's equity. Since the revenue and expenditure accounts are subdivisions of the equity account, the accounting equation becomes

$$A = L + E + R - Ex$$

where the plus sign preceding the argument R reflects the 1:1 positive correspondence between equity and revenue while the minus sign preceding Ex

indicates the 1:1 negative correspondence between equity and expenditures. A slight rearrangement of the equation yields

$$A + Ex = L + E + R \tag{1.5}$$

Again, to increase accounts on the left-hand side of the equation, a debit entry is recorded and to decrease such accounts a credit is entered. To increase an account on the right-hand side, a credit entry is recorded, and to decrease such an account a debit entry is shown. The rules of debit and credit derived from the accounting equation, including the nominal or temporary accounts, may be summarized as follows:

	To Increase	*To Decrease*
Assets	Debit	Credit
Expenses	Debit	Credit
Liability	Credit	Debit
Equity	Credit	Debit
Revenues	Credit	Debit

The same relations also may be summarized by using T accounts, in which the left-hand side corresponds to a debit entry and the right-hand side to a credit:

Asset and Expense Accounts		*Liability, Equity, and Revenue Accounts*	
Debit To Increase	Credit To Decrease	Debit To Decrease	Credit To Increase

1.3.8 Periodic Reporting

The objective of the accounting system is to communicate financial information about the entity in a meaningful way to interested parties. Accounting, then, is the vehicle by which an enterprise seeks to answer the following kinds of questions:

1. How do the revenues and expenditures compare for this period?
2. What is the financial position of the enterprise at the end of the period?
3. What are the sources and applications of the funds received by the enterprise?

To answer these questions, the set of financial statements discussed earlier is prepared at the end of the accounting period. In addition to these, interim reports should be prepared monthly for management purposes.

In general, the fundamental principles described in this chapter are used in accounting for both nonprofit and for-profit organizations. We will consider issues that differentiate accounting for a commercial firm from accounting for a nonprofit organization after reviewing the accounting process which is presented in the next chapter.

Questions for Discussion

1. Define the following terms:

   a. Accounting
   b. Balance Sheet
   c. Assets
   d. Liabilities
   e. Fund Balance (Equity)
   f. Income Statement
   g. Revenue
   h. Expense
   i. Net Income (Loss)

2. Describe briefly and indicate the importance of:

   a. Entity Concept
   b. Continuity Concept
   c. Transaction Concept
   d. Cost Evaluation Concept
   e. Accrual Concept
   f. Matching Concept
   g. Double Entry Accounting

3. Explain the accounting equation.
4. Derive the rules of debit and credit from the accounting equation.
5. Summarize briefly and describe the importance of:

   a. The Realization Rule
   b. The Contribution Rule

Problems for Solution

1. Use the rules of debit and credit to record the following hospital transactions:

   a. it purchases $200 of supplies on account
   b. it receives $400 in cash as a prepayment for the use of service

c. it provides service under Transaction 1(b) valued at $300
d. it provides service to patients on account as follows:

inpatients $800
outpatients $1,200

e. it pays $150 under Transaction 1(a)
f. it receives $1,500 cash under Transaction 1(d)
g. it pays wages and salaries of $500
h. it prepays an annual insurance premium of $240

2. Assess the correctness of each entry in the following and, if any one is incorrect, prepare a correct entry:

a. The institution receives $8,000 on January 1 as a prepayment for the use of service:

Cash	$8,000	
Inpatient Revenue		$6,000
Outpatient Revenue		2,000

b. The hospital provides $3,000 worth of services to patients on account:

Patient Revenue	$3,000	
Accounts Receivable		$3,000

c. The hospital purchases $7,000 worth of supplies on account:

Supplies	$7,000	
Accounts Receivable		$7,000

d. The hospital pays wages and salaries of $8,000:

Wage and Salary Expense	$8,000	
Wages and Salaries Payable		$8,000

3. Use the rules of debit and credit to record the following transactions:

a. Supplies Purchased on Account, $700
b. Payments on Accounts Payable, $200
c. Payment on Mortgage Payable:

Principal	$150
Interest	30

d. Payment of Other Operating Expenses:

Salaries and Wages	$900
Purchases Services	30
Other Expenses	10

Chapter 2

The Accounting Process

An understanding of this text depends to a significant extent on acquiring a knowledge of the fundamentals of accounting. The accounting equation—and the rules of debit and credit that are derived from it—are presented in Chapter 1. It is on these rules that the fundamental principles of financial accounting are based. The purpose of this chapter is to use these rules in describing the process by which accounting information is analyzed, recorded, accumulated, and reported—i.e., a brief review of the accounting process.

2.1 BASIC ELEMENTS OF THE ACCOUNTING PROCESS

Figure 2-1 identifies four phases that comprise the accounting process: (1) journalizing transactions, (2) summarization of data, (3) adjustment of data, and (4) preparation of financial statements and closing entries. This section reviews each of these phases briefly.

2.1.1 Journalizing Transactions

When journalizing or recording transactions, it is necessary to perform the following operations:

1. Select the events that are to be included in the accounting process. Not all events that influence the assets or liabilities of the institution are or can be included at the time they occur.
2. Analyze the events to determine their influence on the financial position of the enterprise.
3. Measure the influence of these events in monetary or financial terms.
4. Classify the effects, as measured in monetary units, in accordance with the revenue, expense, asset, liability, and owner's equity items that are influenced by the event.

Figure 2-1 Phases of the Accounting Process

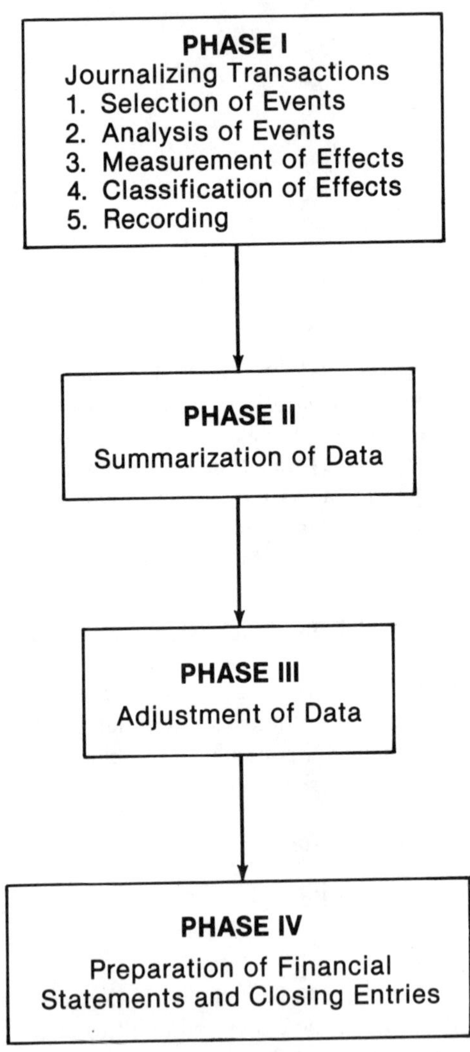

5. Record the effects according to the rules of debit and credit described previously.

Even though these operations are presented in serial fashion, they are not mutually exclusive when viewed from a conceptual perspective and several are performed simultaneously.

As mentioned, the effects of the institution's transactions are recorded according to the rules of debit and credit that emanate from the accounting equation of the form

$$\text{Assets} + \text{Expenses} = \text{Liabilities} + \text{Equity} + \text{Revenue}$$

Recall that

1. to increase (decrease) an asset or an expense, a debit (credit) entry is required; and
2. to increase (decrease) a liability, an equity item, or revenue, a credit (debit) entry is required.

When applying these rules to record transactions, accountants use several journals, each of which has a specific purpose. Most journals are multicolumn forms in which a chronological record of the effects of transactions is entered. Special journals have been designed to permit the efficient recording of different kinds of transactions. The institution may include revenue journals, a cash receipt journal, a cash disbursement journal, a voucher register, and a payroll journal.

2.1.2 Summarization

The second phase of the accounting process in Figure 2-1 is devoted to the summarization of the information contained in the journal system. As noted, the effects of transactions are journalized in chronological order, which indicates that the increases and decreases in a given account are spread throughout the journal. As a consequence, the journal system does not generate the account balances required for the preparation of interim reports or the annual financial statements.

Since the journal system does not indicate account balances, it is necessary to assemble the information that pertains to a single item in one place. This process is accomplished by posting or transferring all information in the journal to the ledger, of which there are several types: the general ledger, a subsidiary accounts receivable ledger, a subsidiary inventory ledger, a subsidiary accounts payable ledger, and a subsidiary plant and equipment ledger.

2.1.3 Adjustment

The third phase of the accounting cycle stems from the need to divide the more or less continuous life of the institution into accounting periods of arbitrary lengths as well as to match revenues and expenses on an accrual basis. Before the preparation of the financial statements, it is necessary to ensure the inclusion of all transactions that pertain to the period and the exclusion of those involving other periods. Once the journal information has been posted or transferred to the ledger, the account balances must be examined to evaluate the extent to which each has been stated properly, since several of the accounts normally will require adjustments. For example, adjustments frequently are required to reflect accurately such items as deferred and accrued revenue, prepaid and accrued expenses, inventory expenses and holdings, depreciation charges, and uncollectable receivables.

To illustrate the need for adjusting entries, suppose that an institution rents a building for three months at $1,000 per month, which it prepays. An asset—the right to occupy space—has been exchanged for another asset, cash. Under the rules of debit and credit, this transaction is recorded in the general journal as follows:

	Dr.	*Cr.*
Prepaid Rent	$3,000	
Cash		$3,000

At the end of the first month, a portion of the asset has been consumed and a rent expense has been incurred. As a consequence, it is necessary to reduce the asset represented by prepaid rent and to recognize the rent expense. Thus, an accurate portrayal of the institution's assets and expenses requires the following entry at the end of the first month:

Rent Expense	$1,000	
Prepaid Rent		$1,000

In this case, the preparation of financial statements based on unadjusted data would understate expenses as well as overstate assets, net income, and the end-of-period fund balance. Hence, to provide an accurate portrayal of operating results and financial position, adjusting entries at the end of the accounting period is required frequently.

2.1.4 Preparation of Financial Statements and Closing Entries

Figure 2-1 shows that the final phase of the accounting process is devoted to the preparation of financial statements and to the elimination of the balances in the temporary accounts by recording and posting the closing entries. As mentioned earlier, the financial reports of an institution consist of statements that depict its financial position and operating results. Operational results are reported in the income statement and in the statement of changes in fund balances. The financial position is portrayed in the balance sheet and in the statement of changes in financial position that depicts the sources and applications of funds.

This final step involves the elimination of the balances in the temporary or nominal accounts. It will be recalled that revenues and expenses represent temporary subdivisions of owner equity. Given the nonprofit orientation of most health care facilities, a periodic review of the extent to which the full costs of operation are returned to the institution in the form of revenue is required to ensure financial viability. Such an evaluation requires a comparison of the revenues earned and the costs incurred during a specific period. Since the focus of evaluation is on the performance of the institution during the current period, previous revenues and expenses are not incorporated in the analysis. As a result, the balances of the temporary or nominal accounts in the annual income statement must be eliminated by a set of closing entries. When these balances are reduced to zero, the operating results achieved during the next period are not confused with those of the current period.

2.2 ILLUSTRATION OF ACCOUNTING CYCLE

To provide a quick review of the accounting process, the rest of this chapter is devoted to a simplified illustration of the accounting cycle for a hypothetical hospital. Table 2-1 presents the general ledger balances of Care City Hospital at the beginning of the accounting period. In an actual situation the ledger balances would have a much larger number of accounts and probably would be grouped by funds. The absence of realism, however, need not detract seriously from the following review.

Table 2-1 General Ledger Balances

CARE CITY HOSPITAL

General Ledger Balances

January 1, 1980

	Dr.	*Cr.*
Cash	$450	
Accounts Receivable	60	
Plant and Equipment	200	
Inventories	50	
Accumulated Depreciation		$100
Accounts Payable		250
Mortgage Payable		175
Fund Balance		235
	760	760

The general ledger of Care City Hospital along with other accounts that will be used in the illustration are summarized in Table 2-2. The account balances in the ledger are those presented in Table 2-1. The opening balances are designated by the notation (OB) so they may be distinguished subsequently from the posting of later transactions.

2.2.1 Journalizing Transactions

During the accounting period, Care City Hospital engages in numerous transactions involving: (1) the provision of service to patients, (2) the purchase of consumable supplies, (3) cash receipts, (4) cash disbursements, and (5) payment of expenses. As indicated in the opening section of this chapter, the first step in the accounting process is to analyze and measure the effects of these transactions and to record them in the journal. The transactions assumed here and the required journal entries are described next.

2.2.1.1 Prospective Payment

Suppose that one of the third party payers assumes the responsibility for financing the costs of care of insured patients by paying this institution $500 before the provision of service and the generation of revenue. Using the rules of debit and credit developed earlier, the receipt of the prepayment increases an asset (cash) and a liability (deferred revenue). As a result, the Cash asset account is debited for $500 and the Deferred Revenue liability account is credited for $500:

Journal Entry # 1

Cash	$500	
Deferred Revenue		$500
To record the receipt of prospective payment from third party.		

2.2.1.2 Purchase of Supplies

During the accounting period, Care City Hospital purchases consumable supplies worth $200 on credit. This example assumes that the acquisition of supplies is recorded initially as an expense of the period. As a result, this transaction increases an expense, which requires a debit entry to the Supply Expense account. In addition, the extension of credit to the institution results in an obligation to pay the vendor at a future date so, as a consequence, the transaction also increases a liability that requires a credit entry to Accounts Payable. Thus, the acquisition of the supply items is recorded by

Journal Entry # 2

Supply Expense	$200	
Accounts Payable		$200
To record the acquisition of supplies on account.		

Table 2-2 The General Ledger

CARE CITY HOSPITAL

General Ledger

January 1, 1980

Cash		*Accounts Receivable*		*Plant & Equipment*	
(OB)* $450		(OB) $60		(OB) $200	

Inventories		*Accumulated Depreciation*		*Accounts Payable*	
(OB) $50			$100 (OB)		$250 (OB)

Mortgage Payable		*Fund Balance*	
	$175 (OB)		$235 (OB)

*OB = opening balance.

2.2.1.3 Provision of Patient Service on Account

Just as suppliers extend credit to customers, health care facilities extend credit to patients and to other third party payers. In such a situation, patient care is provided and revenue is earned before cash is received and, as a consequence, the institution acquires the right to a subsequent payment. Rights to future payments are recorded in an account that is entitled Accounts Receivable. To illustrate, suppose that during the period Care City Hospital provides service on account as follows:

Outpatient Revenue	$400
Inpatient Revenue	200
Total	600

In accordance with the rules of debit and credit, to increase an asset account (e.g., Accounts Receivable) a debit entry is required. On the other hand, to increase a revenue account (e.g., Inpatient Revenue and Outpatient Revenue) a credit entry is needed. Consequently, this revenue-generating activity may be recorded as follows:

Journal Entry # 3

Accounts Receivable	$600	
Inpatient Revenue—Nonplan		$200
Outpatient Revenue—Nonplan		400
To record the provision of service on account.		

In this entry, the Inpatient Revenues—Nonplan and Outpatient Revenues—Nonplan accounts identify the income generated by providing care that is not financed by the prepayment recorded in Journal Entry # 1.

2.2.1.4 Payment on Accounts Payable

As mentioned, the institution is required to disburse cash at a future date in order to extinguish a liability when resources are acquired on account. In such a situation, the disbursement reduces both the cash balance and the liability that is represented by the corresponding account payable. To illustrate, suppose that Care City Hospital pays $200 on an outstanding account. The cash disbursement and the corresponding reduction in the obligations of the institution are recorded as follows:

Journal Entry # 4

Accounts Payable	$200	
Cash		$200
To record payment of outstanding account.		

Here it is assumed that the outstanding accounts payable of the institution are related to transactions involving vendors who provide Care City Hospital with consumable supplies.

2.2.1.5 Provision of Prepaid Services

In the first journal entry, one third party payer reimbursed the institution on a prospective basis. When the $500 was received, the institution assumed an obligation to provide service to patients who were insured by the third party. It now is assumed that Care City Hospital provides care to patients insured by the third party that, when valued at the full established fees of the institution, amount to $500. By providing service, the institution not only earns income but also extinguishes the obligation it assumed when it received the prepayment. In this case, revenue is recognized and the liability is reduced by the following entry:

Journal Entry # 5

Deferred Revenue	$500	
Inpatient Revenue—Plan		$500

To record the provision of service to patients ensured by the prospective third party payer.

Similar to the earlier discussion, the Inpatient Revenue—Plan account identifies the income from providing service that is financed by the prepayment recorded in the first journal entry.

2.2.1.6 Payment on Outstanding Mortgage

Table 2-1 also shows that as of January 1, 1980, the balance of the outstanding mortgage payable amounts to $175. If Care City Hospital disburses $62, of which $12 represents the payment of interest expense and $50 is applied to the outstanding balance, the result is:

1. the cash balance must be reduced by $62;
2. interest expense must be increased by $12; and
3. the outstanding mortgage balance must be reduced by $50.

As a result, the mortgage payment is recorded as follows:

Journal Entry # 6

Mortgage Payable	$50	
Interest Expense	12	
Cash		$62

To record payment on the mortgage payable and interest expense.

In addition to mortgages, health care facilities usually have other long-term obligations, portions of which must be honored during the current period. In such a situation, a record similar to Journal Entry # 6 usually is required.

2.2.1.7 Payment of Salaries and Wages

During the period, it is assumed that the employees of the institution are paid $300. As a result, it is necessary to record the salary and wage expense and the corresponding cash disbursement. A simplified entry to record such a payment is given by

Journal Entry # 7

Salary and Wage Expense	$300	
Cash		$300
To record the payment of wages and salaries.		

It should be noted that this entry is overly simplified. However, a more detailed discussion of payroll accounting and the process of recording labor costs is presented in Chapter 5. At this point, the entries above represent the transactions Care City Hospital engaged in during the period.

2.2.2 Summarization

To obtain the end-of-period balance for each account of Care City Hospital, the entries recorded above must be posted from the journal to the ledger. The transfer of each debit and credit entry, coupled with the opening balances, provides the basis for the development of a preadjusted trial balance (Table 2-3). The transfer of each entry (with the number of the entry in parentheses) is presented in Table 2-3. These calculations provide the basis for developing the preadjusted trial balance presented in Table 2-4. The preadjusted trial balance ensures that the sum of the debits is equal to the sum of the credits. Such an equality is necessary if the accounting entries have been recorded properly.

2.2.3 Adjusting the Accounts

As noted, many of the accounts in the preadjusted trial balance may require adjustment of one kind or another. Frequently, adjustments are required for (1) deferred and accrued revenue, (2) prepaid and accrued expense, (3) inventories, (4) depreciation, (5) uncollectable accounts, and (6) miscellaneous matters. Only a sample of such adjustments is presented here.

2.2.3.1 Prepaid and Accrued Expenses

In general, a prepaid expense arises when a payment is made in the current period on an expense that relates to a future period. Examples are premiums on insurance policies and the payment of rent in advance. When such advance payments are made, the debit is to an asset account (e.g., Prepaid Insurance).

Table 2-3 General Ledger after Transfers of Entries

CARE CITY HOSPITAL

General Ledger

January 1, 1980

Cash

Debit	Credit
(OB)* $450	200 (4)
(1) 500	62 (6)
	300 (7)
388	

Accounts Receivable

Debit	Credit
(OB) $60	
(3) 600	
660	

Plant & Equipment

Debit	Credit
(OB) $200	
200	

Inventories

Debit	Credit
(OB) $50	
50	

Accumulated Depreciation

Debit	Credit
	$100 (OB)
	100

Accounts Payable

Debit	Credit
(4) $200	$250 (OB)
	200 (2)
	250

Mortgage Payable

Debit	Credit
(6) $50	175
	125

Fund Balance

Debit	Credit
	$235 (OB)
	235

Deferred Revenue

Debit	Credit
(5) $500	$500 (1)
	0

Supply Expense

Debit	Credit
(2) $200	
200	

Inpatient Revenue—Nonplan

Debit	Credit
	$200 (3)
	200

Outpatient Revenue—Nonplan

Debit	Credit
	$400 (3)
	400

Interest Expense

Debit	Credit
(6) $12	
12	

Salary & Wage Expense

Debit	Credit
(7) $300	
300	

Inpatient Revenue—Plan

Entry
(5) $500

* OB = opening balance.

Numbers in parentheses refer to journal entries described in Section 2.2.1.

Table 2-4 Pre-adjusted Trial Balance

CARE CITY HOSPITAL

Trial Balance

	Dr.	Cr.
Cash	$388	
Accounts Receivable	660	
Plant and Equipment	200	
Inventories	50	
Accumulated Depreciation		$100
Accounts Payable		250
Mortgage Payable		125
Fund Balance		235
Supply Expense	200	
Inpatient Revenue—Nonplan		200
Outpatient Revenue—Nonplan		400
Inpatient Revenue—Plan		500
Interest Expense	12	
Salary & Wage Expense	300	
	1,810	1,810

As seen previously, the account debited will be overstated at the end of the period and an adjustment is necessary. An inspection of Table 2-1 reveals that Care City Hospital has no prepaid expenses.

As an example of an accrued expense, assume that the last date on which the employees of this hospital were paid and the end of the accounting period do not coincide. In such a situation the institution's work force contributes to operational activity during the interim, which implies that it has incurred a salary and wage expense as well as an obligation to pay its employees for their services. If the employees earn $100 for which no entry has been recorded, the required adjustment is given by

Journal Entry # 8

Salary and Wage Expense	$100	
Salaries and Wages Payable		$100
To record accrued payroll.		

2.2.3.2 Depreciation

Depreciation accounting is simply a process of allocating the cost of plant and equipment to the periods in which these resources contribute to operations. Suppose that the cost of an item of equipment that is expected to contribute to operations for ten years is $75,000. Assume further that the entire $75,000 is recognized as an expense of the first year. In this case, the first-year expenses are overstated while those of subsequent years are understated. To avoid such undesirable consequences, depreciation accounting is used to allocate these costs to the periods in which the resource contributes to operational activity.

Returning to Table 2-1, suppose the depreciation expense of Care City Hospital is $15 per year. The required adjusting entry is given by

Journal Entry # 9

Depreciation Expense	$15	
Accumulated Depreciation		$15
To record depreciation expense.		

The Accumulated Depreciation account is a permanent account, appears in the balance sheet as a contra asset account, and represents the entire amount of depreciation recorded previously. Referring to the second of these characteristics, a contra account is an account the balance of which is subtracted from the balance of an associate account so as to show a more proper amount for the items represented by the associate account. In this case, the subtraction of accumulated depreciation from the balance of the Plant and Equipment account yields the value of the institution's physical plant and capital equipment, net of depreciation. In contrast, the Depreciation Expense account is a temporary or nominal account appearing in the income statement. Similar to other temporary accounts, the balance of the Depreciation Expense account is eliminated at the end of the accounting period. These and related matters are described in Chapter 12.

2.2.3.3 Other Adjustments

Suppose a physical inventory completed on the last day of the accounting period reveals that the inventory holdings of Care City Hospital amount to $70. Table 2-1 shows that, without an adjusting entry, the inventory of the institution will be understated by $20. Since $200 worth of supplies were acquired during the period, the supply expenses incurred may be found as follows:

January 1, 1980, Balance	$ 50
Acquisitions During the Period	200
Supplies Available During the Period	250
Less Ending Inventory	70
Supply Expenses	180

Given that supply expenses of $200 are recognized in the second journal entry, an adjustment is required to reduce this component of expense by $20. Hence, the adjusting entry required at the end of the period is given by

Journal Entry # 10

Inventory	$20	
Supply Expense		$20
To adjust inventory and supply expenses.		

After the adjusting entries are recorded in the journal, they are posted to the general ledger. The accounts influenced by the adjusting entries are presented in Table 2-5. At this point, the adjusted balance of each ledger account is determined and an adjusted trial balance similar to Table 2-6 is prepared.

2.2.4 The Worksheet

As has just been seen, as soon as all transactions are recorded, adjusting entries are made in the journals and posted to the general ledger. After these procedures have been completed, the preparation of the adjusted trial balance provides the basis for developing the financial statements of the period. For small health facilities that have a small number of accounts and few adjustments, such a procedure is satisfactory. However, if the institution has more than a few accounts and adjustments, errors in adjusting the accounts and in constructing the financial statements can be reduced by the use of a worksheet. The worksheet is prepared before recording the adjusting entries in the general journal, posting the adjusting entries to the general ledger, and constructing the financial statements. The worksheet, then, is a mechanism that assists the accountant in (1) assembling information in an orderly fashion, (2) preparing the adjusting entries, (3) constructing the financial statements, and (4) closing the nominal or temporary accounts.

Table 2-7 is the worksheet for Care City Hospital. The worksheet is divided into five pairs of columns. The first pair is titled Trial Balance and, as should

Table 2-5 Adjusted Entries in General Ledger

Salary & Wage Expense		*Salaries & Wages Payable*		*Depreciation Expense*	
(7) $300			$100 (8)	(9) $15	
(8) 100					

Accumulated Depreciation		*Inventories*		*Supply Expense*	
	$100 (OB)	(OB) $50		(2) $200	
	15 (9)	(10) 20			$20 (10)

OB = opening balance.
Numbers in parentheses refer to journal entries described earlier.

Table 2-6 Adjusted Trial Balance

CARE CITY HOSPITAL

End-of-Period Adjusted Trial Balance

	Dr.	*Cr.*
Cash	$388	
Accounts Receivable	660	
Plant & Equipment	200	
Inventories	70	
Accumulated Depreciation		$115
Accounts Payable		250
Mortgage Payable		125
Fund Balance		235
Supply Expense	180	
Inpatient Revenue—Nonplan		200
Inpatient Revenue—Plan		500
Outpatient Revenue—Nonplan		400
Interest Expense	12	
Salary & Wage Expense	400	
Salaries & Wages Payable		100
Depreciation Expense	15	
	1,925	1,925

be verified, reproduces the hospital's unadjusted trial balance. The second set usually is titled Adjustments, where required adjustments to the accounts are recorded. The numbers in the parentheses correspond to the journal entries prepared earlier. General journal entries 8 and 9 require the addition of two account titles that have been written below those listed in the unadjusted trial balance. This is because these accounts did not have balances when the unadjusted trial balance was prepared and, as a consequence, are not included in the trial balance. If proper accounts have been used, the equality of the credit and debit entries in the adjustment section of the worksheet will demonstrate that the adjusting entries have been recorded properly.

The third set of columns is entitled Adjusted Trial Balance. This set combines the trial balance and the adjusting entries in the first and second pairs of columns. For example, the salary and wage expense account has a $300 debit balance in the unadjusted trial balance while the salary and wage payable account has no balance. Combining the $300 debit balance with the adjustment reflected by the $100 debit entry in the adjustment columns results in a $400 debit balance in this account in the adjusted trial balance. Similarly, the balance of the salary and wage payable account in the adjusted trial balance is $100. When no adjustments are made to an account in the

Table 2-7 Worksheet for Care City Hospital

Account Titles	*Trial Balance*		*Adjustments*		*Adjusted Trial Balance*		*Income Statement*		*Balance Sheet*	
	Dr	*Cr*	*Dr*	*Cr*	*Dr*	*Cr*	*Dr*	*Cr*	*Dr*	*Cr*
Cash	$388				$388				$388	
Accounts Receivable	660				660				660	
Plant & Equipment	200				200				200	
Inventories	50		$20(10)		70				70	
Accumulated Depreciation		$100		$15(9)		$115				$115
Accounts Payable		250				250				250
Mortgage Payable		125				125				125
Fund Balance		235				235				235
Supply Expense	200			20(10)	180		$180			
Inpatient Revenue—Nonplan		200				200		$200		
Outpatient Revenue—Nonplan		400				400		400		
Inpatient Revenue—Plan		500				500		500		
Interest Expense	12				12		12			
Salary & Wage Expense	300		100(8)		400		400			
	1,810	1,810								
Salaries & Wages Payable				100(8)		100				100
Depreciation Expense			15(9)		15		15			
			135	135	1,925	1,925	607	1,100	1,318	825
Net Income							493			493
							1,100	1,100	1,318	1,318

Numbers in parentheses refer to journal entries described in Section 2.2.1.

unadjusted trial balance, the trial balance amounts are transferred to the appropriate column of the Adjusted Trial Balance section of the worksheet. Combining the amounts in the trial balance with those in the adjustment's columns results in the adjusted trial balance that was presented initially in Table 2-6.

After combining the unadjusted trial balance with the adjustments, the sum of the debits and the sum of the credits in the adjusted trial balance are compared to prove their equality. Once this has been proved, the adjusted trial balance amounts are transferred to the proper column of the income statement or balance sheet, according to the statement on which they will appear. The transfer process is quite simple and is guided by essentially two questions: (1) Is the item to be transferred a debit or a credit? (2) On which statement will the item appear? As to the first decision, a debit balance in the adjusted trial balance must be transferred to the debit column of either the income statement or the balance sheet section of the worksheet. Regarding the second decision, it is only necessary to remember that revenues and expenses appear in the income statement, and assets, liabilities, and the fund balance on the balance sheet.

Once the amounts have been sorted properly, column totals are obtained. At this point the difference between the debit and credit totals of the income statement section of the worksheet represents the net income or loss for the period. This is because revenues are entered in the credit column and expenses in the debit column. If the sum of the credits exceeds the sum of the debits, the hospital has earned a net income for the period. Conversely, if the sum of the debits exceeds the sum of the credits, a net loss is incurred.

Table 2-7 reveals that Care City Hospital earned a net income of $493. This amount is added to the total of the credit column of the balance sheet section of the worksheet. Such a procedure is required because, with the exception of the fund balance, the amounts in the balance sheet section are carried forward to the next accounting period. Increasing the sum of the credit entries in the balance sheet section by $493 has the effect of adding the net income of the period to the fund balance. Operating losses are added to the debit column because they reduce the fund balance.

Adding the net income or loss to the appropriate column of the balance sheet section provides the basis for proving the accuracy of the worksheet. Obviously, if the sum of the debits and the sum of the credits, including the net income or loss, are equal, it usually is assumed that no errors have been committed. On the other hand, the equality between the two sums does not guarantee that substantive errors have not been committed. For example, even though they may be equal, it is possible that incorrect accounts were used to record one or more of the transactions. If the column totals are unequal, there has been an error and the mistake must be corrected before constructing the financial statements.

When a worksheet is used, both it and the financial statements are prepared before adjusting entries are recorded in the general journal. Once the two have been completed, the general journal entries must be prepared and posted to the general ledger. This is a simple task, however, since the adjusting entries may be obtained directly from the adjustment columns of the worksheet. When this is done, a journal entry is required for each adjustment.

2.2.5 Financial Statements and the Closing Entries

When all of these operations have been completed, financial statements may be prepared directly from the adjusted trial balance or from the worksheet. Table 2-8 is a combination income statement and statement of changes in fund balance; the balance sheet is shown in Table 2-9. The usefulness of these statements is limited somewhat by the assumptions that have been used to simplify this example. However, a set of more realistic and detailed financial statements is considered in Chapters 14 and 15.

The final set of procedures in the accounting process is represented by the entries that eliminate the existing balances in the nominal or temporary accounts and prepare the books for the next accounting period. In closing the books, the objective is to remove from the ledger all balances except those that are retained from period to period. Those that are carried forward are

Table 2-8 Combination of Two Statements

CARE CITY HOSPITAL

Income Statement and Statement of Changes in Fund Balance

Revenue	
Inpatient Revenue	$700
Outpatient Revenue	400
Total Revenue	1,100
Expenses	
Interest Expense	12
Salary and Wage Expense	400
Depreciation Expense	15
Supply Expense	180
Total Expenses	607
Net Income	493
Beginning Fund Balance (Table 2-1)	235
Ending Fund Balance	728

Table 2-9 The Balance Sheet

CARE CITY HOSPITAL		
End-of-Period Balance Sheet		
Assets		
Cash		$388
Accounts Receivable		660
Plant & Equipment	$200	
Less Accumulated Depreciation	115	85
Inventories		70
Total Assets		1,203
Liabilities and Fund Balance		
Accounts Payable		250
Mortgage Payable		125
Salaries & Wages Payable		100
Total Liabilities		475
Fund Balance		728
Total Liabilities and Fund Balance		1,203

called permanent accounts and appear in the balance sheet. Those that are closed are called the nominal or temporary accounts and appear in the income statement. The removal of such balances is accomplished by a series of closing entries.

Closing entries for Care City are seen below. Referring back to Table 2-8, the expense accounts have a debit balance; to eliminate it, an offsetting credit is required. The obverse is true of credit balances in general and of revenues specifically. Here, a temporary account, Revenue and Expense Summary, is used to accumulate the revenues and expenses of the hospital for the period. To close the revenue accounts, the appropriate entry is:

Inpatient Revenue—Nonplan	$200	
Outpatient Revenue—Nonplan	400	
Inpatient Revenue—Plan	500	
Revenue & Expense Summary		$1,100

To close the expense accounts the entry is:

Revenue and Expense Summary	$607	
Interest Expense		$12
Salary & Wage Expense		400
Depreciation Expense		15
Supply Expense		180

After these entries have been recorded, the revenue and expense accounts of the hospital have a zero balance and are ready for the next period. The Revenue and Expense Summary account, however, has been debited for $607 (the total expenses of the period) and credited for $1,100 (total revenues of the period). As a result, the Revenue and Expense Summary has a credit balance of $493, which is the net income of the period. As will be recalled, a net income increases the fund balance, which is recorded as a credit entry. The revenue and expense summary is closed and the net income of the period is transferred to the fund balance by:

Revenue and Expense Summary	$493	
Fund Balance		$493
To close revenue and expense summary to the fund balance.		

Once the closing entries have been journalized, they are posted to the general ledger. At this point the only positive balances in the general ledger are balance sheet accounts. These represent the balances that will be carried forward to the next accounting period.

All the basic operations described in this chapter should be performed on a monthly basis except for the closing entries. Each month, transactions should be journalized and posted, the accounts should be adjusted, and interim financial statements should be prepared. Closing entries, however, are journalized and posted only once a year at the end of the accounting period.

Questions for Discussion

1. List and describe the basic phases of the accounting process.
2. Differentiate between ledgers and journals. Explain what types of journals and ledgers are used by health facilities.
3. Describe why adjusting entries are recorded and reported in the financial statements.
4. Explain the purpose of the closing entries. Describe briefly the entries required to close the books.
5. Differentiate between nominal and permanent accounts.
6. Describe the importance of interim financial statements.
7. Explain the importance of the general ledger.
8. Define a worksheet. Explain its importance to

   a. the preparation of the adjusting entries
   b. the preparation of the financial statements

Problems for Solution

1. On January 1, 198A, the following balances appear in the general ledger of the institution:

Cash	$100	
Inventory	50	
Accounts Receivable	70	
Plant and Equipment	200	
Accumulated Depreciation		$20
Accounts Payable		40
Mortgage Payable		150
Fund Balance		210

Suppose that the institution engages in the following transactions during 198A:

a. It provides service to patients on account:

inpatients	$300
outpatients	100

b. It purchases $100 worth of supplies on account

c. It receives cash:

outstanding receivables	$380
other revenue	20

d. It disburses cash:

outstanding payables	$70
salaries and wages	120
utilities	30
purchased services	10

e. It makes payments on the outstanding mortgage:

principal	$50
interest	15

Required: (1) construct the general ledger of the institution as of January 1, 198A; (2) record the transactions of the period; (3) post journal entries to the general ledger; and (4) prepare an unadjusted trial balance.

2. Assume in Problem 1 that the following information is available at the end of the accounting period:

   a. supply expenses of the period are $90
   b. depreciation expense is $20
   c. unpaid salary and wage expense is $10

   Required: (1) prepare adjusting entries; (2) prepare an adjusted trial balance; (3) prepare the financial statements; and (4) record the closing entries.
3. Use the unadjusted trial balance and the information in Problem 2 to construct a worksheet for the institution.
4. Prepare the financial statements and closing entries from the worksheet developed in Problem 3.
5. Assume that the following data appear in the general ledger accounts of Pine City Hospital at December 31, 198A:

Mortgage Payable	$1,200
Cash	8,000
Accounts Receivable	1,900
Accumulated Depreciation	1,500
Plant and Equipment	3,000
Inpatient Revenue	6,000
Accounts Payable	1,100
Salary and Wage Expense	4,500
Supply Expense	1,500
Outpatient Revenue	7,800
Deferred Revenue	900
Inventory	4,500
Depreciation Expense	300
Salaries and Wages Payable	1,100
Insurance Expense	200
Fund Balance	?

   Required: (1) prepare the closing entries; (2) prepare an income statement; and (3) prepare a balance sheet for Pine City Hospital.
6. Suppose that on January 1, 198A the following data appear in the general ledger accounts of Murder City Hospital:

Cash	$4,000
Accounts Receivable	1,500
Inventory	2,000
Prepaid Rent	300
Plant and Equipment	9,000
Accumulated Depreciation	6,500
Mortgage Payable	2,300
Accounts Payable	4,200
Fund Balance	3,800

Suppose also that the following information pertains to the hospital's transactions of the period:

a. It receives $4,000 as a prepayment for the use of service by patients insured by third party A
b. It provides service to patients on account:

inpatient	$10,000
outpatient	4,000

c. It provides service worth $3,800 to patients insured by third party A
d. It purchases $2,000 worth of equipment for cash
e. It purchases supplies on account of $1,000
f. Its cash receipts on outstanding receivables are $14,000
g. It makes a payment on outstanding payables of $4,700
h. It makes payment on a mortgage:

principal	$900
interest	230

i. It pays operating expenses:

salaries and wages	$3,000
utilities	500
purchased services	850

The following data pertain to the adjustments at the end of the period:

a. rent expense, $100
b. depreciation expense, $250
c. supply expenses, $1,900
d. unpaid wages and salaries, $800

Use a worksheet to complete the accounting cycle.

7. Assume that the total revenue of the period is distributed as follows:

Inpatient Revenues	$950,000
Outpatient Revenues	20,000
Other Revenue	10,000

Suppose further that the expenses of the period are distributed as follows:

Salaries and Wages	$750,000
Supplies Expense	100,000
Other Expenses	100,000

Prepare the closing entries, assuming no deductions in revenue. Explain the influence of operating activity on the equity of the institution.

8. Assume that the institution closes its books on Friday, December 31. Assume also that the last pay period is December 26 and the next pay period is January 7. The following distribution is assumed to be relevant:

Employee	*Hours Worked 12/27 to 12/31*	*Wage Rate*
A	40	$5.00/hr.
B	20	5.00/hr.
C	40	8.50/hr.
D	30	9.00/hr.

Describe what entry is required to record the unpaid wages and how they will be reflected in the financial statements.

Chapter 3

Issues Peculiar to Health Facilities

Thus far, the discussion has covered the phases of the accounting cycle as well as principles and practices that are used for both profit and nonprofit organizations. This chapter considers several issues that differentiate accounting for health facilities from that of other organizations. More specifically, the focus is on the use of fund accounting, the chart of accounts, responsibility accounting, and functional accounting in the health care industry.

3.1 FUND ACCOUNTING

Perhaps the most important feature of accounting in health care facilities is adherence to the principles of fund accounting. Fund accounting may be defined as procedures in which a self-balancing group of accounts is provided for each accounting entity established by legal, contractual, or voluntary action. A fund is a self-balancing accounting entity that is established to record and report the capital or trust monies received for specific purpose(s), the income thereon, the expenditures for designated purposes, and the assets held against the capital of the fund. Consequently, the institution may be viewed as being divided into several subentities that relate to distinct phases of financial activity. Each division is reflected by a fund grouping that contains a set of self-balancing accounts for which financial statements are prepared. Thus, a fund is a subentity within the institutional whole. Assuming three fund groupings—A, B, and C—the accounting system is composed of a series of accounting equations that may be represented by:

Assets of Fund A = Liabilities of Fund A + Equity of Fund A
Assets of Fund B = Liabilities of Fund B + Equity of Fund B
Assets of Fund C = Liabilities of Fund C + Equity of Fund C

In addition, the assets of all funds must equal the sum of the liabilities and the equities of all funds.

Many institutions use fund accounting in response to a need that is created by one of the ways in which they obtain resources. Frequently, hospitals and other health facilities receive gifts or endowments whose use is limited by donor restrictions, such as the acquisition of fixed assets or for teaching or research, or as endowments to provide investment income. By accepting these gifts, the institution is legally obliged to adhere to those restrictions. To fulfill the fiduciary responsibility thus created, a separate set of accounting records for those assets is established. By virtue of receiving donor-restricted gifts, then, the owner's equity of the institution is composed of different sets of claims on several groups of assets. In response to these different claims, the health facility divides owner's equity into a number of fund balances. Each one represents the difference between the assets and liabilities of the fund grouping to which it belongs. As will be seen, one of the approaches to fund accounting is to divide the resources of the institution into restricted and unrestricted fund groupings.

Theoretically, a fund should be established for each project or purpose for which restricted resources have been received. For practical reasons, this practice is not followed since the creation of an accounting entity for each such project or purpose would greatly complicate the system as well as make the financial statements difficult to prepare and understand. Further, since many short-term investment opportunities require large amounts of money, the segregation of investable assets into many fund groupings could deter the allocation of cash for the purpose of earning income. For these practical reasons, it is customary for the institution to establish rather broad groupings of funds that distinguish between restricted and unrestricted funds. Possible fund groupings are discussed next.

3.1.1 The Unrestricted Fund Grouping

Transactions involving resources that donors have not limited to designated purposes should be recorded and reported in an Unrestricted Fund grouping. All of the resources associated with this fund are available for satisfying day-to-day operating needs. More specifically, the Unrestricted Fund includes: (1) the current operating accounts; (2) the plant accounts; and (3) in the case of the hospital, the board-designated accounts.

3.1.1.1 Operating Accounts

The current operating accounts of the institution consist of:

1. unrestricted current assets such as cash, accounts receivable, inventory and investments in marketable securities

2. currently maturing obligations or liabilities
3. the set of nominal accounts that reflects the revenues earned and expenses incurred
4. the unrestricted equity of the institution.

The difference between current assets and current liabilities represents the working capital of the institution while the nominal accounts reflect operational activity during a specified period. Consequently, the revenue accounts show income generated by providing patient service, other operating revenues, deductions in income, and nonoperating income. The expense accounts primarily reflect operating expenditures. In turn, revenues and expenses are recorded and reported in terms of specific accounts that are organized in accordance with the functional units or responsibility centers of the facility.

3.1.1.2 Board-Designated Accounts

In addition to the groupings mentioned above, the board of trustees may decide to earmark or designate otherwise unrestricted resources for use in a special project or in a specified way. In such a situation, a set of board-designated accounts is created to ensure that resources are used in accordance with the board's wishes. Unlike donor-restricted funds, board designations do not carry legal restrictions and may be reversed without external approval. Therefore, unrestricted funds must not be comingled with those limited by donors or by external agencies.

3.1.1.3 Plant Accounts

Plant accounts consist in part of asset accounts that record the actual investment in land, buildings, and equipment. They also include liabilities incurred in acquiring the plant and equipment such as mortgages and leases.

Occasionally plant assets are donated to a hospital. Upon receipt, they should be recorded at fair market value in the Unrestricted Fund, with an offsetting credit entry to the Unrestricted Fund equity account. Conversely, a hospital may receive land, buildings, or items of equipment that are donor-restricted for endowment or other specified purposes. In such cases, the donation is recorded not in the Unrestricted Fund but in the appropriate restricted fund, at fair market value.

Further, resources accumulated for replacement or expansion and not subject to external restrictions should be reflected in the set of board-designated accounts of the Unrestricted Fund. These resources should not be comingled or merged with donor-restricted funds.

3.1.2 Restricted Funds

The major restrictions on funds are of three basic types: (1) specific operating purposes, (2) endowments, and (3) the acquisition of plant assets.

Resources that have been limited to special purposes are recorded in the Specific Purpose Fund while those restricted as endowments are shown in the Endowment Fund. Similarly, resources restricted to the future acquisition of plant and/or equipment are recorded in the Capital Fund. What follows is a brief discussion of the three major restricted fund groupings; an extended discussion is presented in Chapter 11.

3.1.2.1 Specific Purpose Fund

Hospitals receive donations, gifts, and grants whose use is restricted by the donor to a specified purpose other than the future acquisition of capital or an endowment. These resources are recorded in the Specific Purpose Fund. Consider first funds that are limited to a specific purpose such as defraying the costs of a particular project. Once recorded as a restricted resource, these funds remain in the Specific Purpose Fund until the donor restrictions are satisfied. As expenditures are made for the designated project, the previously restricted funds are recorded as revenue in the Unrestricted Fund and used to offset or finance costs of the designated project. If the passage of time satisfies the conditions specified by the donor, funds may be transferred to the Unrestricted Fund and used to satisfy other operating exigencies.

During the period between the receipt of funds and their transfer to the Unrestricted Fund, resources may be available for investment in securities that earn income for the institution. If the donor has restricted the use of such income, any revenues or gains from their investment should be recorded in an appropriately titled Restricted Equity account and losses and expenses should be deducted from it. On the other hand, if the donor imposes no restrictions, revenues and gains from these investments should be recorded in the Unrestricted Fund and made available to meet the operating needs of the health facility.

3.1.2.2 Endowment Fund

Hospitals and other facilities frequently receive endowments, which are donor-restricted resources that may be used for earning income while preserving or maintaining their principal intact. In general, endowments impose legal restrictions that the board cannot alter and that prohibit the expenditure of the principal. Endowments usually are of two types: (1) term endowments that may be spent after a period of time or after the conditions specified by the donor have been satisfied; (2) pure endowments that are permanent and whose principal the institution may not spend. Both types of endowments are recorded in the Endowment Fund when received.

Revenues earned by the investment of endowments may be restricted or unrestricted. As noted, unrestricted investment income should be recorded directly in the Unrestricted Fund while restricted investment income must be reported so as to reflect the donor's conditions.

3.1.2.3 Capital Fund

Cash and other assets that are restricted to the future acquisition of plant and equipment are recorded in accounts created for this purpose. When these assets ultimately are used in obtaining a plant asset, the acquisition is recorded in the Unrestricted Fund, as mentioned earlier. Pledges, less a provision for uncollectables, that are restricted to the purchase of plant assets are recorded as an addition to an appropriately titled Equity Reserve account of the Capital Fund.

Again, during the period between the receipt and expenditure of funds, resources may be available for investment purposes. When the income and gains on the sale of securities resulting from the investment of these funds are unrestricted, the revenue should be recorded in the Unrestricted Fund. When restrictions on investment income exist, the resulting revenue must be recorded in a manner consistent with the donor's conditions.

In summary, this discussion has suggested that the financial activity of the facility should be divided into an Unrestricted Fund and three Restricted Fund groupings. The Unrestricted Fund includes the accounts that pertain to the day-to-day operations of the institution, including both existing plant and equipment. The Restricted Fund grouping usually consists of a Capital Fund, a Specific Purpose Fund, and an Endowment Fund. The Capital Fund includes the accounts pertaining to resources whose use is restricted to the future acquisition of plant and equipment. The Specific Purpose Fund and the Endowment Fund contain all other assets held for special purposes or endowments that have been donated or bequeathed to the institution.

3.2 INTERFUND TRANSACTIONS

Interfund transactions may be either transfers from one fund to another or borrowing by one fund from another. As the following discussion shows, a complete and separate set of entries is recorded in each of the funds involved in the transaction.

3.2.1 Transfers

Perhaps the most frequently encountered interfund transaction is the transfer of previously restricted resources to the Unrestricted Fund. For example, assume that $2,500 is to be transferred from the Specific Purpose Fund to the Unrestricted Fund, where it will be used to offset expenditures incurred in completing the purpose designated by the donor. As seen below, the transfer is recorded as revenue in the Unrestricted Fund, where it is used to offset the incurred cost. In the Specific Purpose Fund, the following entry is recorded:

Transfer to the Unrestricted Fund	$2,500	
Cash		$2,500

In the Unrestricted Fund the following entry is recorded:

Cash	$2,500	
Other Operating Revenue		$2,500

The credit entry to the cash account of the Specific Purpose Fund equals the debit entry to the cash account of the Unrestricted Fund. These elements of the two entries transfer cash from the Specific Purpose Fund to the Unrestricted Fund. The debit to the Transfer account of the Specific Purpose Fund is equal to the credit to the Other Operating Revenues account of the Unrestricted Fund. These are treated as nominal or temporary accounts. Holding other things constant, closing the Transfer to the Unrestricted Fund account will reduce the fund balance of the Specific Purpose Fund by $2,500, while closing the Other Operating Revenue account will increase the fund balance of the Unrestricted Fund by a like amount.

When resources are transferred from the Capital Fund to the Unrestricted Fund, a similar entry is recorded. Assume $1,000 is to be transferred from the Capital Fund to the Unrestricted Fund:

Capital Fund

Transfer to Unrestricted Fund	$1,000	
Cash		$1,000

Unrestricted Fund

Cash	$1,000	
Transfer from the Capital Fund (or revenue account)		$1,000

Again, the transfer accounts are closed to the respective fund balance accounts at the end of the period. In these examples, the transfer accounts should be more descriptive than indicated here.

3.2.2 Interfund Borrowing

Just as the issuance of a promissory note represents a liability to the borrower and an asset to the lender, the fund that borrows resources incurs a liability and the lending fund acquires an asset. As in the transfer of resources, interfund borrowing requires essentially two sets of entries.

In the following situation it is assumed that there are no legal restrictions to interfund borrowing and that management decides that $1,500 is needed for operating purposes that it may borrow from the Specific Purpose Fund. The sets of entries required to record the transaction are as follows:

Unrestricted Fund

Cash	$1,500	
Due to Specific Purpose Fund		$1,500

Specific Purpose Fund

Due from Unrestricted Fund	$1,500	
Cash		$1,500

As before, the credit entry to the cash account of the Specific Purpose Fund is equal to the debit entry to the cash account of the Unrestricted Fund and these elements of the two entries transfer cash from the former to the latter. The account titled Due to Specific Purpose Fund represents a liability of the Unrestricted Fund and must be liquidated by a payment of $1,500 to the Specific Purpose Fund. Clearly, then, the Due from Unrestricted Fund account is an asset of the Specific Purpose Fund and is similar to an account receivable. When the debt is paid, the entry in each of the fund groupings is simply reversed.

3.3 CHART OF ACCOUNTS

In addition to fund accounting, the chart of accounts is a basic element of accounting for the health care facility. The chart of accounts is a systematic listing of categories in which the economic data pertaining to the financial position and operating results of the institution are recorded. The chart should be designed to satisfy the informational needs of the institution as well as facilitate the recording and reporting of its assets, liabilities, income, expenses, and fund balance or equity. The chart identifies categories or accounts through the use of account titles and numerical codes. Thus, the chart's primary purpose is to provide a systematic framework for classifying, recording, and reporting transactions affecting the facility's financial position and operating results.

A related and important purpose of the chart is to provide the framework within which information in a given account is standardized, which of course facilitates a comparison of the performance of the institution during several different time periods. In addition, the chart of accounts must be consistent with the objective of generating the economic data necessary for the determination of the financial support received from third party payers.

Each account in the chart is assigned a numerical code to identify its category. For illustration, suppose the institution uses a primary code consisting of three digits and a supplementary code of a series of digits to identify each account in the chart. With respect to the primary code, let

1. the first digit, represented by the integer values 1, . . . , 9, indicate an asset, liability, equity, revenue, or expense account
2. the second digit denote the fund grouping to which the account belongs
3. the third digit represent the basic account group (e.g., cash, investments, receivables, inventory, prepaid expenses, plant assets, accumulated depreciation, current liabilities, long-term liabilities, and fund balances)

In turn, the supplementary codes can provide additional information about the account.

The secondary codes are of particular value when classifying the revenues and expenses of the organization. Recall that the first digit of the primary code refers to a revenue or an expense account, while the second identifies the corresponding fund grouping. With respect to income, the third digit identifies the source of revenue or the party that assumes the responsibility of financing the use of care. In turn, the supplementary code may be used to classify income in terms of the institution's revenue-generating centers, type of patient, and component of service. For example, the account number 411.20.723 can be interpreted as follows:

4 represents an inpatient revenue account

1 represents the operating fund

1 represents the source of revenue (e.g., Blue Cross, Medicare, etc.)

.

2
0 represents the departmental or functional unit (e.g., laboratory)

.

7
2 represents the type of service (e.g., blood chemistry examination)
3

Similarly, the supplementary codes classify expenses by type of service and object of expenditure. For example, the account number 713.20.723 can be interpreted as follows:

7 represents an expense account

1 represents the operating fund

3 represents the nature of the expenditure (e.g., salary and wage)

.

2
0 represents the departmental or functional unit (e.g., laboratory)

.
7
2 represents the type of service (e.g., blood chemistry examination)
3

The supplementary code thus permits the accumulation of cost and revenue data for each department or functional unit as well as for each service. Consequently, such an approach assists management in controlling the operational performance of each unit as well as in evaluating the extent to which the costs of providing each service are returned to the institution in the form of revenue.

3.4 RESPONSIBILITY ACCOUNTING

The previous section suggested that one of the major considerations in developing a chart of accounts for revenues and expenses is the hospital's organizational structure. Because of differing sizes, functions, and service capabilities, no two institutions are organized in precisely the same way. However, the objective of ensuring financial viability is common to all. If this objective is to be achieved, the chart of accounts must provide the basis for management control through responsibility accounting and budgeting.

A responsibility center is a department, function, or group of functions for which a specific individual is responsible. Each center incurs expenses, and many earn revenue by providing service to patients. To maximize the effectiveness of the internal control system, managers of responsibility centers should be provided with timely reports in which the results of actual operational activity are compared with the standard of performance. Responsibility accounting is a mechanism of accumulating and reporting the results of actual operational activity, as expressed in terms of expenses and, where appropriate, revenues for each responsibility center in the institution. On the other hand, the standard of performance is expressed by the budget of the responsibility center. Comparing the results of actual operational activity, as reported by the responsibility accounting system, with the standard of comparison, as expressed by the responsibility budget, provides the basis for identifying areas in which the results of activity have departed from the standard of performance as well as the individual responsible for eliminating the disparity.

The primary function of responsibility accounting and the responsibility budget is to distribute managerial responsibility and authority to specific individuals who are in charge of designated activities or functions. Associated with budget development are essentially three phases:

1. the specification of objectives and their translation into operational terms
2. an estimation of the workload and the real resources required to achieve stated objectives
3. a translation of real resources into monetary terms that constitute the financial budget.

Thus, the budget constitutes a set of real and financial objectives or standards by which actual performance can be evaluated. Clearly, when a department, function, or group of functions represents the unit of analysis, the budget represents the standard by which the use of real resources and the resulting output, as well as departmental revenues and expenses, may be compared in evaluating the extent to which the organizational entity is achieving its objectives.

To maximize the extent to which management can control institutional activity, the accounting system must be capable of accumulating revenues and expenses in terms that are comparable with the standard expressed in the budget. Just as the budget uses the department or the responsibility center as the unit of analysis, the accounting system must be capable of accumulating the revenues earned and the expenses incurred by the department, function, or group of functions identified as a responsibility center.

The accounting system must accumulate expenses and revenues in a manner that permits a comparison of actual results with the plans or stated objectives as expressed in the budget. Such a comparison frequently identifies areas of activity in which remedial actions are required to reduce or eliminate any imbalance between actual and desired performance.

3.5 FUNCTIONAL ACCOUNTING

On October 25, 1977, Public Law 95-142 was enacted and Section 19 of this legislation mandated a federally imposed system of functional accounting. In general, functional accounting is a mechanism of allocating only those costs that are directly related to the tasks or functions of a given center to the unit. The primary purpose of the system is to provide uniform cost and utilization data that have been classified in terms of functional cost centers.

To illustrate the difference between responsibility and functional accounting, consider the following example. Suppose that a nurse is assigned to a given ward and is paid a salary of $1,000 per month. Suppose further that during the month the nurse devotes 20 percent of the time to stocking floor supplies and 80 percent to providing direct patient care. Under responsibility accounting, the monthly salary of $1,000 is assigned to the nursing ward. Under functional accounting, 20 percent or $200 of the salary is assigned to central supply and 80 percent or $800 to the nursing unit. Thus, under functional accounting and reporting, only expenses that are directly related to the task or functions of a given area are assigned to that unit.

More specifically, the system requires the direct assignment of certain costs to the functional unit responsible for incurring those expenses. The costs that must be recorded directly include:

1. depreciation on buildings and fixtures
2. depreciation on movable equipment
3. salary- and payroll-related benefits
4. drugs
5. medical supplies
6. plant maintenance
7. data processing
8. central patient transportation

Traditionally, these costs have not been assigned directly to functional units. Consequently, it may be necessary to modify the distribution of responsibility in many institutions so that functional units and responsibility centers coincide. Alternatively, the hospital might maintain a responsibility accounting system that corresponds to the existing delegation of responsibility and design a functional accounting system that satisfies the reporting requirements of P.L. 95-142. This text assumes that the responsibility center, the cost center, and the functional unit are synonymous.

Questions for Discussion

1. Define fund accounting. Explain why it is of importance to the health sector.
2. Identify and briefly describe the major funds maintained by most health facilities.
3. Define the chart of accounts and its role in recording transactions.
4. Distinguish between cash and accrual accounting. Explain why accrual accounting is used in most health facilities.
5. Distinguish between statements of financial position and statements of changes in financial position.
6. Discuss the importance of periodic reporting to the management of the health care facility.
7. Define responsibility accounting and explain its importance to the health care industry.
8. Define functional accounting and explain why it is important to the health care industry.

9. Differentiate between responsibility accounting and functional accounting.
10. Distinguish between term endowments and pure endowments.

Problems for Solution

1. Use the rules of debit and credit to record the following transactions:

   a. $6,000 is transferred from the Specific Purpose Fund to the Unrestricted Fund
   b. The Unrestricted Fund borrows $1,800 from the Endowment Fund

2. Use the rules of debit and credit to record the following transactions:

   a. a $10,000 pure endowment is received; its investment income must be used to finance the provision of charity care
   b. income of $2,000 from endowment investment (Problem 2, a) is received; these funds are used for the purpose specified by the donor
   c. $5,000 is received from a donor who restricts the use of the funds to a specific research project
   d. research costs of $2,000 are incurred in using the funds in Problem 2, c

Part II

Accounting for Revenues and Expenses

Chapter 4
Accounting for Revenue

Since most health facilities are nonprofit or not-for-profit, it can be argued that one of the primary objectives of management is to ensure equality between revenues and expenses. On the other hand, it is possible to argue that general inflationary pressures, the rapid advances in medical technology, and the need to maintain or expand the capacity to provide service force the institution to earn revenues in excess of expenses. To ensure that revenues are at least equal to expenses, all income must be recognized, measured, and recorded properly. This chapter discusses the basic principles that should be incorporated in any system of accounting for revenues.

Previously, revenue was defined as the gross increase in assets or the gross decrease in liabilities that results from activities that change owner's equity. In other words, revenue is earned when an asset, usually cash, or a right to receive cash is received or when a liability is liquidated by the sale of goods and services to another entity, usually a patient.

For example, suppose that a hospital provides an x-ray and that credit is extended to the patient or to the third party payer who is responsible for financing the use of this service. If the value of the x-ray is $30, the hospital has earned income by the provision of care; the transaction can be recorded as follows:

Accounts Receivable	$30	
Revenue		$30

Obviously, the transaction involves an exchange of a service (x-ray) for an asset (account receivable). Hence, an asset is received by the hospital and a service is exchanged for the asset.

On the other hand, assume that the hospital receives $100,000 from a third party as a prepayment for services that are to be provided to insured patients during the current or forthcoming accounting period. The receipt of the payment does not result in revenue immediately but rather gives rise to a liability that may be extinguished only by providing service in the future. Just as an account payable constitutes a liability that results from an implied promise to make future payment, the receipt of a payment prior to the provision of service constitutes a deferred revenue or a current liability. As a result, the entry for recording such a receipt is:

Cash	$100,000	
Deferred Revenue		$100,000

Even though an asset has been received, no service has been provided so no revenue is earned when the cash is received. The hospital gains a legal claim to the cash asset only by providing care to plan patients, thus reducing the incurred liability. For example, if the hospital subsequently provides $90,000 worth of service that is the financial responsibility of the prospective payer, the entry

Deferred Revenue	$90,000	
Revenue		$90,000

reduces the liability incurred when the hospital receives cash in advance and recognizes the revenue earned by subsequently providing service.

It is important to note that not all decreases in liabilities or increases in assets result in revenue. Many such decreases are accompanied by a commensurate decline in assets that are given in liquidating the institution's obligations. For example, the payment of a bank loan or of an account payable by a cash disbursement does not result in revenue. Similarly, an increase in an asset (say, cash) that is accompanied by an equal increase in a liability (say, a loan payable or a note payable) does not result in revenue. Further, revenue does not result when an increase in an asset is accompanied by a decrease in another asset. Finally, the receipt of an asset may increase the permanent capital of the enterprise without affecting revenue. The receipt of cash or another asset as an endowment is an example of such a transaction. As a general rule, revenue results from an earning process in which the institution realizes an inflow of assets or a legal claim to assets without an attendant increase in liabilities.

4.1 THE RECOGNITION OF REVENUE

Any enterprise engages in an almost unending stream of economic transactions that produce revenue. This section describes the basic conditions that must be satisfied before revenue is recognized and a credit entry to a revenue account is required.

4.1.1 Revenue Must Be Earned

Revenue normally is recognized and recorded when services have been provided or when goods are sold to patients or other external parties. When services are provided or goods are sold, the institution is said to have earned revenue. This is the first condition that must be satisfied before income is recognized.

Revenue is earned, then, only when service has been provided or goods have been sold to external parties that result in a receipt of cash, a legal claim to the future receipt of cash, or a legal claim to cash received before service is provided. Thus, revenue may be earned before, when, or after cash is received. These situations are discussed next.

4.1.1.1 Before the Receipt of Cash

Under a retrospective system of reimbursement, the institution earns revenue before it receives cash. Under the accrual concept, revenue is recognized at the time service is provided irrespective of when, if ever, cash is received. As seen previously, care that is financed on a retrospective basis generates revenue and involves an exchange of service for an account receivable.

4.1.1.2 When Cash Is Received

Frequently, there is a more or less simultaneous exchange of goods or services for cash. In such a situation, there is little or no time lag between the provision of service and the corresponding cash receipt. As a consequence, under an accrual accounting system, the more or less simultaneous exchange of service for cash results in the recognition of revenue and the corresponding cash receipt. For example, the outpatients of a hospital may use services and pay for them as they leave. In this case, the entry

Cash	$XXXX	
Outpatient Revenue		$XXXX

recognizes the cash receipt and the revenue from providing outpatient care. Thus, under accrual accounting, no formal recognition of an outstanding receivable is required when there is a more or less simultaneous exchange of goods or service for cash.

It is important to note that the receipt of cash or the amount of the money is not the determining factor in the decision to recognize revenue or the sum to be recognized. Rather, revenues are recorded at the time service is provided or goods are sold and are entered at the institution's full established rates, irrespective of the amount of cash received.

4.1.1.3 After Cash Is Received

When prepayment is involved, cash is received before service is provided. As discussed earlier, revenue is not recognized until service has been provided, and the prepayment should be recorded as a deferred revenue or a short-term liability. A deferred revenue is earned when service is provided, and it is at this point that income should be recognized.

Another problem arises in connection with the recognition of revenue from gifts, donations, and grants. Obviously, unrestricted cash receipts for which there are no donor limitations as to use should be recorded immediately as revenue. However, the treatment of donations, gifts, or grants that are donor-restricted is necessarily different. Assume, for example, that in 198A the institution receives a cash donation that may not be used until 198B or until conditions specified by the donor have been satisfied. The donation should not be recorded as a revenue until 198B or until the institution satisfies the specified conditions. Rather, assuming that the donation will be available for operating purposes, the receipt should be recorded as a debit to cash and a credit to a deferred revenue account. On the other hand, if the use of the donation is restricted, the appropriate entry involves a debit to cash and a credit to a restricted fund balance.

4.1.2 Revenue Must Be Secured

Of particular importance to the situation just described is the notion that, before revenue is recognized, the income must be secured or captured. This occurs when external authorities' control over the use of related assets is severed. Obviously, this takes place when the institution provides service to patients or receives an unrestricted gift. On the other hand, restricted gifts, donations, or grants cannot be regarded as secured and recognized as revenue until the donor's conditions have been satisfied.

4.1.3 Revenue Must Be Measured

The recognition of revenue requires the measurement of related assets in monetary terms. Clearly, cash receipts present no measurement difficulties. Other noncash assets may be measured in terms of the net realizable cash value or fair market value as expressed in monetary terms.

From a managerial perspective, it is important to measure and record all revenue generated by providing patient care at the full established rates of the institution. This forms the basis for the uniform measurement of the total revenue earned by providing service. These amounts may be more than the cash receipts from providing care. Therefore, subsequent adjustments that reflect contractual agreements, free care, courtesy discounts, and doubtful accounts are reported as a reduction in revenue in the income statement. Where appropriate, similar adjustments, which reduce receivables to their net realizable cash value, appear in the balance sheet.

4.2 CATEGORIES OF REVENUE: AN OVERVIEW

One of the primary objectives of management is to ensure that the revenues the institution earns are at least equal to the full costs of operation. The extent to which the goal of ensuring financial viability is being met is assessed by inspecting the income statement. As suggested earlier, when total revenues equal total costs, the institution is said to break even since its operational activity results in neither a net income nor a net loss. On the other hand, a net income (loss) is earned (incurred) when revenues exceed (are exceeded by) total costs (Table 4-1).

The framework outlined in Table 4-1 should be used in Table 4-2 to verify that Health City Hospital earned a net income of $4,900 during 198A. This shows that the earned income may be classified as either an operating or a nonoperating revenue. The following discussion describes these categories of

---

Table 4-1 Net Income or Loss from Operational Activity

Inpatient Revenue
+ Outpatient Revenue
Total Patient Service Revenue
Total Patient Service Revenue
− Total Deductions in Revenue
Net Patient Service Revenue
Net Patient Service Revenue
+ Other Operating Revenue
Net Operating Revenue
Net Operating Revenue
− Operating Expenses
Gain (or Loss) on Operations
Gain (or Loss) on Operations
+ Nonoperating Revenue
Net Income (or Loss) for the Year

Table 4-2 Condensed Income Statement

HEALTH CITY HOSPITAL

Condensed Income Statement
198A

Operating Revenues		
Patient Service Revenues		
Inpatient Service	$180,000	
Outpatient Service Revenue	40,000	
Total Patient Service Revenue		$220,000
Less Deductions in Revenue		
Charity Care	500	
Contractual Adjustments	1,500	
Courtesy Discounts	200	
Bad Debts	2,000	
Total Deductions		(4,200)
Net Patient Service Revenue		215,800
Other Nonoperating Revenue		3,200
Net Operating Revenue		219,000
Less Operating Expenses		223,000
Gain (or Loss) on Operations		(4,000)
Nonoperating Revenue		8,900
Net Income, 198A		4,900

income as well as the various deductions in patient service revenue from courtesy discounts, bad debts, contractual adjustments, and the provision of charity care.

4.3 OPERATING REVENUE

As seen in Table 4-2, it is convenient to group operating revenue into: (1) revenues generated by providing inpatient services, (2) revenues from providing outpatient services, and (3) other operating revenue. The patient service revenues are derived from public and private third party payers and, to a lesser extent, from individual patients who assume the responsibility of financing their use of care. On the other hand, the other operating revenues emanate from such activities as selling supplies to a party other than the patient; conducting educational programs; operating gift shops, cafeterias, and snack bars; renting space to physicians; and renting television sets to patients. In addition to these broad income groupings, most hospitals provide classifications in which deductions from revenue are recorded and accumulated. These broad categories are described next.

4.3.1 Inpatient Revenues

The revenues earned by providing inpatient services typically are of three basic types. The first involves the provision of stay-specific services. In general, stay-specific services can be defined as the components of care that depend on the number of days of care provided to a given patient or group of patients or during a specified period of time. Stay-specific services are represented primarily by the provision of room, board, and general nursing care. Income from these services is classified in accordance with the organizational structure of the institution, the source from which the revenue is derived, the type of accommodation the patient occupies, and the individual's financial status. Obviously, the classification system used in a given situation depends on the organizational structure of the institution as well as on the needs of management.

The second type of revenue usually is associated with the hospital sector and is generated by providing nursing care other than general nursing services. For example, the institution might obtain revenue by providing service in the operating room, the recovery room, the delivery room, and other units that are associated organizationally with the nursing services division. Similar to the earlier discussion, revenues from other nursing services can be classified in accordance with the institution's organizational structure, the source of the revenue, etc.

The third source of inpatient revenue in many health care facilities involves ancillary or other professional services. For example, most hospitals operate a laboratory, a radiology department, a pharmacy, and physiology, inhalation therapy, and physical therapy units. As before, revenues from these units are grouped in accordance with the organizational structure of the institution, source of revenue, and financial status of the patient. In addition, from the perspective of managerial control and evaluation, it is desirable to classify the revenue generated by a given department in terms of the type of service provided. As an example, revenue from the laboratory department might be classified in terms of blood chemistry examinations, urinalyses, serological examinations, and so on.

4.3.2 Outpatient Revenue

The second major component of operating revenue involves outpatient service. At least two major categories of outpatient revenue are identifiable. The first is the visit or registration fee charged when patients register for service.

As before, the revenues from registration fees should be recorded in accordance with the full established rates of the institution irrespective of when, if ever, cash is received.

The second major category involves the provision of ancillary or other professional services to outpatients. Similar to the earlier discussion, the revenue from these services should be classified in accordance with the organizational structure of the institution, the type of service, and so on. In addition, the classification scheme should distinguish between revenues from ancillary services to outpatients and service to inpatients.

4.3.3 Deductions in Revenue

As mentioned, net patient service revenue is calculated by subtracting a set of deductions in income from the total generated by providing service. The revenue deductions stem from the fact that health facilities receive an amount that is less than the full established rate when accounts are settled. As emphasized throughout this discussion, income must be recorded in accordance with the established rate structure of the institution which, of course, provides the basis for the uniform measurement of the total revenue earned during a given period. By the same token, listing revenues in accordance with the rate structure provides the basis for measuring income deductions that result from instances in which the full rates are not collected.

Differences between the amount received and the full established rate are recorded as deductions in revenue. Such deductions are equal to the portion of the amount originally recorded as an account receivable, which management decides should not or cannot be collected. As seen in Table 4-2, deductions in revenue usually are divided into four categories:

1. Courtesy Discounts: A courtesy discount is the difference between the full established rate and any lesser rate the hospital charges for service. Deductions from gross revenues that take the form of courtesy discounts usually are offered to such persons as members of the house staff, board of trustees, and others who are formally affiliated with the institution. Courtesy discounts are recorded in accounts that appear in the income statement as deductions in revenue and in the balance sheet as items that permit management to express outstanding receivables in terms of their net realizable cash value.
2. Contractual Adjustments: These usually involve the financial relationship between a hospital and a third party that determines the amount of reimbursement paid on a cost or cost-plus basis. The contractual adjustment is the difference between the value of care, as expressed by the full established rate, and the contractual rate that is based on a cost or cost-plus formula.

3. Charity Care: Free or charity care is a reduction in a patient's account when it is decided that the individual is not, or will not be, in a position to pay the full established rate.
4. Bad Debts: These arise when patients have financial resources to satisfy or liquidate obligations but fail to make payment. At the end of the accounting period, it is necessary to estimate the portion of the outstanding receivables expected to be uncollectable so as to reduce revenue by an appropriate amount and to report outstanding receivables in terms of their net realizable cash value. These issues are considered in Chapter 7.

When presented in the income statement, the deductions in revenue should be reported net of any related gifts, donations, or grants. As an example, large organizations receive gifts or grants from donors who restrict their use to financing the costs of care for indigent patients. Normally, these resources are recorded initially in a Restricted Fund and, as the donor's conditions are satisfied, an appropriate amount is transferred to the Unrestricted Fund in the form of revenue. Special revenue accounts depicting the nature of the transaction should be used to facilitate the preparation of the income statement.

4.3.4 Other Operating Revenue

This classification includes revenues whose use is not restricted by an external authority and result primarily from (1) the sale of goods and services to persons or institutions other than patients; (2) grants received from governmental agencies, universities, or other external sources; and (3) miscellaneous patient billings.

As mentioned, major sources of other operating income include the sale of laundry services, dietary services, and steam or heat; the rental of rooms or other accommodations; and tuition fees for formal educational programs for institutions or persons other than patients. In addition, the institution may operate an ambulance service that earns revenue by transporting patients to the facility, to the patients' home, or to another health care entity. Revenue from these activities is accumulated in an appropriate account such as Revenue—Dietary, Revenue—Laundry, and so on.

Hospitals frequently receive grants from governmental agencies or other organizations to finance research or other operating necessities. These grants should be recognized as revenue once the three conditions mentioned earlier have been satisfied. Income derived by fulfilling the purpose specified in grants should be accumulated in a revenue account such as research and other special purpose.

The final major component of other operating revenues involves miscellaneous charges to patients for items such as television set rentals, long distance calls, etc. Revenues from these activities are recorded in a miscellaneous patient revenue account.

4.4 NONOPERATING REVENUE

The nonoperating revenue component of hospital income is limited to a relatively few items. The following are among the most important.

4.4.1 Unrestricted Investment Income

Unrestricted investment income in the form of interest or dividend payments may be earned by the temporary investment of working capital. As is discussed in Chapter 8, income earned from the investment of endowment funds on which there are no donor restrictions also is regarded as a source of unrestricted investment income.

4.4.2 Contributed Services

Many institutions depend on volunteers to perform day-to-day functions. The question of what value to place on these contributed services often arises. In practice, contributed services are recorded as an amount equal to the difference between the value of the service and any compensation actually paid by the institution. Before contributed services may be recognized as nonoperating revenue, there must be an objective basis for determining their value. Two additional conditions also must be satisfied: (1) management must exert reasonable control over individuals who are providing the contributed service, and (2) the service must be one that is performed in the institution's normal day-to-day operations. As a practical matter, however, contributed services are recognized and reported only in situations in which their omission would distort the financial statements materially.

4.4.3 Contributions in Kind

Occasionally, institutions receive donations in kind—of gifts in a form other than cash or marketable securities, such as food, linen, medicine, and so on. Even though contributions in kind are rarely received, these donations should be recorded at their fair market value if the items are purchased and used by the institution in the course of normal operations.

4.5 ACCOUNTING METHODS

The primary objective of accounting for revenue is to record all income transactions promptly and accurately so as to provide the information required for rational management decisions and external reporting. Since revenue accounting systems vary from institution to institution, no specific system is described here. Rather this discussion outlines the accounting principles and basic elements that should be incorporated in any system of revenue accounting.

4.5.1 Inpatient Service Revenue

This section considers two interrelated aspects of recording the revenue from service to inpatients. The first aspect involves the process of determining the amount of revenue generated by providing inpatient care, the second involves the process by which income is recorded.

4.5.1.1 The Basic Process

As seen earlier, income from inpatient care consists of revenues from daily service, other nursing service, and ancillary service. For illustration, however, this analysis is simplified by assuming that inpatient service revenues emanate from the provision of:

1. routine daily care (i.e., room, board, and general nursing services)
2. ancillary care (other nursing services and other professional services)

Figure 4-1 shows that the process of determining the revenue from direct patient care involves two streams of information: (1) the data required to calculate the revenues from providing routine daily care, and (2) the data on income from ancillary services.

When an individual is admitted as an inpatient, the institution initiates one or more forms on which are recorded the date of admission; the anticipated use of each component of care; the expected charges; personal information such as an identification number, the patient's name, address, and physician; the party responsible for financing the care; and the date of discharge. The primary function of these forms is to provide the data required to determine the daily service revenue from routine daily care as well as information to the organizational units that are influenced by the admission or discharge of the patient.

The revenue earned by providing care to a given inpatient is represented by the daily room charge and the value of the ancillary services as determined by the institution's fee schedule. For example, assume that the following information represents the use of stay-specific and ancillary services on January 1, 198A, by patients to whom the institution extends credit:

Figure 4-1 The Process of Determining the Amount of Inpatient Service Revenue

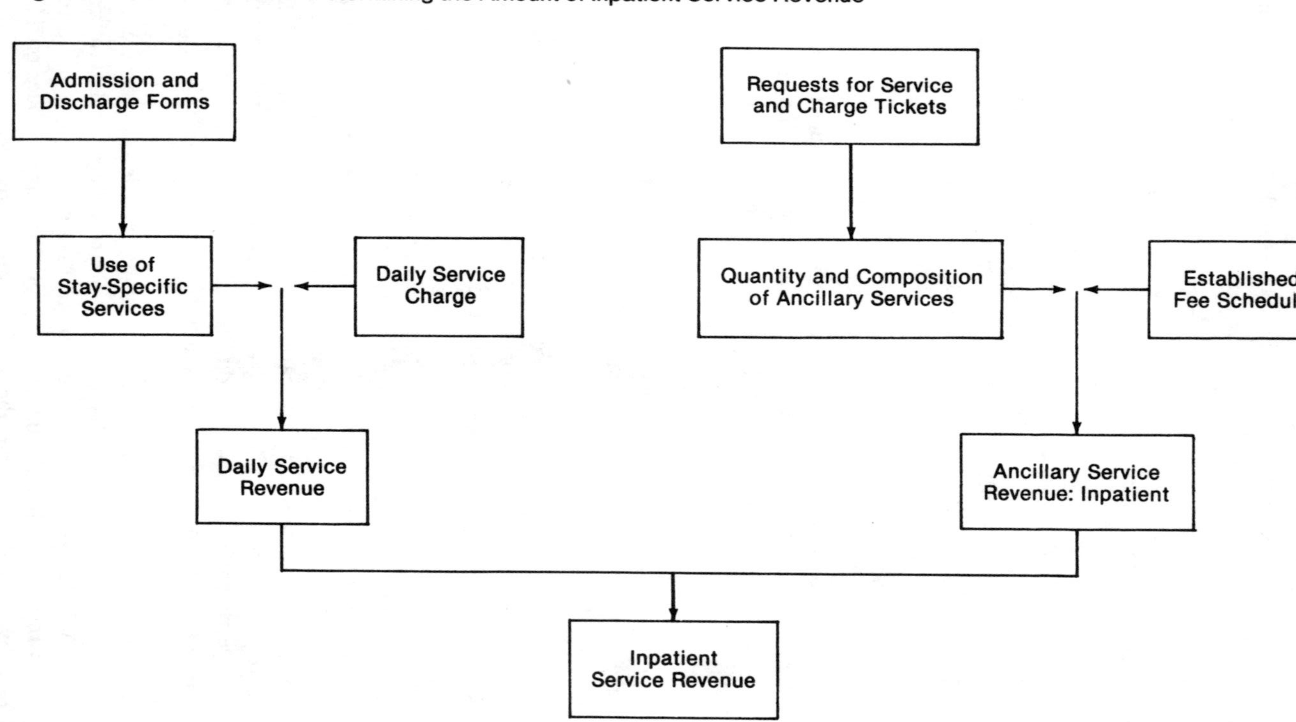

Patient	*Type of Accommodation*	*Units of Ancillary Service*		
		S_1	S_2	S_3
J. Jones	A	1	0	2
H. Brown	B	2	1	0
T. Clement	A	0	2	1
H. Kent	C	0	0	1
B. Allen	B	1	0	1
D. Black	A	3	0	1
E. Cast	C	2	1	1
F. James	A	4	0	1
T. Herbes	B	0	0	2
K. Nichols	A	0	2	0

Suppose further that these individuals represent the patient population of the institution on January 1 and that the charges for the use of stay-specific and ancillary services are as follows:

Component of Care	*Charge*
Stay-Specific Service	
A	\$100/day
B	120/day
C	140/day
Ancillary Service	
S_1	\$5/unit
S_2	10/unit
S_3	15/unit

As can be verified, the revenues earned by providing service are calculated as follows:

Patient	*Daily Service Revenue*	*Ancillary Service Revenue*			*Total*
		S_1	S_2	S_3	
	(1)	(2)	(3)	(4)	(5)
J. Jones	\$100	\$5	\$0	\$30	\$135
H. Brown	120	10	10	0	140
T. Clement	100	0	20	15	135
H. Kent	140	0	0	15	155
B. Allen	120	5	0	15	140
D. Black	100	15	0	15	130
E. Cast	140	10	10	15	175
F. James	100	20	0	15	135
T. Herbes	120	0	0	30	150
K. Nichols	100	0	20	0	120
Totals	1,140	65	60	150	1,415

In this case, the values in the first column correspond to the daily room charge for the type of accommodation occupied by the patient. The values in Columns 2, 3, and 4 are obtained by multiplying the volume of each ancillary service the patient uses by the corresponding charge per unit of service. Finally, Column 5 represents the sum of the charges in the four other columns. In this case, the revenue generated on January 1 by providing stay-specific and ancillary services S_1, S_2, and S_3 amounts to \$1,140, \$65, \$60, and \$150, respectively.

4.5.1.2 Recording Inpatient Service Revenues

As seen earlier, the credit entry that recognizes revenue is accompanied by a debit to a cash account, to an account receivable, or to a deferred revenue account. For example, the calculations of the previous section show that if the institution is forced to extend credit to these patients, these transactions may be summarized by the following entry:

Accounts Receivable—Inpatients	\$1,415	
Daily Service Revenue		\$1,140
Ancillary Service Revenue Unit)		275

The general entry to record revenue earned by providing service on credit always requires a debit entry to accounts receivable and a credit entry to an appropriate revenue account.

The entry just described can be recorded in a general journal in which it is possible to enter any transaction. However, each of these debit and credit journal entries must be transferred to the ledger, which involves a great deal of time and energy. Several methods of reducing the posting time have been devised. They take advantage of the fact that like transactions involve debits and credits to the same accounts. The following discussion assumes that all revenue-generating activity requires an extension of credit and that the institution uses a daily income journal similar to the one in Table 4-3.

The daily income journal is a multicolumn form that permits crediting one or both of the major inpatient revenues and debiting the accounts receivable. The first column identifies the account of the patient to which the debit pertains. As will be seen in Chapter 6, such a specification forms the basis for linking the daily income journal to the subsidiary accounts receivable ledger.

Consider next the process by which the revenue generated on January 1, 198A, may be recorded in the daily income journal. For example, since the institution extends credit to all patients, the revenue earned by providing care to J. Jones may be recorded by the entry

Accounts Receivable	\$135	
Daily Service Revenue		\$100
Ancillary Service Revenue		35

Table 4-3 Daily Income Journal for January 1, 198A: Inpatient Services

	Daily Service Revenue			*Ancillary Service Revenue*			*Accounts Receivable*
Account Debited	*Type A*	*Type B*	*Type C*	S_1	S_2	S_3	
	Credit	*Credit*	*Credit*	*Credit*	*Credit*	*Credit*	*Debit*
J. Jones	$100			$5	$ 0	$30	$135
H. Brown		$120		10	10	0	140
T. Clement	100			0	20	15	135
H. Kent			$140	0	0	15	155
B. Allen		120		5	0	15	140
D. Black	100			15	0	15	130
E. Cast			140	10	10	15	175
F. James	100			20	0	15	135
T. Herbes		120		0	0	30	150
K. Nichols	100			0	20	0	120
Totals	500	360	280	65	60	150	1,415

The first entry in the daily income journal (Table 4-3) also involves:

1. a $135 debit entry to accounts receivable
2. a $100 credit entry to a daily service revenue account
3. a $35 credit entry to the ancillary service revenue accounts

Hence, the daily income journal entries serve the same function as the general journal entry described above.

At the end of each day, column totals should be obtained that, as the table shows, indicate the amount of income earned, by type of revenue, as well as the amount owed by patients to whom credit has been extended. In addition, the amount owed by each patient should be recorded in the subsidiary accounts receivable ledger on a daily basis.

Once the column totals have been calculated, the information in the daily income journal is summarized in the daily income summary presented in Table 4-4. The values corresponding to the January 1 entry correspond to the column totals in Table 4-3. Finally, a similar procedure is used to summarize the revenue and outstanding receivables for the remaining days in January.

The daily income summary provides the basis for determining the income earned during the month by providing service to patients to whom credit has been extended. In Table 4-4, the column totals indicate that the daily service revenue for January amounts to $65,100 and, for the corresponding ancillary service, to $19,375. Accounts receivable of $84,475 are generated.

Table 4-4 Daily Income Summary: January, 198A

Date	*Daily Service Revenue*			*Ancillary Service Revenue*			*Accounts Receivable*
	Type A	*Type B*	*Type C*	*S_1*	*S_2*	*S_3*	
	Credit	*Credit*	*Credit*	*Credit*	*Credit*	*Credit*	*Debit*
1/1	$500	$360	$280	$65	$60	$150	$1,415
1/2	800	480	560	75	90	300	2,305
1/3	1,000	600	700	125	150	450	3,025
1/4	700	1,200	1,400	80	200	465	4,045
.	.	.	.	.	.	.	.
.	.	.	.	.	.	.	.
.	.	.	.	.	.	.	.
1/31	600	1,320	1,540	130	350	45	3,985
Totals	27,900	11,160	26,040	3,100	13,950	2,325	84,475

Subsidiary Revenue Ledger

Daily Service Revenue: A

Date	Dr.	Cr.	Balance
1/31		$27,900	$27,900

Daily Service Revenue: B

Date	Dr.	Cr.	Balance
1/31		$11,160	$11,160

Daily Service Revenue: C

Date	Dr.	Cr.	Balance
1/31		$26,040	$26,040

Ancillary Service: S_1

Date	Dr.	Cr.	Balance
1/31		$3,100	$3,100

Ancillary Service: S_2

Date	Dr.	Cr.	Balance
1/31		$13,950	$13,950

Ancillary Service: S_3

Date	Dr.	Cr.	Balance
1/31		$2,325	$2,325

General Ledger

Daily Service Revenue

Date	Dr.	Cr.	Balance
1/31		$65,100	$65,100

Ancillary Service Revenue

Date	Dr.	Cr.	Balance
1/31		$19,375	$19,375

Accounts Receivable

Date	Dr.	Cr.	Balance
1/31	$84,475		$84,475

At this point it is necessary to introduce the balance column account as a method of presenting the daily income summary in the general ledger and the subsidiary income ledger. The general ledger portion of Table 4-4 shows that a balance column is used to summarize the information in the debit and credit columns. The value in the balance column represents the current balance of the account. On each occasion that the account is debited or credited, a new balance must be calculated and recorded in the balance column. As a result, it is possible to determine the balance of a given account by simply noting the value in the balance column.

Since the column heading does not indicate the nature of the balance in a given account, the recorded balance is assumed to be normal for that account unless otherwise specified. Consequently, the use of the balance column account requires an understanding of normal balances. Fortunately normal balances are easy to understand since an account usually is increased more than it is decreased. Thus, if an account is increased by a debit entry, it normally has a debit balance; if it is increased by a credit entry, it has a credit balance. The normal balances, by type of account, may be summarized as follows:

Type of Account	*To Increase*	*Normal Balance*
Asset	Debit	Debit
Expense	Debit	Debit
Liability	Credit	Credit
Fund Balance	Credit	Credit
Revenue	Credit	Credit
Contra Asset	Credit	Credit

When an account has an abnormal balance, the anomaly usually is indicated by the use of brackets. On the other hand, a situation in which an account has no balance is indicated by placing - 0 - or 0.00 in the balance column.

Consider next the interrelation between the daily income summary, the general ledger, and the subsidiary revenue ledger. Recall that the revenue generated by operational activity is entered in the daily income summary on a daily basis. At the end of the month, the column totals for the revenue categories and outstanding receivables are calculated and the sums of the debit and credit entries are compared to ensure that transactions have been recorded properly. In Table 4-4, the sum of the credit entries ($27,900 + $11,160 + $26,040 + $3,100 + $13,950 + $2,325) is equal to the sum of the debit entries ($84,475). At this point, the column totals are simply transferred to the appropriate column of the corresponding account in the general ledger and the current balance is recorded in the balance column.

In the subsidiary revenue ledger, a balance column account is created for each of the services provided to inpatients. In this case, the revenues from stay-specific services are recorded by type of accommodation and those from ancillary care by type of service. Concerning the balances of the subsidiary revenue accounts, Table 4-4 shows that the revenues generated by providing routine daily care to patients occupying accommodations of Types, A, B, and C are $27,900, $11,160, and $26,040, respectively. The sum of these values is equal to the balance of the daily service revenue account in the general ledger. In a similar fashion, the current balances of the subsidiary revenue accounts of ancillary services S_1, S_2, and S_3 are obtained from the daily income summary section of Table 4-4. In this case, the sum of the current balances in the subsidiary accounts ($3,100 + $13,950 + $2,325) exactly equals the current balance of the ancillary service revenue account in the general ledger.

As indicated, the revenue accounts in the general ledger perform three functions:

1. These accounts indicate the amount of revenue from providing routine daily care and ancillary services.
2. If these accounts are excluded from the general ledger, the sum of the debits will not equal the sum of the credits. As a result, the revenue accounts help keep the general ledger in balance.
3. The revenue accounts in the general ledger represent the basis for verifying and controlling the balances of the individual accounts in the subsidiary revenue ledger. It is for this reason that the accounts of the general ledger are called control accounts.

Thus far, this analysis has been limited to transactions in which the institution extends credit to the patient or to a third party payer. In such a situation, cash is received after the hospital recognizes the revenue earned by providing service. However, when the service is prepaid by the patient or another party, the health care facility receives cash before it provides service and recognizes revenue. Similarly, the recognition of revenue and the receipt of cash frequently occur simultaneously. Although these issues are discussed in Chapter 6, the situation in which cash is received prior to the provision of service deserves brief attention here.

For illustration, suppose the institution receives $100,000 at the beginning of the month to finance inpatient care for insured individuals on a current basis. The entry to record the cash receipt is:

	Debit	Credit
Cash	$100,000	
Deferred Revenue		$100,000
To record prospective payment.		

Obviously, this entry increases the cash assets as well as the liabilities of the institution by $100,000. The entry is recorded initially in a cash receipts journal (which is described in Chapter 6). The liability created by the prepayment may be portrayed by using this balance column account:

Deferred Revenue

Date	*Debit*	*Credit*	*Balance*
1/1		$100,000	$100,000

Recall that liability created by the cash receipt represents an obligation of the institution until service is provided and revenue is earned.

Now, suppose the institution provides routine daily care and ancillary services to insured patients that, when valued at its full established rates, amount to $60,000 and $30,000, respectively. By providing service, the institution earns income and reduces the liability created when the prepayment was received. In this case, the entry to record the revenue generated by providing service to insured patients is:

Deferred Revenue	$90,000	
Daily Service Revenue		$60,000
Ancillary Service Revenue		$30,000

Several aspects of this entry are worthy of note. Obviously, the entry reduces the institution's liability and recognizes the revenue earned by providing care. Also, assuming that the facility engages in no other transactions, the entry results in a credit balance of $10,000 in the deferred revenue account. At this point, the balance column account pertaining to this liability is:

Deferred Revenue

Date	*Debit*	*Credit*	*Balance*
1/1		$100,000	$100,000
1/31	$90,000		10,000

In this case, the current balance is given by the difference between the debit entry of $100,000 and the credit entry of $90,000.

4.5.2 Outpatient Revenue

Similar to the discussion just presented, the major focus of this section is on the process of determining and recording revenues earned by providing service to outpatients. It begins, as before, with a brief analysis of the basic system for determining the amount of outpatient revenue the institution earns, then considers the accounting methods of recording these revenues.

4.5.2.1 The Basic System

In Figure 4-2, the revenues from outpatient services consist of: (1) registration fees and (2) income resulting from providing ancillary services to patients requiring ambulatory care. These components are described next.

Patients requiring ambulatory care usually register at a central desk where their name, address, insurance status, etc., are recorded. In some cases patients may be asked to pay a registration fee. They also may pay for the service they are to receive or arrange to pay for services not insured by a third party payer. Unless specified otherwise, however, the assumption here is that the institution extends credit to outpatients.

Credits to outpatient revenues for the use of service usually emanate from a service requisition form that is sent with the patient or to the department providing the service. That department prepares a medical report and a charge voucher that provides the basis for determining the amount of revenue earned and the entry to the corresponding account receivable. Once the visit is completed, the charge voucher, logs, and other outpatient service records are collected and forwarded to the accounting department for inclusion in the daily income journal. As will be seen in Chapter 6, entries also are recorded in an appropriate account of the subsidiary accounts receivable ledger. As with inpatient revenues, the information in the daily income summary is posted to the institution's general ledger and subsidiary revenue ledger at the end of the month. In addition, at that time the subsidiary accounts receivable ledger is reconciled with the corresponding control account of the general ledger.

4.5.2.2 Recording Outpatient Revenues

As an illustration, suppose that the institution referred to earlier charges outpatients a registration fee of $10 per visit as well as $5, $10, and $15 on each occasion that they use ancillary services S_1, S_2, and S_3, respectively. Suppose further that the data in Table 4-5 represent the use of ancillary care by a group of patients on a given day. These data may be recorded in a daily income journal similar to Table 4-6. In this case, each of the patients is assessed a registration fee of $10 as well as a charge that reflects the use of ancillary services as calculated in Table 4-5. Similar to our earlier discussion, the income generated each day is recorded in a daily income summary from which the amount of income earned during the month is determined.

As indicated earlier, the column totals of the daily income summary pertaining to outpatient revenues are posted to the appropriate column of the corresponding account in the general ledger at the end of the month. Similarly, the revenue earned by providing each ancillary service to outpatients should be distinguished from those generated by providing ancillary care to inpatients, which are entered in the subsidiary revenue ledger.

Figure 4-2 The Process of Determining Outpatient Revenues

Number of Visits
Fee per Visit
Registration Fees
Request for Service and Charge Tickets
Quantity & Composition of Ancillary Service
Fee Schedule
Ancillary Service Revenue: Outpatient
Outpatient Revenue

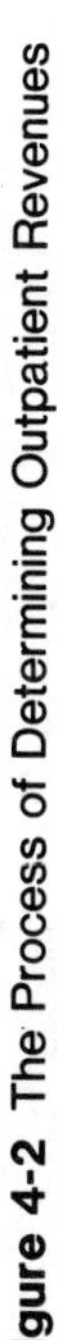

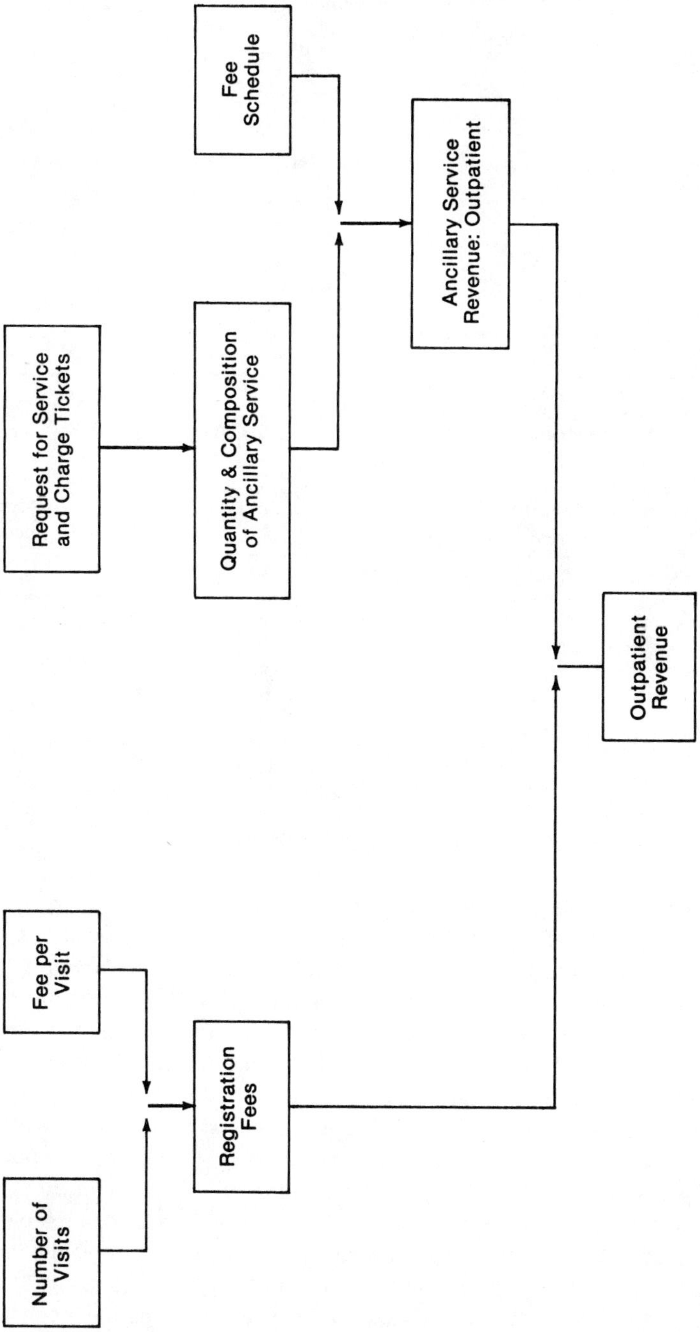

Table 4-5 Revenue from Providing Ancillary Service to Outpatients on January 1, 198A

	Service S_1		Service S_2		*Service S_3*		
Patient	*Quantity*	*Revenue*	*Quantity*	*Revenue*	*Quantity*	*Revenue*	*Total Charge*
S. Clement	0	$0	1	$10	2	$30	$40
C. South	1	5	1	10	1	15	30
L. French	0	0	0	0	1	15	15
J. Smith	0	0	1	10	0	0	10
F. Wader	2	10	0	0	1	15	25
Totals	3	15	3	30	5	75	120

Table 4-6 Daily Income Journal for January 1, 198A: Outpatient Services

Account Debited	*Registration Fee*	*Ancillary Service Revenue*			*Accounts Receivable*
		S_1	*S_2*	*S_3*	
	Credit	*Credit*	*Credit*	*Credit*	*Debit*
S. Clement	$10	$0	$10	$30	$50
C. South	10	5	10	15	40
L. French	10	0	0	15	25
J. Smith	10	0	10	0	20
F. Wader	10	10	0	15	35
Totals	50	15	30	75	170

4.5.3 Deductions in Patient Service Revenue

As mentioned, the revenue from providing patient care is recorded on an accrual basis at the full established rates, irrespective of when, if ever, cash is received. Since the institution occasionally will receive an amount that is less than the full rate when an account finally is settled, adjusting entries reflecting such items as free or charity care, courtesy discounts, contractual allowances, and bad debts are required if the net income of the period and the balance sheet are to be presented accurately.

A failure to recognize the required adjustments will result in an overstatement of the net revenue of the period as reported in the income statement and an overstatement of the receivables and the fund balance in the balance sheet. To avoid such consequences, charity care, courtesy discounts, contractual adjustments, and bad debts are treated as reductions in revenue and are reported as such in the income statement. Similarly, these items are treated as contra asset accounts that reduces the receivables in the balance sheet to their net realizable cash value. Assuming that the revenue reductions pertain to transactions involving an account receivable, the summary adjusting entry is recorded as follows:

Provision for		
Charity Care	$1,500	
Contractual Adjustments	2,500	
Courtesy Discounts	550	
Bad Debts	300	
Allowance for		
Charity Care		$1,500
Contractual Adjustments		2,500
Courtesy Discounts		550
Bad Debts		300

In this transaction, the debit entries are contra revenue accounts and appear in the income statement as deductions in revenue. The credit entries in this transaction are contra asset accounts that appear in the balance sheet and reduce the accounts receivable from the full established rate at which they are recorded to their net realizable cash value.

4.5.4 Other Operating Revenue

As will be recalled, the other major types of operating revenue are recoveries; grants from governmental agencies, universities, or other organizations that may be used for special purposes or other operating exigencies; and miscellaneous patient billings. As a general rule, the principles already discussed govern the accounting for such types of revenue.

For example, assume that the dietary department of the institution provides $17,500 worth of meals to another hospital on account. Obviously, revenue is earned by the sale of the meals that are exchanged for an account receivable. The entry to record the revenue generated by this transaction is:

Accounts Receivable	$17,500	
Other Operating Revenue—Dietary		$17,500

Grants normally are recorded as revenues when they are received. However, when they are obtained prior to their use, they should be recorded in an equity account. In the first case, assume that the cash receipt and the recognition of revenue coincide. The entry to record a $24,500 research grant is:

Cash	$24,500	
Special Research Grant		$24,500

On the other hand, if the cash had been received prior to its use, the entry in the Specific Purpose Fund is:

Cash	$24,500	
Appropriated Equity		$24,500

When the funds are used in support of the designated research, the revenue should be recognized and recorded in the following fashion:

Specific Purpose Fund

Transfer to Unrestricted Fund	$24,500	
Cash		$24,500

Unrestricted Fund

Cash	$24,500	
Special Research Grant		$24,500

As an example of miscellaneous patient billings, suppose that a patient made a $15 long distance telephone call, rented a television set for $30, and obtained a $3 meal for a guest. The following entry is required to record the resulting revenue:

Accounts Receivable	$48	
Miscellaneous Patient Revenue		$48

4.5.5 Nonoperating Revenue

As noted, the major sources of nonoperating revenue recognized by most institutions are unrestricted investment income, contributed services, contributions in kind, and ancillary operations. The hospital also may receive donations, bequests, and grants in the form of cash or marketable securities. The accounting treatment of each of these forms of nonoperating revenue is discussed next.

4.5.5.1 Investment Income

The principal source of the institution's nonoperating revenue consists of unrestricted income earned by the investment of Specific Purpose Funds or Endowment Funds and all investments of unrestricted funds. Investment income usually is earned in the form of interest or dividends and may be accounted for on either a cash or accrual basis.

When unrestricted investment income is recorded on a cash basis, its receipt is recorded in the daily cash report, resulting in an entry similar to

Cash	$62.50	
Investment Income		$62.50

where it is assumed that the investment income is recognized when the cash payment of $62.50 is received. If the investment income had been recorded on an accrual basis, two entries would have been required. On the date it is reasonably certain that a cash flow will result from the investment, the entry recorded is:

Investment Income Receivable	$62.50	
Investment Income		$62.50

When the cash is received, the entry

Cash	$62.50	
Investment Income Receivable		$62.50

records the cash receipt and eliminates the accrued receivable associated with the earlier recognition of investment income.

4.5.5.2 Contributed Services

The value assigned to contributed services is the difference between the value of the service and the compensation actually paid by the institution. The value of the service is recorded as a debit to the appropriate salary and wage expense and is offset by a credit to cash and to the revenue account for contributed services. For example, assume that volunteer services would have cost the institution $22,500 if performed by paid employees. Further, suppose that the health facility actually paid $2,500 for these services. The entry to record such a transaction is:

Salary and Wages	$22,500	
Cash		$2,500
Contributed Services		20,000

4.5.5.3 Donations

Donations in kind, which normally are purchased and used in support of the day-to-day activities, are recorded at fair market value in an appropriate expense category. For example, if the institution is given linen that has a fair market value of $2,000, the donation in kind is recorded thus:

Supply Expense	$2,000	
Donations and Bequests		$2,000

The debit entry to the expense account is offset exactly by the credit entry to the revenue account Donations and Bequests which, other things held constant, leaves the fund balance or the equity of the institution unchanged.

The facility also may receive donations and bequests that may be used for any purpose. Their receipt should be recorded as revenue in the unrestricted or operating fund. The treatment of restricted donations and bequests is discussed in Chapter 11.

4.5.5.4 Other Operations

Typically, the revenue earned through other activities such as the operation of a gift shop, a snack bar, and so on is recorded on a cash basis. Thus, revenue is recognized and recorded when cash receipts are turned in for deposit. If the cash receipts of the gift shop for a given day are $570, the revenue is recorded as follows:

Cash	$570	
Ancillary Income		$570

When the revenue from these operations exerts a material influence on the financial statements, they are recorded so as to reflect the activity earning the income.

4.6 INTERNAL CONTROL OVER REVENUE

The basic objective of accounting for revenue is to ensure, to the extent possible, that all income is recorded at the full established rates in the proper income account. This is accomplished by:

1. the preparation of revenue budgets that are based on the expected number of units of service to be provided and expressed in monetary terms
2. the implementation and use of sound admitting and discharge procedures
3. the proper development and use of census reports, charge vouchers, and other documents

4. adherence to the principles of responsibility accounting
5. the maintenance of a sound recording system
6. the reconciliation of recorded revenue with the quantity of care provided

One of the most important features of an accounting system that satisfies the goal of properly recording all revenue involves the implementation and use of effective admission, registration, and discharge procedures. The admission process should provide information that permits a proper classification of revenues by type of patient, type of service or accommodation, and the individual's insurance status. In determining inpatient revenues, the institution's census must be taken accurately and compared with admission and discharge records to validate the data. In addition, statistics on occupancy, discharge and admission dates, length of stay, and patient days of service should be accumulated in accordance with established definitions.

Clearly, the system of accounting for service revenue must be designed to ensure that proper source documents are executed properly and that all care provided is reflected in the revenue accounts of the institution. The system should be designed to provide safeguards against oversights and incorrect pricing in charge vouchers, which should be compared with established rates to ensure the accurate calculation of revenue. This consideration is of primary importance in determining outpatient income.

The control over outpatient revenues is complicated by the fact that the person receiving the cash frequently is the same one who is responsible for recording cash receipt. When this is the case, effective controls over cash and receivables must be exercised. These matters receive attention in Chapter 6.

Questions for Discussion

1. Explain why is it important to record and report revenues accurately.
2. Define the term revenue.
3. Describe conditions under which revenue should be recognized.
4. Define deductions in revenue and describe how they are reported in the financial statements.
5. Differentiate between operating and nonoperating revenue.
6. Discuss the major sources of operating and nonoperating revenue.
7. Describe the basic system by which the amount of inpatient revenue is determined.
8. Describe the basic system by which the amount of outpatient revenue is determined.
9. Describe the relation between the daily income journal and the subsidiary income ledger.
10. State the factors that contribute to the various deductions in revenue.
11. Explain how revenues are controlled.

12. Explain why special journals are used to record revenue.
13. Define a balance column account and the meaning of a normal balance.
14. Describe the normal balance of:

    a. an asset
    b. an expense
    c. a liability
    d. a revenue
    e. the fund balance
    f. a contra asset account

15. Explain conditions under which contributed services are recorded and reported.

Problems for Solution

1. Suppose the following information pertains to the provision of inpatient services on January 1, 198A:

Patient	*Type of Accommodation*	*Use of Ancillary Services (In Units)*		
		S_1	S_2	S_3
A	A	10	6	2
B	A	15	3	0
C	B	9	7	1
D	C	10	3	1
E	B	6	4	4
F	C	5	6	9
G	A	0	1	2
H	B	3	8	2

Suppose further that the following charges pertain to the use of these services:

Type of Accommodation		*Ancillary Services*	
A	\$100/Day	S_1	\$1.50 per unit
B	130/Day	S_2	2.00 per unit
C	150/Day	S_3	3.50 per unit

If the hospital extends credit to these patients, prepare the journal entries required to record these transactions. Explain how much revenue the institution earns.

2. Use the results of the calculations in Problem 1 to record the income the institution earns in a daily income journal and a subsidiary revenue ledger. Assuming no other transactions during the month, show how the information recorded in Problem 1 will appear in the general ledger.
3. Assume that the following information pertains to the use of outpatient services on January 1, 198A:

	Use of Ancillary Service		
Patient	S_1	S_2	S_3
A	1	0	2
B	0	1	1
C	2	2	0
D	1	0	0
E	1	1	1
F	1	0	2
G	0	3	2

Suppose further that these services are provided on credit and that the institution charges the following fees:

Registration Fee :	\$15.00
S_1 :	\$3.00 per unit
S_2 :	4.00 per unit
S_3 :	5.00 per unit

Determine the amount of revenue earned and record the required journal entries.

4. Record the outpatient revenue earned in Problem 3 in a daily income journal and a subsidiary revenue journal. Assuming that no other services are provided to outpatients during the month, explain how these balances will appear in the general ledger.
5. Suppose that on January 2 the institution is certain that investment income of \$7,000 will be paid on February 14. Record these transactions on an accrual basis.
6. Assume that volunteer services would have cost the institution \$30,000 if provided by paid employees. However, the facility pays \$4,000 for these services. Describe what general journal entry is required to record this transaction.
7. Assume a donation in kind has a fair market value of \$10,000. Show what journal entry records the receipt of this donation.
8. The hospital gift shop earns \$10,000 in sales on August 10. Show what entry is required to record these sales.

Chapter 5

Accounting for Expenses

A substantial portion of the costs of providing health care consists of recurring annual expenditures that, because of inflation and rapid technological advances, have reached unprecedented levels that many believe will continue to increase without abatement. Health administrators are responsible for huge sums of money, so a high order of expense accounting is necessary if they are to use funds intelligently and thereby achieve their institution's objectives.

In a commercial enterprise, the extent to which a company has achieved the objective of earning a profit is evaluated by examining the difference between revenues and expenditures. If revenues exceed expenses for an extended time, the firm's financial viability is assured and it will expand and prosper. On the other hand, if expenses exceed revenues for a prolonged period, the enterprise faces extinction.

In the health care industry, however, no single measure of success exists. Clearly, the excess of revenues over expenses does not necessarily imply that the facility has been successful in achieving its goal of providing the community with required services. No final conclusions regarding the performance or effectiveness of an institution can be gained solely from financial statements; however, accounting information, when presented in a clear and concise fashion, is of assistance in an overall evaluation. Certainly, this evaluation requires that expenses be recorded and reported in accordance with sound accounting practice.

The purpose of this chapter is to examine the problems of accounting for the operating expenses of a health care facility. It specifically covers accounting for employee costs and nonlabor expenditures such as supplies, utilities, rent, and purchased services. An extended discussion of accounting for depreciation as well as the acquisition and disposal of plant equipment is deferred to Chapter 12.

5.1 COSTS VS. EXPENSE

The terms cost and expense have been used in a variety of ways and, thus frequently are a source of confusion. Basic to the notion of cost is the sacrifice or exchange of one thing for another in an economic transaction. Thus, the term cost refers to an outlay of cash or other assets or services, or the incurring of a liability in exchange for goods or services. Costs generally are measured in terms of the cash that is disbursed or will be disbursed in exchange for an item. They also are measured in terms of the fair market value of noncash assets or the services that are given or will be given in an exchange transaction.

An expense, on the other hand, is an expired cost. Expenses are costs that are associated directly or indirectly with the revenue of a given period. The expiration of costs and the resultant recognition of expenses normally is governed by one of the following principles:

1. Association of Cause and Effect: Since certain cost items are directly related to the generation of revenue (or are presumed to be so) they are recognized as an expense. Consequently, the recognition of revenue is accompanied by the recognition of the related expense.
2. Systematic and Rational Allocation: When costs are not directly related to the generation of a specific item of revenue, they are allocated to the time periods that benefit from the use of the corresponding resources.
3. Immediate Recognition: Some costs can be recognized immediately because the use of the corresponding resource does not contribute to a future period or to the generation of future revenue.

Costs that have not expired and have not been recorded as an expense are carried in the books as an asset.

A simple example illustrates the differences between cost and expenditure. Suppose the institution purchases an insurance policy requiring the prepayment of an annual premium of $60,000. Such a transaction is recorded as follows:

Prepaid Insurance	$60,000	
Cash		$60,000

With the prepayment of the premium, the facility acquires an asset that is carried on the books at a cost of $60,000. Each month, a portion of this cost expires and is recognized as an expense by

Insurance Expense	$5,000	
Prepaid Insurance		$5,000

Obviously, the debit to the Insurance Expense account serves to recognize the expiration of a portion of the original cost that was incurred when the insurance asset was acquired. Thus, the first of these entries refers to the concept of cost, the second to the concept of expense. Despite these differences, however, the terms cost and expense are used interchangeably in this discussion.

5.2 CLASSIFICATION OF EXPENSES

In health facility accounting, two methods of classifying costs may be identified. The first, and perhaps most basic system, categorizes cost according to purpose or function; the second classifies expenses according to the object or nature of the expenditure.

5.2.1 Classification of Expense by Function

As implied earlier, the classification of expenses that most health facilities use conforms to their organization chart. The institution can be envisioned as being composed of a set of separate but integrated units, each of which performs a specific function. A responsibility center can be defined as a unit or a group of units for which an identifiable individual is accountable. For purposes of control, expenses traditionally have been classified in accordance with the distribution of responsibility and authority in the institution.

However, as mentioned in Chapter 2, the reporting requirements imposed by P.L. 95-142 force hospitals to classify costs in terms of functional centers. In this regard, cost centers can be defined in terms of a well-defined function or set of functions. In performing the function, the center incurs costs that are associated with acquiring the real resources used in productive activity. The classification of expense by function, then, is the basis for grouping costs in terms of the unit providing a standardized service or a set of more or less standardized tasks.

From a theoretical perspective, a functional cost center should be established for each identifiable and distinguishable service provided by the institution. Under such a scheme, expenses are recorded and assembled for each of the services. From a practical perspective, however, such a detailed level of disaggregation is impossible. As an apparent compromise, P.L. 95-142 requires the hospital to report costs on a functional basis. Accordingly, recall that functional accounting requires the collection of information that depicts the use of resources in performing a set of specific tasks. In turn, these data provide the basis for assigning an appropriate amount of cost to the unit responsible for performing the set of functions.

As indicated, there appears to be a conflict between responsibility accounting and functional accounting. This text assumes that the conflict has been resolved by assigning costs on a functional basis. To simplify the analysis, it is assumed further that the responsibility center and the functional unit are synonymous. However, as noted, it may be possible to define the responsibility center as one or more functional units for which an identifiable individual is accountable. Such an approach implies that the financial data reported to external authorities are classified in terms of the functional unit. On the other hand, from the perspective of internal control, financial information is classified in terms of the responsibility center. In addition, data that have been grouped in terms of functions or tasks for purposes of external reporting can enhance the extent to which management exerts control over operational activity.

5.2.2 Classification of Expense by Nature

The second method of classification within each functional unit or responsibility center categorizes expenditures according to the object of the expense. Major categories of expenditure in this classification are:

1. Cost of Employment: This includes salaries, wages, and employee benefits such as health insurance, pensions, unemployment insurance, and worker compensation.
2. Cost of Purchased Services: This involves expenditures incurred in obtaining services from outside agencies that otherwise would have been performed by employees of the institution, such as auditing, as well as consultant and laboratory services provided by employees of agencies other than those of the health facility.
3. Cost of Consumable Supplies: This involves the stock and other consumable material used in providing patient care or general support service.
4. Cost of Physical Facilities: This includes depreciation expenses, rent, taxes, heat, light, power, etc.
5. Cost of Financing: This includes interest, bond amortization, and the cost of issuing debt instruments.
6. Miscellaneous: This includes expenditures that are not included conveniently in any of the other expense categories, such as membership fees in professional organizations, travel expenses, and bank charges (other than interest).

As mentioned, responsibility centers may be defined in terms of the functional unit(s) for which an identifiable individual is accountable. From the perspective of internal reporting and control, the line manager should be provided with reports that specify expenses over which significant control is exerted. Controllable expenses should be classified in a manner designed to associate costs with individuals who are responsible for their incurrence.

Similarly, anticipated costs, as expressed by the budget, also should be classified so that the results of operational activity can be compared with budgetary expectations and thereby provide the basis for evaluating the performance of the institution at each level of managerial responsibility. In this way, the performance of a given responsibility center or functional unit is evaluated in terms of only those costs over which the manager exerts significant control. Thus, when the results of operational activity and the budget are expressed in terms of the same unit of analysis, differences between actual and desired performance are traceable to a single individual who is responsible for investigating factors contributing to the variance and, where appropriate, implementing remedial action.

5.3 WAGE AND SALARY EXPENSES

Since the costs of employment represent 50 percent to 60 percent of the operating costs of most health care facilities, particular emphasis must be devoted to the development of a sound system by which payroll and related costs are determined and recorded. This section describes the accounting methods by which employment costs are determined and assigned to the institution's functional units or responsibility centers. It also considers methods of recording payroll taxes imposed on the employer and the payment of payroll deductions.

5.3.1 Determination of Payroll Expenses

The calculation of payroll expenses and other related costs involves two interrelated steps: (1) the calculation of the gross payroll and (2) the determination of each employee's net pay, which requires the calculation of several payroll deductions. These steps are described next.

5.3.1.1 Computing the Gross Payroll

The calculation of the gross payroll is accomplished in the following fashion. For other than salaried personnel, the number of hours worked is validated by an employee who is independent of the timekeeping function. The gross pay of individuals compensated on an hourly basis is composed of a regular component that is given by the product of the number of hours worked and the authorized wage rate and, when appropriate, an overtime premium. For salaried employees, the gross pay per period is a fixed amount that, once calculated, does not change unless the annual salary is altered. All changes in wage rates or salaries that result from promotions, merit increases, union-mandated raises, and so on should enter into the calculations of gross pay only when authorized in writing by the manager of the responsibility center or functional unit.

Each pay period, the information necessary for compiling gross pay as described above is summarized in a Payroll Register. The portion of the Register pertaining to the calculation of the gross weekly pay of individuals employed in the laboratory department is shown in Table 5-1. The columns headed Daily Hours show the number of hours worked during the week by each employee. The number of overtime hours worked is entered in the column so identified. The total number of hours worked during the week is recorded for each employee in the Total Hours column while the Regular Pay Rate column lists the authorized pay rate for each individual.

In the computation of each employee's regular pay and overtime premium, it is assumed that the institution's normal work week is 40 hours. The Regular Pay column presents the results obtained when the number of hours worked are multiplied by the regular pay rate. Table 5-1 shows that A. Maier worked 48 hours (eight of them overtime) during the week and was paid $8.00 per hour. The regular weekly pay of this individual is $384 (48 hours × $8.00/hour). The overtime premium of time and a half in the next column is computed by multiplying half of the regular pay rate by the number of overtime hours worked. Maier worked eight overtime hours during the week; when multiplied by half the regular pay rate of $8.00, this results in an overtime premium of $32.00.

The gross pay of each employee is simply the sum of the regular pay and the overtime premium. The gross pay in the last column is the base on which the amount withheld from the pay of each individual is determined.

5.3.1.2 Payroll Deductions and Net Pay

The employees' net pay is obtained by subtracting a number of deductions from the gross figure. The amounts withheld by employers include:

- Taxes that support the federal Old Age and Survivors Insurance (OASI) benefits program of the Social Security Act
- federal, state, and municipal income taxes
- insurance premium payments
- other deductions that might be authorized by the employee such as union dues, credit union, savings bonds, and charitable donations.

The portion of the Payroll Register pertaining to the withholdings or deductions from the gross pay of each employee is presented in Table 5-2.

Table 5-1 Calculation of Gross Pay

Employee	M	T	W	TH (1)	F	S	S	Total Hours (2)	Overtime Hours (3)	Regular Pay Rate (4)	Regular Pay (5)	Overtime Premium (6)	Gross Pay (7)
	Daily Hours												
A. Maier	8	8	8	8	8	8		48	8	$8.00	$384.00	$32.00	$416.00
H. Tallent	8	4	8	4	8	8		40	—	7.00	280.00	—	280.00
P. Griswold	8	8	8	8	8	—		40	—	6.50	260.00	—	260.00
S. Ohlm	8	4	8	—	8	4	8	40	—	6.00	240.00	—	240.00
J. Coleman	8	8	8	8	8	8		48	8	7.50	360.00	30.00	390.00
L. Corrillia	8	8	8	8	8	—	4	44	4	5.50	242.00	11.00	253.00
													1,839.00

Table 5-2 Calculation of Net Pay

Employee	Gross Pay	Deductions: Social Security Taxes (1)	Deductions: Federal Income Taxes (2)	Deductions: Hospital Insurance (3)	Deductions: Other Deductions (4)	Deductions: Total Deductions (5)	Payment: Net Pay (6)	Payment: Check No. (7)
A. Maier	$416.00	$29.12	$12.50	$11.00	$0.00	$52.62	$363.38	950
H. Tallent	280.00	19.60	8.00	14.00	10.00	51.60	228.40	951
P. Griswold	260.00	18.20	9.50	9.00	0.00	36.70	223.30	952
S. Ohlm	240.00	16.80	7.00	8.00	20.00	51.80	188.20	953
J. Coleman	390.00	27.30	6.50	6.00	0.00	39.80	350.20	954
L. Corrillia	253.00	17.71	10.00	4.50	0.00	32.21	220.79	955
Totals	1,839.00	128.73	53.50	52.50	30.00	264.73	1,574.27	

As this suggests, the first deduction to be considered involves the Social Security taxes under the Federal Insurance Contributions Act (F.I.C.A.). In general, the employer not only must deduct Social Security taxes from employees' pay but also must pay a tax equal to the amount withheld. That amount is obtained by applying a tax rate, expressed in percentage terms, to the gross pay of each employee. The tax applies to annual earnings up to a specified amount, so additional income earned during the year is exempt from the levy.

Since the tax rate and the maximum amount of earnings subject to the levy have been increasing steadily, it is assumed here that an F.I.C.A. rate of 7 percent is applied to the first $15,000 paid to each employee during the year. Table 5-2 assumes further that none of the employees have earned $15,000 or more to date and, as a result, the gross pay of each is subject to Social Security taxes. As a consequence, Column 1 shows that 7 percent of the gross pay has been deducted from each individual's earnings. For example, the gross pay of Maier is $416.00; the Social Security deduction is 7% × $416.00, or $29.12. The Social Security deductions for all employees total $128.73, which also represents a tax liability of the employer.

Column 2 lists employee income tax deductions that employers (with few exceptions) are required to calculate, collect, and remit to the Internal Revenue Service. Hospitals and other health care facilities thus are required to act as tax collectors for the federal government.

In general, the amount of federal income tax withheld depends on the employee's earnings and the number of exemptions claimed. In determining this amount, employers use a withholding table that indicates how much taxes they must withhold for any combination of earnings per period and number of exemptions claimed. It should be noted that the income tax withholdings in Table 5-2 are assumed data.

Health care facilities also are required to withhold state and municipal income taxes from employees' pay. These are treated in the same way as are federal income taxes.

In Columns 3 and 4 are the remaining deductions. Column 3 contains a set of assumed withholdings that are used to pay hospital insurance premiums; those in Column 4 refer to the ones authorized by the employee and can be related to the purchase of savings bonds, the payment of accident or life insurance, the repayment of loans, union dues, credit union, and donations to charitable organizations.

Each entry in Column 5 reflects the total of the deductions from individuals' pay. For example, the total withholdings deducted from the pay of A. Maier is given by the sum

$$\$29.12 + \$12.50 + \$11.00 = \$52.62$$

The total amount withheld from the pay of all employees represents a liability to the institution until payment is remitted to the appropriate party.

Each individual's net pay is determined by subtracting total deductions from gross earnings. In Column 6 each value represents the net pay of one of the employees. For example, consider the first worker, A. Maier, whose weekly earnings amount to \$416.00. Since \$52.62 is withheld from this individual's gross pay, the net pay is given by \$416.00 − \$52.62, or \$363.38. Consequently, the values in Column 6 represent the amounts for which individual paychecks are prepared while the column's total is the sum that will be paid to all employees. Column 7 indicates the number of the payroll check issued to the employee.

A final observation concerning Table 5-2 is worthy of note. The sum of the total deductions and the net pay of all employees (i.e., \$264.73 and \$1,574.27, respectively) is exactly equal to the gross payroll of the unit (i.e., \$1,839). A comparison of these employees' gross pay with the sum of their net pay and total deductions validates the payroll calculations.

5.3.2 Allocation of Wage and Salary Expenses

Wage and salary expenses should be allocated (assigned) on a functional basis. For illustration, assume that the primary function of the unit referred to earlier is to provide services S_1, S_2, and S_3. To verify that the wage and salary expenses calculated in Sections 5.3.1.1 and 5.3.1.2 should be charged to the unit, assume further that the distribution of the hours worked by each of the employees in Table 5-3 is available for analysis. A comparison of the values in Column 2 of Table 5-1 with the total hours in Table 5-3 shows that, with the exception of A. Maier and L. Corrillia, the hours worked by all employees are devoted to performing the functions of the unit. It is assumed that the values in the Idle Time column represent the capacity to provide service during periods of peak demand. It also is assumed that these hours of work represent an acceptable use of labor in performing the functions of the unit.

Column 2 of Table 5-1 indicates that the gross wages of Maier and Corrillia are based on a total of 48 and 44 hours of work, respectively. However, as indicated in Table 5-3, they devote 6 and 11 hours, respectively, to the preparation and presentation of a seminar. Consequently, the objective now is to allocate an equitable share of their gross wages to the laboratory unit and to an appropriate administrative cost center.

The assignment of the labor costs associated with these employees can be based on the percentage of the total work time they devote to these two areas

Table 5-3 Distribution of Hours Worked, by Employee and Type of Service

	Distribution of Worktime (in Hours)				
	Service				
Employee	S_1 *(1)*	S_2 *(2)*	S_3 *(3)*	*Idle Time*	*Total*
A. Maier	38	0	4	0	42*
H. Tallent	0	15	24	1	40
P. Griswold	0	20	18	2	40
S. Ohlm	0	18	21	1	40
J. Coleman	0	44	3	1	48
L. Corrillia	0	11	22	0	33†

* 6 hours are devoted to educational activity.
† 11 hours are devoted to educational activity.

of activities. As should be verified, the relevant percentages that pertain to this example are given by:

Employee	*Laboratory Unit*	*Educational Activities*
A. Maier	87.5	12.5
L. Corrillia	75.0	25.0

In this case, Maier devotes 87.5 percent of the total number of hours worked to the laboratory unit and 12.5 percent to educational activities. Consequently, 87.5 percent of Maier's gross wage should be charged to the laboratory unit and 12.5 percent to the appropriate administrative cost center. After performing the required calculations, the allocation of the gross wages earned by these two employees is as follows:

Employee	*Laboratory Unit*	*Educational Activities*	*Gross Wage*
A. Maier	$364.00	$52.00	$416.00
L. Corrillia	$189.75	$63.25	$253.00

At this point in the analysis, it is possible to determine the labor costs that ought to be charged to the laboratory unit. Recall that the gross wages earned by all of the employees assigned to the laboratory total $1,839. Consequently, the costs that should be charged to the unit may be expressed in the form

$$\text{Expense of Unit} = \text{Gross Wages of Employees Assigned to the Unit} - \text{Cost of Performing Functions Not Assigned to the Unit}$$

Returning to the example, we find that

$$\text{Expense of Laboratory Unit} = \$1{,}839 - (\$52.00 + \$63.25)$$

or $1,723.75. On the other hand, the sum represented by the term ($52.00 + $63.25) should be charged to an appropriate administrative cost center.

5.3.3 Recording the Payroll

Generally, the Payroll Register is a supplementary memorandum and, as a result, the information it contains is recorded first in a general journal and then posted. The entry to record the payroll calculated in Tables 5-1 and 5-2 is:

Salary and Wage Expenses*	$1,839.00	
Social Security Taxes Payable		$128.73
Federal Income Taxes Payable		53.50
Insurance Payable		52.50
Other Deductions Payable (Classified)		30.00
Accrued Payroll Payable		1,574.27

* Classified by functional unit and object of expenditure (see Section 5.3.2).

The debit entry to salary and wage expense is obtained directly from Table 5-1, where gross wages are calculated, while the amount of each of the credit entries is derived from Table 5-2. The credit to accrued payroll payable represents the amount that must be paid to the employees.

5.3.4 Paying the Employees

Once the payroll has been recorded, the institution must disburse cash to individual employees in the amount of the net pay they earned during the period. Typically, a single check is drawn on the facility's general cash account in the amount of the net payroll. The check is deposited in a special payroll checking account. Returning to Table 5-2, the net pay earned by all employees totals $1,574.27. The transfer of this sum from the general cash account to the special payroll account is accomplished by the entry

Cash—Payroll	$1,574.27	
Cash—General		$1,574.27

This entry simply alters the composition of the institution's assets and does not extinguish the liability represented by the credit entry to accrued payroll payable.

After transferring funds, individual checks are drawn on the special payroll account and recorded separately in a Check Register similar to Table 5-4. In this illustration, each check produces a debit to the accrued payroll payable account and, as a result, the payment of the payroll eliminates the institution's $1,574.27 liability. In summary form, the payment of employees' net earnings may be recorded by the entry:

Accrued Payroll Payable	$1,574.27	
Cash—Payroll		$1,574.27

All of the payroll checks should clear the special cash account quickly, resulting in a zero balance. In such a situation, the reconciliation of this bank account is unnecessary. If the account does not have a zero balance, management should determine which checks are outstanding by comparing the identification numbers of those returned in the bank statement with those appearing in the Check Register. The balance of the special payroll account should equal the sum of the checks that remain outstanding. As can be imagined, the use of a special payroll account facilitates the reconciliation of general checking accounts that are not complicated by a large volume of payroll checks.

5.3.5 Payroll Taxes Levied on the Employer

As noted, Social Security taxes are levied in identical amounts on employee and employer. Consequently, the institution is required to deduct those taxes from employees' checks and also to pay a levy equal to the sum of the Social Security taxes withheld from all employees. In the example in Table 5-2, the Social Security taxes imposed on the institution total $128.73. Furthermore,

Table 5-4 Check Register—Payroll

Date	*Check No.*	*Employee*	*Account Debited*	*Accrued Payroll Payable Debit*	*Cash—Payroll Credit*
Oct. 12	950	A. Maier	Accrued Payroll Payable	$363.38	$363.38
12	951	H. Tallent	Accrued Payroll Payable	228.40	228.40
12	952	P. Griswold	Accrued Payroll Payable	223.30	223.30
12	953	S. Ohlm	Accrued Payroll Payable	188.20	188.20
12	954	J. Coleman	Accrued Payroll Payable	350.20	350.20
12	955	L. Corrillia	Accrued Payroll Payable	220.79	220.79
				1,574.27	1,574.27

since the taxes on employer and employee are paid simultaneously, the liabilities for both normally are recorded in the Social Security Taxes Payable account.

The institution also is required to pay federal and, frequently, state unemployment taxes. To avoid presenting obsolete information here, the relevant provisions of the Federal Unemployment Tax Act are expressed in general terms. This act requires employers to pay an excise tax, as expressed in percentage terms, on the first $X earned by employees during the year. It is important to note that the federal unemployment taxes imposed on the employer are used to finance administration of the federal-state unemployment program rather than for the payment of unemployment benefits, which is a function of state programs.

Suppose that a tax of .5 percent is imposed on the first $4,200 earned by employees during the year. Returning to Table 5-1, and assuming that none of the employees have earned $4,200 or more to date, we find that the federal unemployment insurance tax on the employer is given by .005 × $1,839.00 (gross pay), or $9.20.

All states finance their unemployment insurance programs by a payroll tax on employers and, in isolated instances, on employees. Similar to the federal program, states impose a payroll tax, expressed in percentage terms, on the first $X earned by employees. In addition, the employer can obtain a merit rating by not dismissing employees during slack periods, which in turn reduces the basic tax rate. In some cases, the merit rating may reduce the basic payroll tax rate to zero.

For illustration, suppose the state in which the institution is located imposes a tax of 2.7 percent on the first $4,200 earned by employees during the year. Table 5-1 assumes that none of the employees earned $4,200 or more to date, so the state unemployment taxes on the institution are given by .027 × $1,839 (gross pay), or $49.65. This discussion may be summarized as follows:

Type of Tax Imposed on the Employer	*Amount*
Social Security	$128.73
Federal Unemployment Insurance	9.20
State Unemployment Insurance	49.65
Total	187.58

Most employers use a single journal entry to record these three taxes when preparing the payroll to which the taxes relate. In terms of this example, the entry to record the payroll taxes of the institution is given by

Payroll Tax Expenses	$187.58	
Social Security Taxes Payable		$128.73
Federal Unemployment Taxes Payable		9.20
State Unemployment Taxes Payable		49.65

The debit entry of $187.58 represents the sum of the employer-specific payroll expenses. The credit entry of $128.73 to Social Security taxes payable is equal to the amount deducted from the pay of all employees for F.I.C.A. taxes. Similarly, the other credit entries to the state and federal unemployment taxes payable are liabilities of the employer and are based on the assumptions introduced earlier.

Under tax laws, the institution must pay the liabilities in the previous entry. In general, the amount of income taxes withheld coupled with the sum of the Social Security levies on both employer and employee determine when the institution must remit required amounts. On the other hand, the federal unemployment taxes are payable annually on January 31, state unemployment taxes on a quarterly basis. These payments are recorded in the same manner as any other liability.

5.3.6 Other Payroll-Related Costs

This section considers other costs related to payroll—specifically, the techniques of computing and recording vacation pay and the accounting methods that pertain to workers' compensation programs.

5.3.6.1 Vacation Pay

After a specified period of employment, employees of the health care facility usually are entitled to an annual vacation with pay, generally two weeks per year, which means that they work for 50 weeks but are paid for 52. Vacation pay is earned by employees and incurred as a cost by the institution during each of the 50 working weeks. Recognition of vacation pay and the associated liability should not be deferred until the employee takes the two weeks annual vacation. Rather, vacation pay should be charged to an appropriate expense account in the payroll periods during which it is earned by employees.

Returning to Table 5-1, note that the first employee, A. Maier, earns $8.00 per hour that, when multiplied by the normal work week of 40 hours, results in a weekly pay of $320. Since it is assumed that employees are entitled to two weeks of paid vacation per year, Maier will have accrued vacation pay of $640 (2 × $320) during the year, earned at the rate of $12.80 per week ($640 ÷ 50). Presented below is the computation of the weekly vacation pay earned by each employee in Table 5-1:

Employee	*Earnings/ Week*	*Annual Vacation Pay*	*Weekly Vacation Pay*
A. Maier	$320	$640	$12.80
H. Tallent	280	560	11.20

Employee	*Earnings/ Week*	*Annual Vacation Pay*	*Weekly Vacation Pay*
P. Griswold	$260	$520	$10.40
S. Ohlm	240	480	9.60
J. Coleman	300	600	12.00
L. Corrillia	220	440	8.80
Total			64.80

The proper weekly payroll entry to record the vacation pay for this group of employees (disregarding withholdings) is:

Salary and Wage Expense*	$64.80	
Accrued Vacation Pay Payable		$64.80

* Classified by functional unit and object of expense.

The liability recorded in this entry is extinguished when employees take their vacation.

5.3.6.2 Worker Compensation

Legislation in all states provides for payments to employees for an injury or disability arising out of or in the course of their work. In effect, the employer is required to insure employees against injury or disability that may result from occupational hazards. Premiums usually are based on the degree of risk involved and on the total payroll. The procedures for payment may be summarized as follows:

1. At the beginning of each year, every covered employer is required to submit to the Worker Compensation Board an estimate of the expected payroll for the coming year.
2. Premiums are established, by the insurance carrier.
3. Premiums normally are payable in three to six installments per year and are borne by the employer.
4. At the end of the year, actual payrolls are submitted to the board and final assessments are made, depending on the difference between actual and expected payrolls.

Assume, for example, that the institution is subject to a program that requires payments in four installments per year and the following data are available:

Employee Group	*Estimated Annual Payroll*	*Estimated Quarterly Payroll*	*Assessment per $100*	*Quarterly Advance Premium*
A	$8,000	$2,000	.90	$18.00
B	12,000	3,000	.60	18.00
C	32,000	8,000	.35	28.00
Total				64.00

The advance quarterly premium is determined by the product of the estimated payroll and the assessment per $100, which reflects the relative risk of each of the three groups. In this case, the higher the risk, the higher the employer assessment.

Given these estimates, assume the following data pertain to the first quarter of the year:

Employee Group	*Actual Payroll*	*Assessment Rate per $100*	*Expired Portion of Advance Premium*
A	$1,500	.90	$13.50
B	2,950	.60	17.70
C	7,000	.35	24.50
Total			55.70

The journal entries to record this information are:

Prepaid Worker Compensation	$64.00	
Cash		$64.00
Worker Compensation Expense	55.70	
Prepaid Worker Compensation		55.70

At the end of the year, the prepaid worker compensation account will probably have either a debit or a credit balance. A debit balance indicates an overpayment, a credit balance an underpayment that represents a liability for premium due.

5.4 ACCOUNTING FOR SUPPLIES AND OTHER EXPENSES

As much as 30 percent of the annual operating costs of health care facilities are related to the acquisition of supplies. Since substantial amounts are expended each year for supplies, heat, light, and other purchased services, the effective management of these costs requires that they be recorded and reported accurately.

As indicated throughout the discussion of payroll accounting, wages and salary expenses should be recorded on a functional basis. Under functional accounting, the supply expenses incurred during a given period also should be recorded on a functional basis. However, as will be seen in Chapter 9, the amount of supply expense recognized during a given period depends on the method of valuing inventories as well as on the system by which they are recorded. Consequently, it is convenient to discuss the assignment of supply expenses to functional units when examining the accounting techniques that pertain to inventories. The following discussion provides a brief analysis of the accounting problems and the general principles associated with recording expenses of acquiring and using consumable supplies.

5.4.1 Purchasing

Any system of purchasing and inventory management consists of the basic steps of requisitioning, ordering, receiving, controlling, and issuing goods. Figure 5-1 is a basic system by which the process of purchasing and issuing inventory can be controlled and is discussed next.

Authority to order and requisition goods or equipment should be limited to specific individuals in the institution. Once it is found that an item is required in operational activity, the manager of the center or some other responsible employee initiates a request for it by preparing a supply requisition form that contains the date of the requisition, the number and nature of the item(s) requisitioned, the date(s) they will be needed and the organizational unit(s) requesting them. A copy of the supply requisition is forwarded to the stores section or central supply where the request for reorders is initiated.

If an item is out of stock or if a requisition reduces the supply below a predetermined rcorder point, a purchase requisition is prepared by central supply and sent to the purchasing department. The purchasing department uses the requisition form to prepare a purchase order that authorizes the vendor to ship the item(s) ordered. Upon receipt of a copy of the purchase order, the supplier ships the goods along with an invoice that describes them.

When the goods are delivered, the receiving department should count, weigh, and otherwise inspect the shipment. The department prepares a receiving report containing information on its inspection and forwards it to the accounting department. At this point in the process, the accounting department should be in possession of the requisition slip, the purchase order, the invoice, and the receiving report. The accounting department then can compare the information on these forms.

A comparison of the goods requisitioned with the goods ordered provides an internal check on the institution's purchasing practices while a comparison of the purchase order with the invoice and the receiving report constitutes the basis for validating the quantities and prices of goods ordered and received. On the basis of these comparisons, the accounting department is in a position to approve the invoice for entry in the books and ultimate payment.

5.4.2 Recording Purchases

Once a supply item has been obtained and all relevant forms have been validated, the institution may use either a periodic or a perpetual accounting system to record the purchase. Under the periodic inventory system, supplies may be recorded in either an expense or an inventory asset account. Conversely, in a perpetual inventory system, a supply acquisition must be recorded

Figure 5-1 Basic Elements of an Inventory Control System

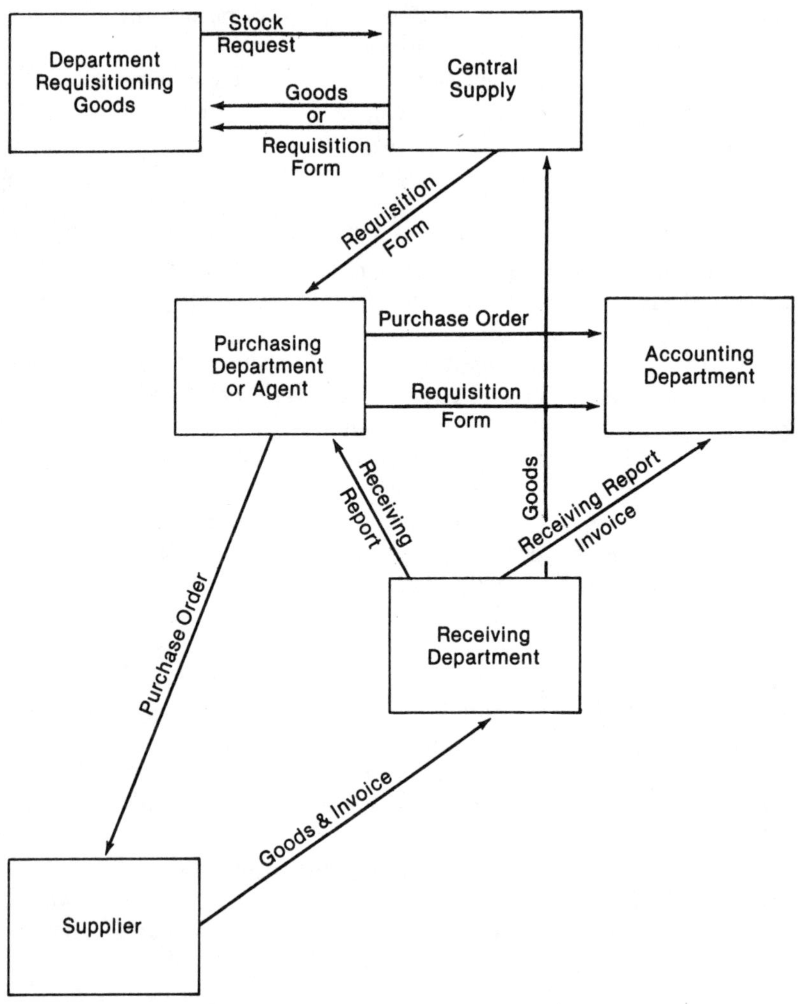

in an inventory asset account. Although this is considered in Chapter 9, the general entry to record the acquisition of consumable supplies is given by

Supply Expense* (or Inventory)	$XX,XXX	
Accounts Payable		$XX,XXX

* Classified by functional unit.

where it is assumed that the vendor extends credit to the institution.

Where the institution receives trade credit, a slight complication arises in the process of recording supply acquisitions. In general, trade discounts allow the purchaser to deduct a specified percentage from the gross invoice cost if payment is made on or before a given date. For example, terms of trade credit specified by 2/10/30 mean that 2 percent of the gross invoice cost may be deducted by the purchaser if payment is made on or before 10 days after the invoice date. Otherwise, the full cost is due and payable 30 days after the invoice date.

Some institutions use gross invoice costs to record acquisitions while others prefer net invoice costs (i.e., gross invoice cost less the discount offered by the vendor) to record purchases. These methods are described next.

5.4.2.1 Gross Invoice Cost Method

To illustrate the gross invoice method, suppose that the hospital purchases $10,000 of supplies on terms 2/10/30. Under the gross invoice cost method, the journal entry to record the acquisition is:

Supply Expense (or Inventory)	$10,000	
Account Payable		$10,000

If the institution elects to ignore the discount and pay the account on, say, day 29, the entry to record payment is:

Account Payable	$10,000	
Cash		$10,000

In these two entries, it is important to note that the supply expense (or inventory) and the related liability are recorded at gross invoice cost without consideration of the discount opportunity. Hence, no formal record is made of the fact that the invoice is paid after the discount date and that a 2 percent discount ($200) is foregone because of the failure to pay obligations promptly.

Conversely, if the hospital decides to take advantage of the discount and pay on day 9 of the discount period, the entry to record payment is:

Account Payable	$10,000	
Purchase Discount Earned		$200
Cash		9,800

Consequently, under the gross invoice cost method, the discount receives accounting recognition only when taken.

5.4.2.2 Net Invoice Method

In the net invoice cost method, purchased supplies are recorded net of the 2 percent discount. Returning to the last example and assuming that the net invoice method is used, the value assigned to the inventory acquisition is \$9,800 (\$10,000 − .02[\$10,000]), which is recorded as follows:

Supply Expense (or Inventory)	\$9,800	
Account Payable		\$9,800

If the invoice is paid promptly (for example, on day 9) and the hospital takes advantage of the discount, the entry to record the payment is:

Account Payable	\$9,800	
Cash		\$9,800

No formal record is made of a discount earned. However, should the institution pay on day 29 and fail to take advantage of the discount, the entry would be:

Account Payable	\$9,800	
Discount Lost	\$200	
Cash		\$10,000

The Discount Lost, rather than Purchase Discount Earned, is recorded to indicate to management the additional expenses incurred as a result of failing to pay the invoice within the stated discount period.

As can be seen, then, the gross invoice method tends to conceal the costs of inefficiencies in processing and paying obligations. In addition, the gross method tends to overstate both the cost of purchased items and the related liabilities. These considerations suggest that the net invoice cost method is perhaps more desirable than the gross method.

5.4.3 Storing and Issuing Supplies

Once the receiving department has completed the process of counting, weighing, or otherwise inspecting the incoming shipment, the items are moved to central supply, where they remain until used.

As seen earlier, supplies are issued in response to requisitions initiated by other organizational units. If the item is on hand and the supply requisition does not violate a reorder point, the item is issued. Assuming that a perpetual inventory accounting system is used, the supply requisition mentioned earlier is the basis for journal entries such as the following:

Supply Expense*	$1,500	
Inventory		$1,500

* Classified by functional unit and item.

The general entry just presented usually is recorded in a special journal that is described in Chapter 9. To anticipate this discussion somewhat, the values that represent the use of supplies depend on the institution's method of evaluating inventory. The health sector uses several techniques such as average weighted pricing, LIFO (Last In, First Out), and FIFO (First In, First Out), each of which receives detailed attention in the same chapter.

Questions for Discussion

1. Differentiate between a cost and an expense.
2. Discuss the conditions that must be satisfied before an expense is recognized.
3. Describe which methods are used to classify expenses.
4. Describe the process of calculating gross payroll and net pay.
5. List the major deductions in calculating net pay and the employer liabilities that emanate from the payroll.
6. Describe the process of calculating worker compensation premiums.
7. Describe the system by which purchases and inventory can be controlled.
8. Differentiate between the gross and net invoice cost methods of recording inventory acquisitions.

Problems for Solution

1. Suppose the following information is available:

			Percent of Gross Pay Withheld			
				Unemployment		*Federal Income*
Employee	*Hours Worked*	*Wage Rate*	*FICA*	*State*	*Federal*	*Taxes*
A	48	$10.00	8%	2.5%	.4%	18%
B	40	12.00	8	2.5	.4	20
C	40	6.00	8	2.5	.4	16
D	44	8.00	8	2.5	.4	15

Use these data to (1) calculate the gross and net pay of each employee and (2) record the required journal entries.

2. Record the payment of the net wages in Problem 1, using the check register.
3. Suppose that each of ten employees are (1) paid $200 per week and (2) entitled to a two-week vacation each year. Calculate and record the accrual pertaining to the vacation pay of these employees.
4. Assume that the institution is required to pay an advance premium to the Worker Compensation Board on January 1, 198A, and that the following information is available:

Class of Employee	*Estimated Annual Payroll*	*Assessment Rate (per $100)*
A	$900,000	$.80
B	800,000	.70
C	400,000	.60
D	600,000	.50

Suppose that the actual payroll for January is as follows:

Class of Employee	*Actual Payroll*
A	$80,000
B	70,000
C	30,000
D	40,000

Record the journal entries for January 1 and January 31.

5. Use the gross and net invoice cost methods to record the following transactions:

June 1: purchase of $60,000 in supplies; terms 2/10/30.
June 5: purchase of $40,000 in supplies; terms 2/10/30.
June 9: payment of June 1 invoice.
June 27: payment of June 5 invoice.

6. Suppose that the employees in Problem 1 work in Department D_1, which provides services S_1, S_2, S_3, and S_4. Also suppose that the distribution of hours worked by these employees is as follows:

Employee	*Provision of Service* S_1	S_2	S_3	S_4	*Nursing Administration*	*Total*
A	30	5	5	0	8	48
B	20	0	0	20	0	40
C	0	20	20	0	0	40
D	10	10	10	10	4	44

Describe how the wages paid to these employees should be distributed to nursing administration and Department D_1.

7. Suppose that in Problem 6, the volume of service provided during the period is as follows:

Service	*Volume (in Units)*
S_1	60
S_2	40
S_3	100
S_4	200

Give the total direct labor costs of providing each of the services. Provide the direct labor costs associated with each unit of service S_1, S_2, S_3, and S_4.

Part III

Accounting for Assets and Liabilities

Chapter 6

Accounting for Cash

Cash is used universally to purchase goods and services and, as a result, represents general purchasing power to its possessor. The importance of cash stems from essentially two characteristics.

First, cash is important because of its obvious value in financing the operational activity of the health facility. Clearly, cash represents the vehicle by which the institution may acquire the real resources it uses in the production process. Consequently, cash may be viewed as the other side of the coin of liabilities, expenses, revenues, and other noncash assets required in providing health care. The importance of cash also stems from its susceptibility to misappropriation. Cash is small in bulk and can be high in value. When coupled with these characteristics the absence of special identification marks that indicate ownership makes cash a prime candidate for theft or misappropriation.

On the other hand, idle cash is unproductive and managers of health facilities recognize that excessive cash balances should be avoided. In fact, the earning power of idle cash is negative during periods of increasing prices. Consider the policy of maintaining a minimum cash balance of $200,000 during a period in which the general purchasing power of money declines by 10 percent because of a general rise in the price level. The $20,000 ($200,000 × .10) decline in purchasing power is quite real, even though the "loss" is not reflected in the institution's financial statements.

These considerations suggest that management must devise and implement an effective cash control system so as to avoid theft or misappropriation. In addition, accurate cash accounting and reporting is a prerequisite to effective management that seeks to ensure that neither too little nor too much is allowed to remain in idle balances. Cash is received or disbursed daily by health care facilities, so cash flows must be recorded accurately and promptly. Indeed, effective cash management depends upon the accounting records. Since one of management's primary objectives is to hold neither too much nor too little cash, the purpose of this chapter is to describe the accounting procedures and techniques that are conducive to the attainment of this goal.

6.1 CASH ACCOUNTS

Even the smallest health facility will find it desirable to establish several cash accounts. For example, most institutions use three types of unrestricted cash accounts:

1. Cash on hand: This group includes petty cash funds, change funds, and check-cashing funds.
2. General Purpose Bank Account: This group involves any cash on deposit with a bank for the purpose of meeting nonlabor operating exigencies.
3. Special Payroll Cash: This involves the facility's establishing a special account upon which payroll checks are drawn (see Section 5.4.4).

In large institutions, special checking accounts also are established for each major type of cash disbursement. One or more special payroll checking accounts simplifies the reconciliation of bank statements and provides control over the amount that may be disbursed from a given account. A similar procedure can be used for any other major cash disbursement that is encountered with a frequency that warrants such treatment.

6.2 CASH CONTROLS

For the reasons stated at the beginning of this chapter, controls are essential wherever and whenever cash is received or disbursed. Safeguards must be implemented and integrated into the accounting system if the cash resources of the institution are to be recorded and protected from error and misappropriation. This section identifies elements or components that are or should be key parts of any cash control system.

6.2.1 General Guidelines

Some of the typical procedures that are incorporated in the cash control system are:

- All employees who have access to or routinely handle cash should be bonded.
- The number of imprest funds (e.g., petty cash and change funds) as well as the number of persons who have access to cash should be limited.

- The facility's various bank accounts should be reconciled by responsible employees who do not have access to cash.
- There should be a distinct separation of responsibility for cash handling and cash accounting. For example, persons who handle incoming cash should not have access to or control over records for outstanding receivables.
- Definite responsibility should be assigned for handling cash and the custody of cash funds.
- All cash received should be deposited daily and intact.
- All forms pertaining to cash receipts and cash disbursements should be prenumbered and accounted for in numerical sequence.
- In large institutions, internal audits and surprise checks should be made by responsible employees at irregular intervals.
- In large facilities, the business office should be organized so that an error or misappropriation by one employee will be discovered by another.
- All personnel who handle cash should be required to take an annual vacation.
- Physical protection in the form of vaults, cash registers, and locked cashier facilities are imperative.
- Specific methods of handling routine receipts and disbursements of cash should be established in writing. Decisions regarding nonroutine cash transactions should be made by the chief financial officer of the institution.
- The system by which cash is controlled should be the subject of continuous evaluation and review.

The observance of sound internal controls is conducive to promoting efficiency and effectiveness in the business office. Sound internal cash controls make daily and monthly reports more timely and accurate since errors or imbalances are minimized. More importantly, any system of internal control will deter theft and other forms of misappropriation. It should be noted that no system is foolproof but even the simplest controls can discourage misappropriations.

In designing the control system, management should be aware of the techniques used to misappropriate cash. Some of these methods are:

- disbursing cash to nonexistent companies

- altering the dollar amount of vouchers, checks, or other business documents
- collecting patient accounts and listing them as uncollectable
- creating ghost payrolls, in which nonexistent persons are added to the register, or padding the payroll by overstating time worked or payable
- diverting payment on one account to personal use and recording payment on other accounts to the first

Only when management is aware of the means by which funds can be misappropriated can the internal cash control system discourage theft and at least force the dishonest to devise new methods of embezzlement.

6.2.2 The Control of Cash Receipts

Attention turns next to the basic systems by which cash receipts and cash disbursements can be controlled. The cash receipts of the institution are divisible into two main categories: (1) mail receipts and (2) over-the-counter cash receipts. To maximize the effectiveness of the internal control system, it is necessary to recognize and accommodate the peculiarities of each type.

6.2.2.1 Mail Receipts

Figure 6-1 presents a basic system by which mail receipts can be controlled. The system begins with the arrival of cash and the preparation of a mail remittance form by a bonded employee who is independent of the accounting department and the general cashier. Checks received through the mail should be endorsed immediately and entered by amount and payer name in a mail remittance report.

In this system, the mail clerk prepares a prenumbered cash receipt, which is sent to the payer, and a mail remittance report in triplicate, which is distributed as follows:

1. The original and any relevant correspondence are forwarded to the accounting department where they are used as the basis for recording the cash receipt in the cash receipt journal, the accounts receivable subsidiary ledger, and the eventual posting to the general ledger. At the end of the day, or on a periodic basis, an employee in the accounting department compares mail remittance reports with bank deposit slips to verify the prompt and accurate deposit of all cash receipts.
2. The duplicate copy and the cash receipts are sent to the chief cashier, who compares the cash with the mail remittance report. The purpose

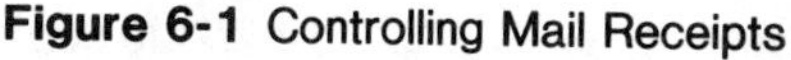
Figure 6-1 Controlling Mail Receipts

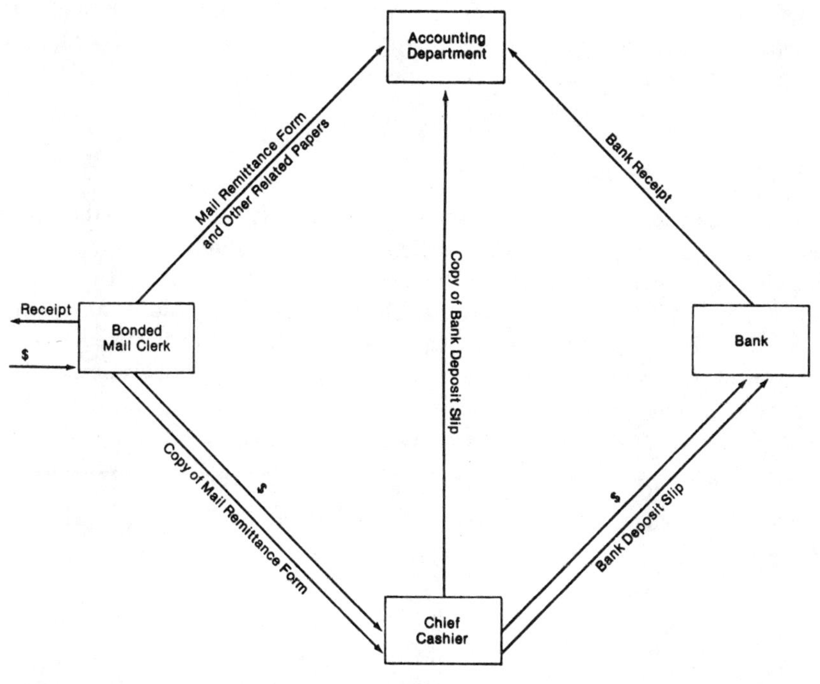

of the comparison is to ensure that the cash items in the report are listed correctly.

3. The third copy, which should be certified and signed by the chief cashier, is retained by the mail clerk.

Once the chief cashier has validated the mail remittance report, a daily bank deposit slip is prepared in duplicate. The original and the cash as well as endorsed checks are transmitted to the bank. The duplicate is sent to the accounting department, where the mail remittance report and the bank deposit slip are compared. At a later point, the bank sends a deposit receipt to the accounting department, where it is compared with the mail remittance report and bank deposit slip. Obviously, such a comparison is likely to reveal the presence of errors or the misappropriation of funds.

This system makes misappropriation difficult unless several employees act in collusion. The mail clerk cannot appropriate cash if the corresponding receipt is omitted from the mail remittance report. If the receipt is omitted, the appropriate account will not be credited by the accounting department and subsequent billings will lead patients or other third parties to file complaints with the institution. Mail receipts cannot be misappropriated by the chief cashier since the accounting department verifies all such receipts by an independent comparison of the mail remittance form with bank deposit slips. Employees in the accounting department cannot misappropriate funds since they have no access to the cash.

6.2.2.2 Over-the-Counter Receipts

Cash received over the counter presents more serious difficulties than mail receipts. This is because a major portion of over-the-counter cash frequently is collected in several locations in the institution—for example, the cafeteria, gift shops, and snack bar. The number of such locations should be minimized and, to the extent possible, the receipt of cash should be centralized.

A basic system of controlling over-the-counter cash receipts is depicted in Figure 6-2. This assumes that cash is received in only one location. The control process begins with ensuring that each transaction is recorded prop-

Figure 6-2 Control of Over-the-Counter Cash Receipts

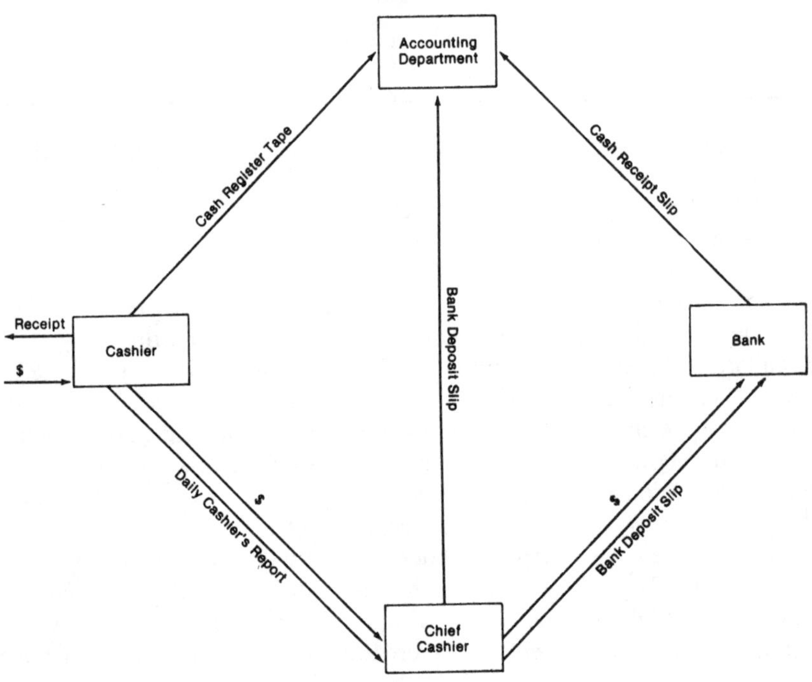

erly on a cash register tape. Ideally, the cashier, who has access to the cash, should not have access to the tape. The system here assumes that the cashier is required to count the cash in the register at the end of each day and prepare a cashier's report recording the results of the count. The cash and daily cashier's report are sent to the head cashier, who also has access to the cash but not to the register tape. The chief cashier compares the cash items with the daily cashier's report and, in the absence of discrepancies, prepares a bank deposit slip in duplicate. The original and the cash go to the bank for deposit and the duplicate to the accounting department. Concurrently, an employee from the accounting department, who does not have access to cash, receives the cash register tape and compares it with the deposit slip and the bank receipt to ensure that cash has been accurately and promptly deposited in the bank.

In the system in Figure 6-2, the accounting department employee has access to the cash register tape but not to the cash. As a result, this individual cannot misappropriate cash without the participation of the sales clerk and the chief cashier. Conversely, the two latter individuals have access to cash but not to the register tape. Since the tape, bank deposit slip, and bank receipt are compared by employees in the accounting department, the sales clerk and the chief cashier cannot misappropriate cash unless they secure the assistance of others. As in the case of mail receipts, the implementation of a control system similar to the one just described makes the misappropriation of funds difficult in the absence of collusion.

6.2.3 The Control of Cash Disbursements

The key to controlling cash disbursements is determining the authenticity of liabilities and of the amounts owed at the time they are entered in the books. The proper recording of liabilities usually leads to the proper disbursement of funds, while their improper recording is just as likely to result in an improper disbursement of cash. Therefore, much care must be exercised to ensure that liabilities are recorded properly.

With the exception of imprest funds, all cash disbursements should be made by prenumbered checks that are written on protective paper. Definite authority and responsibility for signing checks should be given to only a few individuals and, in certain circumstances, it may be desirable to require two signatures in disbursing cash.

As in controlling cash receipts, there should be a division of duties in disbursing cash. Figure 6-3 is an example of the segregation of duties in the process of disbursing cash.

The first step involves the validation of the liability and the preparation of the voucher. The voucher is the central control document that authorizes the

Figure 6-3 Controlling Cash Disbursements

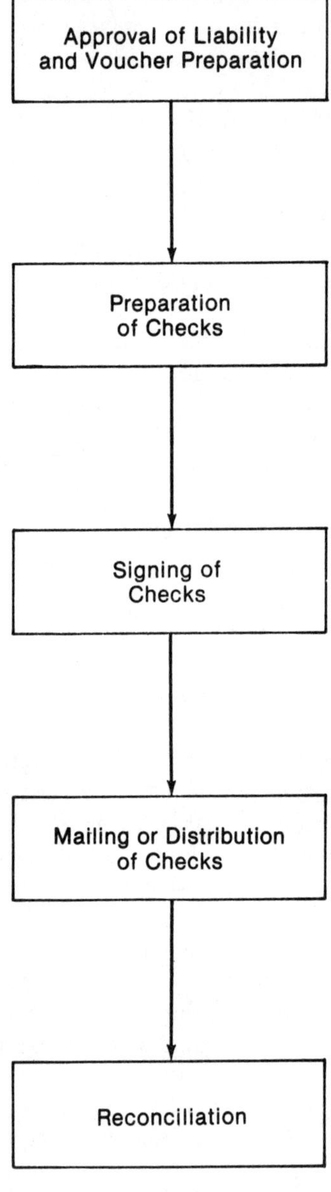

disbursement of funds. No disbursement should be made without the proper execution of a voucher that requires the examination of all supporting documents such as the purchase orders, invoices, and receiving reports that were discussed in Section 5.4.1. The voucher bears witness to the fact that all authorizations, prices, quantities, and extensions have been examined and, to the extent possible, have been found to be correct and accurate.

Once the voucher has been completed, it constitutes the basis for preparing the check and disbursing the authorized amount of cash. The voucher, attached papers, and the check are presented to the disbursing authority, who reviews all documents to ensure that the check is prepared properly. Once satisfied that all is in order, the disbursing officer signs the check, which should be mailed to the payee directly from the disbursing office. The voucher and related documents should be perforated and marked "paid" so they cannot be presented again for payment. These documents are sent to the accounting department, where the transaction is recorded in the Check Register or the Cash Disbursement Journal.

Regarding cash disbursements related to the payroll, the person responsible for signing checks should have nothing to do with the compilation, validation, preparation, or recording of employee earnings. Before signing payroll checks, the disbursing officer should make a random examination of all of them to ensure that they have been prepared properly.

Signed payroll checks should be distributed by someone independent of both the accounting department and the process by which payrolls are approved. Giving the payroll manager the responsibility of distributing checks is not desirable because nonexistent persons might be included on the list.

6.2.4 Reconciliation

As noted in Figure 6-3, a major element of any cash control system is the reconciliation of the facility's various bank accounts. Typically, the cash balance on the institution's books will not agree with the balance on the bank's books. The disparity results from the time lag between transactions initiated by the institution and the ensuing effect on the bank, and vice versa. For example, there usually is a period of time between the issuance of a check and its presentation at the bank for payment and between then and its clearance and return to the hospital. Because of the financial importance of cash balances, it is essential to evaluate the accuracy of the bank account. Its periodic reconciliation is one process by which that accuracy is assured.

There are basically two types of factors in reconciling the bank statement: (1) transactions recorded in the institution's books that have not been entered by the bank; (2) transactions listed by the bank that have not been recorded by the facility. Examples of each type are:

1. Checks issued and recorded by the institution may not have been presented at the bank for payment. From the perspective of the bank reconciliation, these transactions involve outstanding checks.
2. Similarly, deposits presented after the bank's cut-off time on the reconciliation date will appear on the institution's books but will not have been recorded by the bank.
3. Bank service charges and other fees entered by the bank have not been recorded by the institution because it has not been notified of their assessment.
4. Collections on patients' accounts may have been listed by the bank but, because the institution has not been notified, have not been recorded by the health facility.

Practice varies somewhat, but the reconciliation process should involve, at least on a sample basis, the following procedures:

1. Checks returned from the bank should be arranged in numerical order and compared with the list of outstanding checks from the prior month's reconciliation and with the cash disbursements of the period. This process identifies the value of outstanding checks as of the reconciliation date.
2. Outstanding checks should be identified and listed by date, payee, amount, and identification number.
3. The institution then should examine the list to determine whether payment should be stopped on any checks.
4. A sample of cancelled checks should be inspected to uncover any irregularities that may exist in their endorsement.

The reconciliation process requires a comparison of the deposits recorded by the institution with those of the bank. If a deposit was in transit on the prior month's reconciliation, the institution must ensure that it appears on the current month's statement. On the basis of the comparison, a list of deposits in transit at the end of the current period should reflect the dates and the amounts outstanding. When the reconciliation is complete, it should be reviewed and approved by the chief financial officer, who will authorize any adjusting entries required to reflect errors, bank service charges, and collections and otherwise bring the book and bank cash balances into agreement.

Sometimes the reconciliation is accomplished by adjusting the bank balance so it agrees with the balance in the institution's books or by adjusting the book balance so it agrees with the bank balance. Both methods will result in a satisfactory reconciliation. The method in Table 6-1 is called a proof of cash and involves the adjustment of two incorrect balances to reflect the correct one. This procedure is preferred because it provides the basis for reporting cash assets accurately in the balance sheet.

It also provides for adjustments to the bank's and health care facility's balances. Adjustments to the hospital books involve transactions that have been recorded by the bank but not by the institution. Adjustments to the bank balance involve transactions that have been entered by the hospital but not by the bank. Table 6-1 assumes that on the reconciliation date, the cash balance on the hospital's books is $25,300 while the bank reports a credit balance of $28,000. It further assumes that as of the reconciliation date, the hospital has recorded a $500 deposit that the bank has not received or listed. Hence, this value is added to the amount of cash on the bank balance. Similarly, the hospital has issued $3,000 in checks that, as of the reconciliation date, have not been presented for payment. The value is subtracted

Table 6-1 Example of Proof of Cash Statement

SAMPLE HOSPITAL
Proof of Cash
January 31, 198A

	Hospital Books		*Bank Books*	
Item	*Dr.*	*Cr.*	*Dr.*	*Cr.*
Balance Jan. 31, 198A	$25,300			$28,000
Deposit in Transit Jan. 31, 198A				500
Checks Outstanding			$3,000	
Bank Service Charge		$100		
Note Collected by Bank	1,000			
NSF* Check Returned		700		
Totals	26,300	800	3,000	28,500
Adjustment	(800)			(3,000)
Adjusted Cash Balance Jan. 31, 198A	25,500			25,500

* NSF = Not sufficient funds.

from the bank balance by the $3,000 entry in the debit column of the bank's portion of the reconciliation.

Turning next to the required adjustments in the hospital books, suppose that the institution incurs bank service charges of $100 that have not been recorded as of the reconciliation date. This obviously reduces the cash balance on the hospital's books. Further, assume that a payment of $1,000 on a receivable with a principal value of $900 and interest charges of $100 is received by the bank, which later notifies the hospital of the transaction. As seen in Table 6-1, the payment of the $900 note receivable and $100 in interest increases the cash balance on the hospital books by $1,000. Finally, assume that a check originally recorded by the hospital in settlement of a $700 account receivable is returned by the bank to the maker because of insufficient funds in the individual's account. The return of the check reduces the cash balance on the hospital's books, as evidenced by the $700 credit entry in its portion of the reconciliation.

The final step is to determine the adjusted balance per the hospital and bank books as of the reconciliation date. As Table 6-1 shows, the adjusted cash balance is $25,500 and, as a result, the figure on the hospital's books must be increased by $200. It also is necessary to:

1. recognize the $100 bank service charge
2. recognize payment of the $900 note and the related $100 interest charges
3. reverse an earlier entry that recorded the receipt of the $700 check that later was returned because of insufficient funds

These tasks are accomplished by the entry

Cash	$200	
Accounts Receivable	700	
Sundry Expense	100	
Note Receivable		$900
Interest Income		100

where the $100 debit entry to the sundry expense account recognizes the bank service charge and the $200 debit entry increases the cash balance to reflect a correct balance of $25,500. The $700 debit entry to the outstanding receivable account reflects the amount owed to the hospital by the individual whose check was returned by the bank. Finally, the credit entries eliminate the note receivable from the institution's books and recognize the interest income associated with the note received earlier.

As mentioned previously, the use of special accounts for different types of disbursements facilitates the reconciliation of bank statements. As might be imagined, the reconciliation process would be cumbersome indeed if all checks were drawn on a single account. By establishing a payroll checking account, the large volume of such checks is removed from the general cash account; this, of course, simplifies the reconciliation of both types of accounts.

6.3 RECORDING CASH RECEIPTS

The receipt of cash usually is related to income-generating activities or the issuance of either a long-term or short-term debt instrument. Concerning the first of these two possibilities, recall that cash may be received

1. before service is provided and revenue is recognized
2. at the time service is provided and revenue is recognized
3. after service is provided and revenue is recognized

This section illustrates the process of recording the recognition of revenue and the receipt of cash for each of these three situations.

6.3.1 Prepayment

Suppose the institution routinely receives payment from third party payers A, B, and C before it provides service and recognizes revenue. To simplify the discussion, assume further that these funds are intended to finance the use of inpatient services on a current basis and that the cash received from the three third party payers is summarized as follows:

Date of Cash Receipt	*Third Party Payer*	*Amount of Cash*
1/1	A	$9,000
1/1	B	10,000
1/2	C	20,000

As seen earlier, the entry

Cash	$9,000	
Deferred Revenue		$9,000

is used to record the cash received from third party payer A.

Even though the receipt of cash could be recorded in general journal form, accounting procedures may be simplified and the time required to transfer information from the general journal to the general ledger may be reduced by recording cash inflows in a cash receipts journal similar to the one in Table

6-2. The mechanics of using the journal shown in the example to record the cash received from the third party payers are as follows.

After entering the date and party responsible for financing the use of care on a current basis, the obligations of the institution are increased by the credit entries in the column headed Deferred Revenue. In the last column, the receipt of funds is given accounting recognition by recording debit entries to the cash account. At this point, the similarity between the general journal entry and the mechanics of recording the receipt of funds prior to the provision of service in the cash receipts journal should be obvious.

Table 6-2 also shows the relation between the cash receipts journal and the general ledger. Assume, for a moment, that the institution receives no additional cash during the period. At the end of the month, the entries in the Deferred Revenue and Cash columns are totaled and compared to ensure

Table 6-2 Cash Receipts Journal: Prepayment of Service

Date	*Deferred Revenue Account Credited*	*Deferred Revenue*	*Cash*
		Credit	*Debit*
1/1	Third Party A	$ 9,000	$ 9,000
1/1	Third Party B	10,000	10,000
1/2	Third Party C	20,000	20,000
.	.	.	.
.	.	.	.
.	.	.	.
1/31			
Totals		39,000	39,000

Subsidiary Ledger

Third Party A

Date	*Dr.*	*Cr.*	*Balance*
1/1		$9,000	$9,000

Third Party B

Date	*Dr.*	*Cr.*	*Balance*
1/1		$10,000	$10,000

Third Party C

Date	*Dr.*	*Cr.*	*Balance*
1/2		$20,000	$20,000

General Ledger

Cash

Date	*Dr.*	*Cr.*	*Balance*
1/31	$39,000		$39,000

Deferred Revenue

Date	*Dr.*	*Cr.*	*Balance*
1/31		$39,000	$39,000

that the transactions are recorded properly. These amounts then are transferred to the appropriate control account in the general ledger.

Table 6-2 also reveals that a subsidiary account has been created for each of the entities that finance the use of care on a current basis. The example shows that the prepayment is recorded in the subsidiary account of the third party on the day cash is received. For example, the receipt of $9,000 is recorded in the subsidiary account of third party payer A on January 1, with a similar procedure on each occasion that cash is received from the other third parties. If no other prepayments are received during the reporting period, the sum of the credit balances in the subsidiary accounts ($9,000 + $10,000 + $20,000) is equal to the credit balance of the corresponding control account in the general ledger.

Finally, assume that the revenues earned during the month by providing care to insured patients are as in Table 6-3. In summary of these revenue-generating activities, the following entry can be recorded:

Deferred Revenue	$35,615	
Daily Service Revenue		$27,110
Ancillary Service Revenue S_1		3,280
Ancillary Service Revenue S_2		2,985
Ancillary Service Revenue S_3		2,240

which, in addition to recognizing the income earned by providing care to insured patients, reduces the obligation created when the institution received funds.

Table 6-3 Revenues for Insured Patients' Care

Date	Third Party	Daily Service Revenue	*Ancillary Service Revenue* S_1	S_2	S_3	Total
1/3	A	$1,800	$ 50	$ 75	$ 75	$2,000
1/4	A	2,650	0	30	40	2,720
1/5	A	2,450	75	0	50	2,575
1/15	B	2,100	400	120	110	2,730
1/16	B	1,790	700	600	100	3,190
1/17	B	2,400	400	550	625	3,975
1/27	C	2,650	180	140	160	3,130
1/28	C	5,300	625	730	470	7,125
1/29	C	5,970	850	740	610	8,170
Totals		27,110	3,280	2,985	2,240	35,615

Under normal circumstances, the facility provides care to insured patients on each day of the reporting period, and the recognition of revenue as well as the corresponding reduction in the deferred revenue account is recorded in a daily income journal. Under the simplifying assumptions here, however, the revenue from providing service to insured patients can be recorded directly in the daily income summary in Table 6-4. After entering the date and identifying the party responsible for financing the use of care, the daily service revenue and the ancillary service revenue, by type of service, are recorded in the appropriate columns of the journal. The obligation created when funds are received from one of the third party payers is reduced by a debit entry in the Deferred Revenue column.

Consider next the relation between the daily income summary and the subsidiary ledger section of the example. On each day that all or a portion of the obligation to one of the third party payers is satisfied, the corresponding liability is reduced by an appropriate amount. For example, on January 3, $2,000 worth of service is provided to patients insured by third party payer A. Accordingly, on that date the balance of the subsidiary account is reduced from $9,000 to $7,000, which of course represents the current obligation of the institution to this third party.

Similar to the earlier discussion, the revenues generated and the total reduction in the obligations of the institution are transferred to the appropriate control account in the general ledger at the end of the month. The general ledger section of Table 6-4 shows ancillary service revenues of $8,505 ($3,280 + $2,985 + $2,240) and daily service revenues of $27,110 have been transferred to the appropriate control account. Accordingly, the corresponding obligations of the institution are reduced by $35,615 ($8,505 + $27,110). After transferring this amount to the control account in the general ledger and adjusting the balance, the table indicates that an additional $3,385 worth of service must be provided to satisfy the institution's obligation to these third party payers. The credit balance of the deferred revenue account in the general ledger ($3,385) is equal to the sum of the credit balances in the subsidiary ledger ($1,705 + $105 + $1,575).

In general, a credit balance in the deferred revenue account indicates that the funds received before service is provided exceed the value of the care used by insured patients. Conversely, a debit balance in the deferred revenue account indicates that the prepayment is less than the value of services used by insured patients and such a balance should be recovered from the responsible third party payer.

6.3.2 Cash Transactions

As mentioned earlier, the recognition of revenue and the receipt of cash frequently occur simultaneously. In such a situation, the cash inflow and the recognition of revenue are recorded directly in the cash receipt journal.

Table 6-4 Daily Income Summary: Prepaid Inpatient Services

Date	Deferred Revenue Account Debited	Daily Service Revenue	Ancillary Service Revenue			Deferred Revenue
			S_1	S_2	S_3	
		Credit	*Credit*	*Credit*	*Credit*	*Debit*
1/3	Third Party A	$1,800	$50	$75	$75	$2,000
1/4	Third Party A	2,650	0	30	40	2,720
1/5	Third Party A	2,450	75	0	50	2,575
1/15	Third Party B	2,100	400	120	110	2,730
1/16	Third Party B	1,790	700	600	100	3,190
1/17	Third Party B	2,400	400	550	625	3,975
1/27	Third Party C	2,650	180	140	160	3,130
1/28	Third Party C	5,300	625	730	470	7,125
1/29	Third Party C	5,970	850	740	610	8,170
Totals		27,110	3,280	2,985	2,240	35,615

Subsidiary Ledger

Third Party A

Date	*Dr.*	*Cr.*	*Balance*
1/1		$9,000	$9,000
1/3	$2,000		7,000
1/4	2,720		4,280
1/5	2,575		1,705

Third Party B

Date	*Dr.*	*Cr.*	*Balance*
1/1		$10,000	$10,000
1/15	$2,730		7,270
1/16	3,190		4,080
1/17	3,975		105

Third Party C

Date	*Dr.*	*Cr.*	*Balance*
1/2		$20,000	$20,000
1/27	$3,130		16,870
1/28	7,125		9,745
1/29	8,170		1,575

General Ledger

Daily Service Revenue

Date	*Dr.*	*Cr.*	*Balance*
1/31		$27,110	$27,110

Ancillary Service Revenue—Inpatient

Date	*Dr.*	*Cr.*	*Balance*
1/31		$8,505	$8,505

Deferred Revenue

Date	*Dr.*	*Cr.*	*Balance*
1/31		*$39,000*	*$39,000*
1/31	$35,615		$3,385

For illustration, assume that the cash transactions of the institution emanate from the provision of outpatient care only and that the following information pertains to the use of these services during January:

Date	Patient	Registration Fee	Ancillary Service Revenue S_1	S_2	S_3	Cash Receipt
1/2	J. McCure	$10	$ 5	$10	$15	$40
1/4	M. Prot	10	0	0	0	10
1/12	E. Perry	10	10	0	30	50
1/30	C. Cayen	10	5	20	30	65
1/31	A. Buger	10	5	10	15	40
Totals		50	25	40	90	205

In summary of these transactions, the entry

Cash	$205	
Registration fee		$50
Ancillary service revenue S_1		25
Ancillary service revenue S_2		40
Ancillary service revenue S_3		90

can be recorded in the general journal.

As before, the process of recording cash transactions may be simplified by the use of a cash receipt journal. As seen in Table 6-5, a credit entry to the appropriate revenue account is recorded for each of the cash transactions. In addition, each of the credit entries is accompanied by an appropriate debit to the cash account. The revenues earned by providing ancillary service are classified by type of service and recorded in greater detail in the subsidiary revenue ledger referred to earlier.

Table 6-5 reveals that the registration fees and the revenue generated by providing ancillary services to outpatients during the period amounted to $50 and $155, respectively. At the end of the month, these values are transferred to the appropriate control account in the general ledger. In addition, the general ledger section indicates that, at this point in the analysis, the cash balance of the institution amounts to $39,205, which, of course, includes the $39,000 in payments received from third party payers A, B, and C (see Section 6.3.1) as well as the cash receipts from providing ambulatory care.

6.3.3 Retrospective Reimbursement

This section considers transactions in which cash is received after the provision of service and the recognition of revenue. In such a situation, the institution extends credit to either the patient or to a third party who assumes the responsibility for financing the costs of care. For example, assume that the revenue from providing inpatient services on January 1 is summarized as follows:

Responsible Party	*Daily Service Revenue*	*Ancillary Service Revenue*		
		S_1	S_2	S_3
Third Party D	$950	$100	$200	$100
L. Calvet	120	30	10	40
Third Party E	700	140	100	100
P. Fitt	100	20	30	10
Third Party F	580	50	110	50

Assume that the institution extends credit to a set of self-responsible patients as well as the third party payers D, E, and F.

As before, the revenues from inpatient services can be recorded in a daily income journal as in Table 6-6. The Account Debited column identifies the patient or third party that assumes the financial responsibility for the costs of care. Similar to the earlier discussion, the revenue earned by providing service is recorded by a credit entry to the appropriate revenue account. In the last column of the daily income journal, the amount listed as a debit to accounts receivable is simply the sum of the credit entries associated with a given transaction. For example, the daily service revenue and the ancillary service revenue from providing care to patients insured by third party payer D totals $1,350 ($950 + $100 + $200 + $100). Consequently, the debit entry of $1,350 represents the increase in the outstanding receivables that emanates from the transaction.

Consider next the relation between the daily income journal and the subsidiary accounts receivable ledger that also is presented in Table 6-6. The basic purpose of the subsidiary ledger is to identify specific patients and third party payers to whom credit has been extended as well as the value of the corresponding receivables. Thus, the subsidiary accounts receivable ledger represents the mechanism for determining the amount owed to the institution by each patient or third party payer. Consequently, each entry in the last column of the daily income journal is transferred to the appropriate account in the subsidiary accounts receivable ledger on a daily basis. For example, Table 6-6 shows that on January 1, L. Calvet incurred charges of $200. The subsidiary ledger indicates that on January 1 the account of L. Calvet has been debited for this amount. Since a similar procedure is applied to the other values in the last column of the daily income journal, the amount currently owed to the institution by a given patient or third party payer may be determined by simply inspecting the subsidiary accounts receivable ledger.

Table 6-5 Cash Receipts Journal

		Ancillary Service Revenue						
		S_1	S_2	S_3	Registration Fees	Accounts Receivable	Sundry Accounts	Cash
Date	*Account Credited*	*Credit*	*Credit*	*Credit*	*Credit*	*Credit*	*Credit*	*Debit*
1/2	Outpatient Revenue	$5	$10	$15	$10			$40
1/4	Outpatient Revenue	0	0	0	10			10
1/12	Outpatient Revenue	10	0	30	10			50
1/30	Outpatient Revenue	5	20	30	10			65
1/31	Outpatient Revenue	5	10	15	10			40
Totals		25	40	90	50			205

General Ledger

Daily Service Revenue*

Date	*Dr.*	*Cr.*	*Balance*
1/31		$27,110	$27,110

Registration Fees

Date	*Dr.*	*Cr.*	*Balance*
1/31		$50	$50

Cash*

Date	*Dr.*	*Cr.*	*Balance*
1/31	$39,000		$39,000
1/31	205		39,205

Ancillary Service Revenue*
—Inpatient

Date	*Dr.*	*Cr.*	*Balance*
1/31		$8,505	$8,505

Deferred Revenue

Date	*Dr.*	*Cr.*	*Balance*
1/31		$39,000	$39,000
1/31	$35,615		3,385

Ancillary Service Revenue—
Outpatient

Date	*Dr.*	*Cr.*	*Balance*
1/31		$155	$155

* For explanation of these control accounts, see Section 6.3.1 and the discussion of Table 6-4.

Table 6-6 Daily Income Journal for January 1, 198A: Inpatient Services

Account Debited	*Daily Service Revenue*	*Ancillary Service Revenue*			*Accounts Receivable*
		S_1	S_2	S_3	
	Credit	*Credit*	*Credit*	*Credit*	*Debit*
Third Party D	$950	$100	$200	$100	$1,350
L. Calvet	120	30	10	40	200
Third Party E	700	140	100	100	1,040
P. Fitt	100	20	30	10	160
Third Party F	580	50	110	50	790
Totals	2,450	340	450	300	3,540

Subsidiary Accounts Receivable Ledger

Third Party D

Date	*Dr.*	*Cr.*	*Balance*
1/1	$1,350		$1,350

Third Party E

Date	*Dr.*	*Cr.*	*Balance*
1/1	$1,040		$1,040

L. Calvet

Date	*Dr.*	*Cr.*	*Balance*
1/1	$200		$200

P. Fitt

Date	*Dr.*	*Cr.*	*Balance*
1/1	$160		$160

Third Party F

Date	*Dr.*	*Cr.*	*Balance*
1/1	$790		$790

To simplify the illustration, assume that the transactions in Table 6-6 represent the occasions on which the institution extended credit during the month. As before, the revenues earned as well as the sum of the outstanding receivables are posted to the corresponding control account in the general ledger at the end of the month. Since the institution extended credit only to patients or third party payers identified in Table 6-6, the general ledger account that controls the outstanding receivables of the facility has the following balance on January 31:

Accounts Receivable

Date	*Dr.*	*Cr.*	*Balance*
1/31	$3,540		$3,540

The account that controls outstanding receivables in the general ledger serves three basic purposes:

1. The balance of the control account indicates the total amount owed to the institution by patients and other agents who assume the responsibility of financing the use of care.
2. The use of the control account is a necessary but not a sufficient condition for maintaining an equality between the sum of the debits and the sum of the credits in the general ledger.
3. The balance of the control account represents the basis for validating the accuracy of the amounts owed by individual patients or other agents as recorded in the subsidiary accounts receivable ledger.

Table 6-6 shows that the balance of the control account in the general ledger ($3,540) is equal to the sum of the balances in the subsidiary accounts receivable ledger ($1,350 + $200 + $1,040 + $160 + $790). Such a comparison provides the basis for ensuring the accuracy of the set of subsidiary accounts.

To complete the example, suppose that the institution receives payment on these outstanding receivables during the month:

Date	*Party*	*Cash Payment*
1/15	L. Calvet	$40
1/18	Third Party E	1,040
1/31	P. Fitt	75
Total		1,155

These cash receipts can be summarized by recording the following entry in the general journal:

Cash	$1,155	
Accounts Receivable		$1,155

Suppose further that the institution issues a note to the bank in exchange for $30,000 on January 28. The general journal entry

Cash	$30,000	
Note Payable		$30,000

records the transaction.

Although each of the cash receipts can be recorded in the general journal, the accounting process is simplified by the use of the cash receipts journal in Table 6-7. On each day that cash is received, the date is entered and the party responsible for financing the use of care is identified in the second column of the journal. The receipt of payment requires a credit entry in the Accounts Receivable column and a debit entry in the Cash column. As seen earlier, the credit entry reduces the balance of the outstanding receivable while the debit entry increases the balance of the cash account. Also recall that the institution exchanged a note payable for $30,000. As seen in Table 6-7, the transaction is recorded by the debit entry to the cash account and the credit entry that appears in the Sundry Accounts column.

As before, the column totals are transferred to the appropriate control accounts in the general ledger at the end of the month. The credit entries to the individual accounts also are recorded in the subsidiary accounts receivable ledger on a daily basis and new balances are computed to reflect the current status of each account. At this point, the amounts owed by individual patients or their agents should be verified by comparing the sum of the balances in the subsidiary accounts receivable ledger with the balance of the control account in the general ledger. The general ledger portion of Table 6-7 shows that the balance of the control account ($2,385) is equal to the sum of the balances in the subsidiary accounts receivable ledger ($1,350 + $160 + $85 + $790). Such a comparison provides the basis for ensuring the validity of the amounts owed by individual patients or specific third party payers.

6.4 RECORDING CASH DISBURSEMENTS

The major cash disbursements of most health facilities are related to wage and salary payments as well as to the cash outlays associated with the acquisition of supplies and other nonlabor resources. Since payroll accounting and cash disbursements for payment of wages and salaries were discussed in Section 5.4, this section focuses on the acquisition of supplies and their related cash outlays.

In recording the acquisition of a supply item that is subject to periodic inventory accounting methods, the purchase may be recorded as a debit either to a supply expense account or to an inventory asset account and as a credit

Table 6-7 Cash Receipts Journal

Date	Account Debited	Ancillary Service Revenue			Registration Fee Credit	Account Receivable Credit	Sundry Accounts Credit	Cash Debit
		S_1 Credit	S_2 Credit	S_3 Credit				
1/15	L. Calvet					$40		$40
1/18	Third Party E					1,040		1,040
1/28	Note Payable						$30,000	30,000
1/31	P. Fitt					75		75
Totals						1,155	30,000	31,155

Subsidiary Accounts Receivable Ledger

Third Party D

Date	Dr.	Cr.	Balance
1/1	$1,350		$1,350

L. Calvet

Date	Dr.	Cr.	Balance
1/1	$200		$200
1/15		$40	160

Third Party E

Date	Dr.	Cr.	Balance
1/1	$1,040		
1/18		$1,040	-0-

P. Fitt

Date	Dr.	Cr.	Balance
1/1	$160		$160
1/31		$75	85

Third Party F

Date	Dr.	Cr.	Balance
1/1	$790		$790

General Ledger

Cash

Date	Dr.	Cr.	Balance
1/31	$39,205		$39,205
1/31	31,155		70,360

Note Payable

Date	Dr.	Cr.	Balance
1/28		$30,000	$30,000

Accounts Receivable

Date	Dr.	Cr.	Balance
1/31	$3,540		$3,540
1/31		$1,155	2,385

to an appropriate accounts payable. On the other hand, when perpetual inventory accounting methods are used, the debit entry always is made to an inventory asset account. Assume that the facility operates under a perpetual inventory system, so the acquisition of supplies requires a debit entry to an inventory asset account.

Before proceeding, one further assumption must be made explicit. It has been argued in Section 5.4.2 that the net invoice cost method of recording supply acquisitions is preferred to the gross invoice cost method. As a consequence, the former is used in this discussion.

For illustration, supply acquisitions are grouped into four major categories: (1) medical and surgical, (2) drug, (3) food, and (4) other general supplies. These major groupings constitute a general ledger account by which subsidiary inventory records are controlled.

In January, assume that the institution acquires consumable supplies as summarized here:

			Gross Invoice		
Date	*Item*	*Vendor*	*Cost*	*Terms*	*Net Invoice Cost*
1/1	Medical & Surgical Supplies	M & F Inc.	$10,204.08	2/10/30	$10,000
1/10	General Supplies	Goods Inc.	8,163.26	2/10/30	8,000
1/15	Food Supplies	Schaarf & Son	4,081.63	2/10/30	4,000
1/22	Medical & Surgical Supplies	Bandages Inc.	6,122.45	2/10/30	6,000
1/30	Drugs	Sticks & Stones	7,142.85	2/10/30	7,000

In this case, the net invoice costs in the last column are determined by subtracting the dollar value of the discount (.02 × gross invoice cost) from the gross invoice cost.

Normally, the acquisition of consumable supplies and the related liabilities are recorded in a Supply Acquisition Journal similar to Table 6-8. For example, consider the supplies acquired on January 1. The date of the acquisition is recorded in the Date column and the account credited in the subsidiary accounts payable ledger is indicated in the second column. The net invoice cost of $10,000 for the acquisition is recorded as a debit entry to the appropriate inventory account. The net invoice cost also is entered in the Accounts Payable column. At the same time that the acquired inventory item is recorded in the supply acquisition journal, the net invoice cost is credited to the M & F account in the subsidiary accounts payable ledger, which indicates the amount owed to each of the vendors and is controlled by the accounts payable account in the general ledger. As seen in Table 6-8, a similar procedure is followed in recording the remaining supply acquisitions.

For items that are maintained on a perpetual inventory basis, all acquisitions are entered immediately in subsidiary inventory records. As is discussed

Table 6-8 Supply Acquisition Journal

Date	Account Credited	Medical & Surgical Inventory	Drug Inventory	Food Inventory	General Inventory	Accounts Payable
		Debit	Debit	Debit	Debit	Credit
1/1	M & F Inc.	$10,000				$10,000
1/10	Goods Inc.				$8,000	8,000
1/15	Schaarf & Son			$4,000		4,000
1/22	Bandages Inc.	6,000				6,000
1/30	Sticks & Stones		$7,000			7,000
1/31	Totals	16,000	7,000	4,000	8,000	35,000

Accounts Payable Ledger

M & F Inc.

Date	Dr.	Cr.	Balance
1/1		$10,000	$10,000

Goods Inc.

Date	Dr.	Cr.	Balance
1/10		$8,000	$8,000

Schaarf & Son

Date	Dr.	Cr.	Balance
1/15		$4,000	$4,000

Bandages Inc.

Date	Dr.	Cr.	Balance
1/22		$6,000	$6,000

Sticks & Stones

Date	Dr.	Cr.	Balance
1/30		$7,000	$7,000

General Ledger

Accounts Payable

Date	Dr.	Cr.	Balance
1/31		$35,000	$35,000

Medical & Surgical Inventory

Date	Dr.	Cr.	Balance
1/31	$16,000		$16,000

Drug Inventory

Date	Dr.	Cr.	Balance
1/31	$7,000		$7,000

Food Inventory

Date	Dr.	Cr.	Balance
1/31	$4,000		$4,000

General Inventory

Date	Dr.	Cr.	Balance
1/31	$8,000		$8,000

in Chapter 9, the primary purpose of the subsidiary inventory records is to indicate the number of units of a specific supply item that are on hand at any moment in time.

As suggested above, the total of each column is calculated and posted to the appropriate control account in the general ledger. For example, medical and surgical, drug, food, and general supplies of $16,000, $7,000, $4,000 and $8,000, respectively, are acquired during the month. As Table 6-8 demonstrates, these totals have been posted to the appropriate control account in the general ledger at the end of the month. In addition, the sum of the values in the last column represents the value of the accounts payable incurred during the month. At the end of the month, this value also is posted to the appropriate control account of the general ledger.

Now assume that the institution disburses cash in settlement of these accounts during the month as follows:

Date	*Payee*	*Account Payable Settlement*	*Discount Lost*	*Cash Outlay*
1/4	M & F Inc.	$10,000	—	$10,000.00
1/23	Goods Inc.	8,000	$163.26	8,163.26
1/24	Bandages Inc.	2,000	—	2,000.00

It is assumed that, with the exception of the Goods Inc. account, the institution pays within the discount period and, as a result, cash in the amount of the net invoice cost is disbursed.

Cash payment in settlement of these accounts is recorded in a cash disbursement journal as in Table 6-9. Consider first the $10,000 payment to M & F Inc. The date of the cash disbursement is recorded in the first column and the identification number of the check used to pay each supplier is recorded in the second. The payee and the account payable are listed in the next two columns, respectively, and the amount of the payment in the Accounts Payable Debit column. The reduction in cash associated with the payment is shown in the Cash Credit column. As payments are made, the creditor's account in the subsidiary accounts payable ledger is debited in the amount of the payment and new balances are calculated. The discount that was lost by paying the Goods Inc. account after day 10 is recorded as a debit in the Discount Lost column. A freight bill of $200 is shown in the Sundry Accounts Debited column and posted immediately to the control account of the general ledger. A similar process should be followed when posting entries in the Sundry Account Debit column.

At the end of the month, the totals of the debits to the Accounts Payable and Discount Lost columns as well as the sum of the credits to the Cash

Table 6-9 Cash Disbursement Journal

Date	Ch. No.	Payee	Account Debited	Sundry Account Debit	Account Payable Debit	Discount Lost Debit	Cash Credit
1/4	26	M & F Inc.	M & F Inc.		$10,000.00		$10,000.00
1/23	27	Goods Inc.	Goods Inc.		8,000.00	$163.26	8,163.26
1/24	28	Bandages Inc.	Bandages Inc.		2,000.00		2,000.00
1/30	29	L & R Rail	Freight In	$200.00			200.00
Totals				200.00	20,000.00	163.26	20,363.26

Accounts Payable Subsidiary Ledger

M & F Inc.

Date	Dr.	Cr.	Balance
1/1		$10,000.00	$10,000.00
1/4	$10,000.00		—

Goods Inc.

Date	Dr.	Cr.	Balance
1/10		$8,000.00	$8,000.00
1/23	$8,000.00		—

Schaarf & Son

Date	Dr.	Cr.	Balance
1/15		$4,000.00	$4,000.00

Bandages Inc.

Date	Dr.	Cr.	Balance
1/22		$6,000.00	$6,000.00
1/24	$2,000.00		$4,000.00

Sticks & Stones

Date	Dr.	Cr.	Balance
1/30		$7,000.00	$7,000.00

General Ledger

Accounts Payable

Date	Dr.	Cr.	Balance
1/31		$35,000.00	$35,000.00
1/31	$20,000.00		15,000.00

Cash

Date	Dr.	Cr.	Balance
1/31	$39,205.00		$39,205.00
1/31	31,155.00		70,360.00
1/31		$20,363.26	49,996.74

Freight In

Date	Dr.	Cr.	Balance
1/30	$200.00		$200.00

Discount Lost

Date	Dr.	Cr.	Balance
1/31	$163.26		$163.26

column are calculated and compared to ensure their equality. These calculations and comparisons are as follows:

	Debits	Credits
Sundry Accounts	$200.00	
Accounts Payable	20,000.00	
Discounts Lost	163.26	Cash $20,363.26
	20,363.26	20,363.26

As soon as the validation of the credits and debits is completed, the totals are posted to the control accounts in the general ledger.

Similar to the earlier discussion, the control account pertaining to outstanding payables is used to validate the balances in the subsidiary accounts payable ledger. As Table 6-9 shows, the balance of the accounts payable account in the general ledger is $15,000, which equals the sum of the balances in the individual accounts of the subsidiary ledger ($4,000 + $4,000 + $7,000).

6.5 IMPREST FUNDS

No institution should keep unnecessary cash on hand. All cash receipts should be deposited promptly and cash should never be disbursed directly from receipts. Rather, checks that have been duly authorized and properly executed should be used.

As a practical matter, however, most health facilities provide special funds from which cash can be disbursed when the proper authorization and execution of checks is not feasible. For example, the institution might maintain a petty cash fund, a change fund, and a check-cashing fund. These are accounted for on an imprest basis that implies that each fund is established in a fixed amount and replenished when exhausted. The responsibility for each imprest fund should be assigned to a single individual who exercises sole control over the resources of the fund.

6.5.1 The Establishment of Imprest Funds

When an imprest fund is established, a check for the amount of the fund is drawn and made payable to the custodian who cashes the check and assumes responsibility for the fund. An entry such as the following serves to create the imprest fund:

Petty Cash Fund	$15.00	
Cash—General		$15.00

If the facility uses a cash disbursement journal, the entry to transfer the $15.00 from the general cash account to the petty cash fund is:

Cash Disbursement Journal

Date	*Ch. No.*	*Payee*	*Account Debited*	*Sundry Accounts Debit*	*Cash Credit*
1/1	78	J. Jones—Petty Cashier	Petty Cash	$15.00	$15.00

The petty cash fund is created by the entry in the Account Debited column. This record simply transfers cash from the institution's general cash account to its petty cash fund. The debit entry to the Petty Cash Fund account is recorded *only* when the fund is established or increased. Conversely, a credit entry to the account is recorded *only* when the fund is decreased. For example, if the fund is exhausted and requires replenishment frequently, consideration should be given to increasing its size. This results in an additional debit entry to the petty cash fund and a credit entry to the general cash account. On the other hand, if the fund is too large, a portion of petty cash should be returned to the general cash account by recording a credit entry to the petty cash fund and a debit entry to the general cash account.

6.5.2 Cash Disbursements from Imprest Funds

During the first month of operation, suppose that cash is disbursed from the fund as follows:

1/3	Purchased pencils	$1.50
1/7	Collected telegram	2.00
1/10	Purchased postage stamps	2.50
1/11	Paid for window cleaning	1.00
1/12	Paid for meal for person working overtime	2.50
1/17	Paid for repair of typewriter	1.00
1/20	Paid for repair of hall clock	2.00
1/28	Purchased paper clips	.65
1/30	Purchased postage stamps	1.70
Total		14.85

As each amount is disbursed, a petty cash voucher or receipt must be signed by the person receiving the payment. Each voucher is recorded in the petty cash record as shown in Table 6-10, where the disbursements assumed above are recorded.

The petty cash record is a supplementary record rather than a book of original entry from which information is transferred to the general ledger. A supplementary record is one in which information is summarized but not

Table 6-10 Petty Cash Record

Date	Explanation	Voucher No.	Receipts	Payments	Distribution of Payments				
								Misc. Payments	
					Postage	Freight	Misc. General Expense	Account	Amount
1/1	Established fund		$15.00						
1/3	Purchased pencils	1		$1.50				Off. supp.	$1.50
1/7	Paid for collect telegram	2		2.00			$2.00		
1/10	Purchased postage stamps	3		2.50	$2.50				
1/11	Paid for window cleaning	4		1.00			1.00		
1/12	Paid for meal for person working overtime	5		2.50			2.50		
1/17	Paid for repair of typewriter	6		1.00			1.00		
1/20	Paid for repair of hall clock	7		2.00			2.00		
1/28	Purchased paper clips	8		.65				Off. supp.	.65
1/30	Purchased postage stamps	9		1.70	1.70				
	Totals		15.00	14.85	4.20		8.50		2.15
	Balance			.15					
	Totals		15.00	15.00					
	Balance		.15						
1/31	Replenished Fund		14.85						

posted. The information summarized is used as a basis for an entry in a general journal or register that, in turn, is transferred to the general ledger.

6.5.3 Replenishing the Imprest Fund

Table 6-10 also shows that on January 30, only $0.15 remains in the fund. The petty cashier, recognizing that this is insufficient to cover another disbursement, turns in the $14.85 paid petty cash vouchers in exchange for a $14.85 check that is used to replenish the fund. When the check is received, the petty cash record is balanced as seen in the example. In addition, the check is cashed and the amount of the reimbursement is recorded in the petty cash record.

The check by which the petty cash fund is reimbursed is recorded in the cash disbursement journal with the following entry:

Cash Disbursement Journal

Date	*Ch. No.*	*Payee*	*Account Debited*	*Sundry Accounts Debit*	*Cash Credit*
1/1	78	J. Jones—Petty Cashier	Petty Cash	$15.00	$15.00
1/31	130	J. Jones—Petty Cashier	Postage Expense	4.20	
			General Expense	8.50	
			Office Supply Expense	2.15	14.85

The cash disbursements journal records that the accounts in the Account Debited column refer to expense items financed by disbursements from the petty cash fund. A debit to these accounts is required to record the amount of expense in an original book of entry from which information is transferred to the general ledger. Consequently, the petty cash fund must be reimbursed at the end of the accounting period as well as whenever it is exhausted. Obviously, if this fund is not reimbursed at the end of the period, its assets will be overstated and the expenses of the period will be understated in the institution's financial statements.

In the example, the petty cash fund is in balance. However, regardless of the care exercised, too much or too little change may be disbursed from the fund. In such a situation, the Cash Over and Short account is used to reflect the discrepancy. Returning to Table 6-10, suppose that only $0.10 remains in the petty cash fund rather than the $0.15 required to balance it. The entry to replenish the fund is:

Sundry Accounts Debited	$14.85	
Cash Over and Short	.05	
General Cash		$14.90

If, at the end of the period, $1.10 is found in the petty cash fund, an entry similar to the following is required to replenish it:

Sundry Accounts Debited	$14.85	
Cash Over and Short		$1.10
Cash—General		13.75

Clearly, any frequent and large errors reflected in the Cash Over and Short account constitute the basis for changing the fund custodian.

Questions for Discussion

1. Describe the cash accounts maintained by most health facilities.
2. Discuss what procedures should be present in any system of controlling cash and what role each plays.
3. Describe the system by which cash receipts can be controlled.
4. Describe the system by which cash disbursements can be controlled.
5. Describe a bank reconciliation and the process by which it is reconciled.
6. Discuss the relationship between the subsidiary accounts receivable (payable) ledger and the corresponding account in the general ledger.
7. Describe the importance and use of imprest funds.
8. Describe the process of

    a. creating an imprest fund
    b. changing the size of an imprest fund
    c. replenishing the fund

Problems for Solution

1. Suppose the institution receives $15,000 as a prepayment for the use of service by patients insured by a third party payer. Assume that the following revenue is earned by providing service to insured patients during the month:

Date	*Daily Service Revenue*	*Ancillary Service Revenue*
3/1	$400	$900
3/2	700	400
3/3	800	300
3/4	1,200	1,500
3/27	600	500
3/28	500	300

Record these transactions in the daily income summary, the subsidiary income ledger, and the general ledger.

2. Assume that the cash transactions from providing outpatient services during December are:

Date	*Patient*	*Registration Fee*	*Ancillary Service Revenue*
1	A	$15	$0
3	B	15	20
10	C	15	40
20	D	15	10
28	E	15	30
30	F	15	45
31	G	15	20

Record these transactions in:

a. the cash receipts journal
b. general journal form

Also post relevant totals to the general ledger.

3. Suppose the following transactions pertain to the provision of service on account:

Date	*Responsible Party*	*Daily Service Revenue*	*Ancillary Service Revenue (Inpatients)*	*Ancillary Service Revenue (Outpatients)*	*Registration Fee*
5/1	Patient A			$20	$10
5/3	Patient B			40	10
5/10	Third Party A	$5,000	$3,500		
5/12	Third Party B	10,000	6,000	50	40
5/13	Third Party A	20,000	8,000	120	60
5/20	Third Party B	60,000	7,000		
5/21	Patient C			30	10
5/27	Third Party A	30,000	12,000	150	50
5/30	Patient D	120	150		

Suppose further that the institution receives payments on these accounts:

Date	*Responsible Party*	*Amount*
5/5	Patient A	$20
5/8	Patient B	50

Date	*Responsible Party*	*Amount*
5/15	Third Party A	$8,000
5/17	Third Party B	16,050
5/20	Third Party A	20,000
5/28	Third Party B	67,000
5/31	Patient C	30

Record these transactions using the daily income summary, the cash receipts journal, the general ledger, and the subsidiary accounts receivable ledger.

4. Suppose that during the month, the institution acquires supply items as follows:

Date	*Vendor*	*Supply Class*	*Amount*	*Terms*
8/1	F & G Food	Food	$20,000	2/10/30
8/8	Bandages Co.	Medical	120,000	2/10/30
8/12	Jones & Smith	Drugs	60,000	2/10/30
8/15	Finch Food	Food	49,000	2/10/30
8/17	Bandages Co.	Surgical	30,500	2/10/30
8/20	Jones & Smith	Drugs	70,000	2/10/30
8/31	Pens & Pencils	General	9,500	2/10/30

Payments on these accounts during the month are as follows:

Invoice Date	*Date of Payment*	*Vendor*
8/1	8/9	F & G Food
8/8	8/17	Bandages Co.
8/12	8/25	Jones & Smith
8/15	8/25	Finch Food
8/17	8/30	Bandages Co.

Assuming the institution uses the net invoice method, record these transactions in the supply acquisitions journal, the cash disbursements journal, and the subsidiary accounts payable ledger, and post the information to the appropriate control accounts in the general ledger.

5. Suppose the institution decides to create a petty cash fund of $15.00. During the month, the fund disburses cash as follows:

Item	*Amount*
Office Supplies	$4.00
Postage	3.00
Transportation	5.00
Miscellaneous	1.50

Suppose further that, at this point, $1.50 in cash remains in the fund and that it is replenished. Record all transactions concerning this fund.

6. Suppose it is decided to increase (reduce) the fund in Problem 5 by $5.00. List the entries required to effect these changes.
7. Suppose that, as of May 31, the bank statement reports a cash balance of $170,000 while the cash balance on the hospital books is $160,850. Also suppose that the institution obtains the following information:

   a. A deposit in transit amounts to $17,000.
   b. Outstanding checks total $7,000.
   c. The bank collects $20,000, of which $19,000 is a payment on the principal of an outstanding note and $1,000 an interest payment.
   d. An $800 check that had been accepted in settlement of an outstanding receivable is returned to the maker because of insufficient funds in that individual's account.
   e. Bank service charges are $50.

   On the basis of these data, prepare a bank reconciliation and the necessary adjusting entry.

Chapter 7

Accounting for Receivables

That health facilities rely on third party payers and, to a lesser extent, self responsible patients for reimbursement is well recognized. Given that most third party payers reimburse the institution retrospectively and since administrators cannot refuse service because patients are unable to pay on a cash basis, the extension of credit in the health industry is an operating necessity. The basic process by which accounts receivable are recorded was discussed in Chapter 6. This chapter deals with a number of issues related to outstanding receivables.

7.1 VALUATION OF RECEIVABLES

The term receivable refers to the institution's claims against patients, third party payers, and others. As seen in Chapter 6, these claims arise primarily from the provision of service to patients and other third party payers to whom the institution extends credit as well as from the sale of goods or services to external entities other than patients. Collections on these accounts usually are not received until some time after service has been provided or the goods and services have been sold. In the meantime, the institution has a legal claim against the patient, the third party payer, and/or the entity to whom goods or services have been provided.

A unique characteristic concerning the receivables of the health care facility as compared with those of other organizations is that the full established charges may not be collected in a number of instances. Charges incurred by patients may be settled by the payment of an amount that is less than full established rates because of contractual agreements, charity service, courtesy discounts, and bad debts. As a consequence, the valuation of receivables requires special attention.

Theoretically, notes and accounts receivable should be reported in the balance sheet at their net realizable cash value. In other words, outstanding receivables that have been recorded at full established rates should be reduced to the net amount that the institution reasonably expects to collect in the form of cash. As indicated below, expected uncollectables should be estimated and reported in the income statement as well as in the balance sheet. As for the adjustment in the balance sheet, the gross value of the outstanding receivables is reduced by the sum of the balances appearing in a series of contra asset accounts.

Recall that the balance of a contra account is subtracted from the balance of the associate account; this, in turn, permits the construction of a more accurate set of financial statements. Such a treatment results in an estimate of the net realizable cash value of outstanding receivables and tends to avoid the problem of overstating current assets. On the other hand, the estimated value of the uncollectable accounts also should be reported as a contra revenue account in the income statement. In this case, the use of the contra revenue account results in a more accurate measure of the net income or net loss of the period as well as a more accurate statement of the end-of-period fund balance in the balance sheet. In summary, the procedures described in this section are required to obtain a proper matching of revenues and revenue deductions on an accrual basis as well as a proper valuation of the receivables reported in the balance sheet.

7.1.1 Bad Debts

It is reasonable to expect that the institution will not be able to collect a portion of the outstanding receivables from providing service for which patients are responsible. At the time of admission or as soon as practical thereafter, the patient's financial status should be determined so that uncollectables, resulting from the individual's unwillingness to pay (bad debt) may be distinguished from uncollectables that are a result of inability to pay (charity care). A commercial enterprise usually will not extend credit unless collection is reasonably assured but, because of the nature of medical care, health facilities do not enjoy this luxury. Even though health care institutions usually are unable to exercise complete discretion when extending credit, the avoidance of bad debts is just as important in the health industry as it is in the profit-oriented sector of the economy.

7.1.1.1 Estimating Bad Debts

At the end of the accounting period, management should develop an estimate of the value of outstanding receivables that ultimately will prove to be uncollectable and will result in bad debts. Such an adjustment process is necessary to avoid an overstatement of assets in the balance sheet and to provide for the proper matching of revenue and deductions in revenue in the income statement of the period in which the receivables are created.

Suppose that the outstanding receivables at the end of 198A amount to $50,000 and that total revenue of $970,000 is earned during the period. Assume further that the operating expenses of the period amount to $940,000. In the absence of an adjustment reflecting the value of uncollectable receivables, a net income of $30,000 ($970,000 − $940,000) and accounts receivable of $50,000 are reported in the financial statements.

Suppose, however, that $40,000 of the accounts receivable prove to be uncollectable during the ensuing year. Assume further that as these accounts are deemed uncollectable by the credit manager, they are at that time recognized as losses. Such a procedure obviously results in a recognition of bad debt losses in the wrong year. The $40,000 of bad debts should be given accounting recognition in the year in which the revenue is recorded. Clearly, the procedure results in a mismatching of revenues and reductions in revenue and, as a consequence, the net income and the assets of the first period are overstated. Had the reduction in revenue been recorded in the first year, the income statement would have reported a net loss of $10,000 rather than a surplus of $30,000 and the receivables reported in the balance sheet would have reflected a net realizable cash value of $10,000 rather than $50,000.

The problem, of course, is that it is impossible to ascertain precisely which accounts will prove to be uncollectable. It also is impossible to predict the exact total dollar amount of the uncollectables. However, reasonable estimates can be developed and the amount of the misstatement may thereby be reduced to acceptable levels.

There are essentially three methods by which bad debts are estimated. The institution may:

1. apply the historic percentage of accounts receivable that result in bad debts to the balance of those receivables that are reported at the end of the period
2. apply a historic percentage of accounts that result in bad debts to the total of the outstanding receivables that are acquired during the period
3. analyze accounts receivable by considering the length of time they have remained unpaid (this is called the aging of accounts receivable)

As a practical matter, management may use all three methods, and a comparison of the results of each may lead to the most accurate estimate of probable bad debts.

The percentages referred to earlier represent a probability that an account will result in a bad debt. That probability is based on past experience as tempered by expectations regarding economic conditions that might exist during the collection period. It may be found, for example, that in recent years 15 percent of the accounts outstanding at the end of the period proved uncollectable. If factors influencing collections are expected to remain unchanged during the next period, it might be expected that a similar 15 percent will prove uncollectable.

The aging procedure is likely to give the most accurate estimate of bad debts and is perhaps the most useful from a managerial perspective. Under the aging process, accounts are classified into "age" groups reflecting the number of days that have elapsed since the date of discharge or the date on which payment was last received. Totals are obtained for each age group and appropriate probabilities based on past experience are applied to these sums to obtain an estimate of probable bad debts.

For example, assume that the institution referred to earlier uses the aging process in estimating bad debts and that the information is summarized as in Table 7-1. The ages of the accounts are grouped into the categories 1–30 days, 31–60 days, etc. In the second column are the number of accounts in each group that, when divided into the corresponding value in Column 3, yield the average value of the receivables in the age group. This provides a criterion by which collection efforts can be directed. The accounts in the age group 181–364 days and 61–90 days have the highest average value. As a result, management may decide to place a greater emphasis on collecting these accounts than on the much larger number of smaller valued ones.

In the Probability of Bad Debt column is the proportion of accounts in each age group that historically have proved worthless. As a general rule, the older an account, the less likely it is to be collected; this tendency is reflected by the probabilities in Table 7-1. The Value of Bad Debt column is simply the product of the probability of bad debt and the total value of the accounts associated with each age group. For example, the estimated bad debts involving accounts aged 1–30 days is given by the product of the value of all accounts in the group ($8,000) and the probability of bad debt (.10). The total of the Value of Bad Debt column is the value of all accounts that are expected to prove uncollectable. This process involves nothing more than an application of the principles of mathematical expectation to the problem of estimating the value of outstanding receivables that will prove uncollectable.

As seen in the last column of Table 7-1, the bad debts of the period are expected to total approximately $12,000, so the appropriate entry at the end of the period is:

Provision for Bad Debt	$12,000	
Allowance for Bad Debt		$12,000

To record provision for bad debt as estimated in the aging schedule.

At this point no specific accounts are recognized as bad debts since, at the time the entry is recorded, it is not known which ones will prove uncollectable.

Table 7-1 Aging of Outstanding Receivables

Age of Account (1)	*Number of Accounts (2)*	*Total Value of Accounts (3)*	*Average Value of Accounts (4)*	*Probability of Bad Debt (5)*	*Value of Bad Debt (6)*
1-30	1,000	$8,000	$8	.10	$800
31-60	200	2,000	10	.18	360
61-90	50	5,000	100	.22	1,100
91-180	1,000	15,000	15	.25	3,750
181-364	100	20,000	200	.30	6,000
Totals		50,000			12,010

Rather, as seen above, a contra revenue account (i.e., Provision for Bad Debt) and a contra asset account (Allowance for Bad Debt) are used to record expectations of the bad debts of the period.

The balance of the Provision for Bad Debt account appears in the income statement as a reduction in revenue. Returning to the example, the contra revenue account might appear in the condensed income statement of the institution as follows:

	Revenue	$970,000
Less	Provision for Bad Debt	(12,000)
	Net Operating Revenue	958,000
Less	Expenses	940,000
	Net Income	18,000

The adjustment for bad debts results in a net income of $18,000 rather than $30,000, which would have been reported if potential bad debts had received no formal accounting recognition.

Consider next the presentation of the contra asset account in the balance sheet. Referring to the example, the Allowance for Bad Debt account is presented in the balance sheet as follows:

	Accounts Receivable	$50,000
Less	Allowance for Bad Debt	(12,000)
		38,000

The balance of the contra asset account is subtracted from the balance of the associate account, reducing the value of outstanding receivables to a net realizable cash value of $38,000.

7.1.1.2 Collections and Write-Offs

Referring to the example, assume that in 198B $30,000 of the 198A accounts receivable are collected and recorded as described earlier. A summary entry recording these collections is:

Cash	$30,000	
Accounts Receivable		$30,000

Also assume that during 198B the credit manager notifies the accountant that the remaining $20,000 is uncollectable and should be written off as bad debts. As a result, the following entry is required:

Allowance for Bad Debts	$20,000	
Accounts Receivable		$20,000

At this point, specific accounts that have proved uncollectable are removed from the subsidiary accounts receivable ledger or eliminated from active files. The last entry results in the following T account balances:

Accounts Receivable	
$50,000	$30,000
	20,000
0	

Allowance for Bad Debts	
$20,000	$12,000
Debit $8,000	

If payments are received on accounts that have been written off previously, it is necessary to record a debit entry to cash and a credit to a Recovery of Written Off Account. The recovery is reflected in the income statement as a reduction in the provision for bad debts. In addition, an appropriate notation of such payments should be recorded in the subsidiary accounts receivable ledger to maintain an accurate credit history.

7.1.1.3 Subsequent Adjustments for Bad Debts

Now, assume that the required provision for bad debts at the end of 198B is $23,000, as determined in the manner just described. A problem arises in that the allowance for bad debts has a debit balance of $8,000. In other words, the bad debts emanating from the receivables outstanding at the end of 198A are $8,000 greater than estimated. This implies that the reported net income for the period is overstated by $8,000 and should be $10,000 rather than the reported $18,000. Moreover, the December 31, 198A, receivables reported in the balance sheet of that date are overstated by $8,000.

Even though the net income and the net realizable cash value of the outstanding receivables on the balance sheet are overstated, no revision or adjustment of the data reported for 198A is necessary. Rather, normally recurring adjustments of this type should be reflected in the income statement of the current period. Thus, if an allowance for bad debt of $23,000 is required at the end of 198B, the entry is:

Provision for Bad Debt	$31,000	
Allowance for Bad Debt		$31,000

In this case, the required adjustment is calculated as follows:

Desired Credit Balance	$23,000
Current Debit Balance	8,000
Allowance for Bad Debts	31,000

The accounting treatment of errors in projections on bad debts is equivalent to saying that "two wrongs make a right." Referring to the example, the understatement of bad debts and the resulting overstatement of net income and accounts receivable in 198A are offset by an intentional overstatement of bad debts as well as an intentional understatement of the net income and accounts receivable reported at the end of 198B. While errors have been made in 198A and 198B, the net income and the receivables associated with the two years are correct since the errors offset one another.

At this point, assume that receivables of $23,000 are recognized as uncollectable in 198C. The entry

Allowance for Bad Debts	$23,000	
Accounts Receivables		$23,000

provides formal accounting recognition of the decision to write off these receivables as uncollectable and eliminates the credit balance of the allowance for bad debts account.

7.1.2 Valuation of Other Reductions in Revenue

A loss in revenue resulting from bad debts can be expected. Revenue losses also may result from the contractual agreements, courtesy discounts, and charity care mentioned earlier. Since operating revenues should be credited and accounts receivable should be debited for service to all patients at full established rates, the matching principle requires that these additional reductions in revenue be given accounting recognition on an accrual basis.

By way of illustration, assume that gross revenues earned by providing service to all patients amount to $900,000 during 198C. Further, assume that the operating expenses of 198C are $750,000 and accounts receivable of $200,000 are acquired, of which $150,000 actually are collected in 198D. Suppose that the uncollected balance of $50,000 is distributed as follows:

Bad Debts	$10,000
Free or Charity Care	15,000
Contractual Adjustments	8,000
Courtesy Discounts	17,000
Total Revenue Losses	50,000

If no losses in revenue are anticipated and recorded, a net income of $150,000 ($900,000 − $750,000) is reported in the income statement for 198C and the assets in the balance sheet will include accounts receivable valued at $200,000. Thus, when potential deductions in revenue are not given formal accounting recognition, the financial statements for the year will be incorrect.

As a result, it is necessary to analyze accounts receivable at the end of the reporting period to estimate the proportion that is likely to be uncollectable for the reasons indicated. As in the process of estimating the bad debt expense, the deductions in revenue resulting from charity care, courtesy discounts, and contractual arrangements may be projected by analyzing individual accounts, or by applying percentages based on a sample of the accounts, or on past experience. Based on this analysis, the deductions in revenue and the allowance for bad debts can be recorded thus:

Provision for		
Bad Debts	$10,000	
Charity Care	15,000	
Contractual Adjustments	8,000	
Courtesy Discounts	17,000	
Allowance for		
Bad Debts		$10,000
Charity Care		15,000
Contractual Adjustments		8,000
Courtesy Discounts		17,000

The effect of this entry is to record the estimated reductions in revenue associated with the accounts receivable reported on December 31, 198C, as follows (figures in parentheses represent probabilities that an account will be uncollectable).

Bad Debts (.05)	$10,000
Charity Care (.075)	15,000
Contractual Adjustments (.04)	8,000
Courtesy Discounts (.085)	17,000
	50,000

When it is possible to determine precise revenue deductions, credits may be made directly to accounts receivable rather than to the allowance accounts.

The effect of this entry on the operating results in the income statement for 198C is:

Gross Revenues		$900,000
Less Deductions from Revenue		
Provision for Bad Debt	$10,000	
Free or Charity Care	15,000	
Contractual Adjustments	8,000	
Courtesy Discounts	17,000	50,000
Net Revenue		850,000
Less Operating Expenses		750,000
Net Income		100,000

After the deductions in revenue have been incorporated into the statement of revenues and expenses, a net income of $100,000 is reported rather than the $150,000 that would have been shown if no deductions had been anticipated. The balance sheet for December 31, 198C, should report accounts receivable of \$200,000 and the corresponding net realizable cash value of \$150,000.

7.2 ACCOUNTING FOR NOTES RECEIVABLE

A promissory note is an unconditional promise to pay a definite sum of money on demand or at a fixed future date. For example, if Hospital A promises to pay Hospital B a definite sum of money on a fixed future date, Hospital A is the maker of the note and Hospital B is the payee. To Hospital A, it is a note payable and to Hospital B a note receivable. The purpose of this section is to discuss the accounting procedures by which notes receivable are recorded. Notes payable are discussed in Chapter 10.

A note may be interest bearing or it may be noninterest bearing. To the borrower (maker of the note), an interest payment is an expense, while to the lender it represents a revenue. When the note is interest bearing, the rate of interest is stated and usually is expressed as a percentage of the principal. If a note is noninterest bearing, no interest is collected unless it is not paid when due. If a noninterest-bearing note is not paid when due, interest at the full legal rate may be collected from the legal due date to the time when final payment is made.

Unless otherwise specified, the rate of interest on a note is the amount charged for use of the principal for one year of 365 days. The formula for calculating interest is expressed in the form

$$\text{Interest} = \begin{matrix}\text{Principal}\\\text{of Note}\end{matrix} \times \begin{matrix}\text{Rate of}\\\text{Interest}\end{matrix} \times \begin{matrix}\text{Time}\\\text{of Note}\end{matrix}$$

The time is expressed as a ratio in which the numerator is the life of the note, including a three-day grace period, and the denominator is 365 days (366 days in a leap year). For example, the interest on a \$2,000, 7 percent, one-year note is calculated as follows:

$$\$2{,}000 \times .07 \times \frac{368}{365} = \$141.15$$

Similarly, the interest on a \$6,000, 8 percent, 90-day note is computed as follows:

$$\$6{,}000 \times .08 \times \frac{93}{365} = \$122.30$$

Notes receivable are recorded in an account so titled. Each note may be identified by naming the maker as an explanation to the record of the account. Only one account is needed since individual notes are on hand and the maker, rate of interest, due dates, and any other information desired by management may be obtained by examining each document.

When accepting a note in granting an extension on a past due account, the institution should attempt to collect part of the outstanding receivable in cash. This reduces the debt and makes possible a note for a smaller amount. For example, suppose that on September 1, Hospital B agrees to accept $1,000 and a $7,000, 6 percent, 90-day note from Hospital A in settlement of an $8,000 past due account. When Hospital B receives the cash and the note, the entry is:

Cash	$1,000	
Note Receivable	7,000	
Accounts Receivable—Hospital A		$8,000

Received note and cash from Hospital A in settlement of outstanding account.

This entry changes the composition of hospital assets from an $8,000 account receivable to a $7,000 note receivable and $1,000 in cash.

The interest on the note is

$$\$7{,}000 \times .06 \times \frac{93}{365} = \$107.01$$

which is distributed over the life of the note as follows:

$$\text{September } \$7{,}000 \times .06 \times \frac{30}{365} = \$34.52$$

$$\text{October } 7{,}000 \times .06 \times \frac{31}{365} = 35.67$$

$$\text{November } 7{,}000 \times .06 \times \frac{30}{365} = 34.52$$

$$\text{December } 7{,}000 \times .06 \times \frac{2}{365} = \underline{2.30}$$

$$107.01$$

The interest income on this note is earned by the passage of time and should be recorded by Hospital B as earned income through a series of monthly accruals:

Accrued Interest Receivable	$34.52	
Interest Income		$34.52
Accrued Interest Receivable	35.67	
Interest Income		35.67
Accrued Interest Receivable	34.52	
Interest Income		34.52

When Hospital A pays the note, the entry is:

Cash	$7,107.01	
Accrued Interest Receivable		$104.71
Interest Income		2.30
Note Receivable		7,000.00

This entry eliminates the note receivable from the books of Hospital A. It also gives formal accounting recognition to the cash receipt as well as to the last two days of interest.

Occasionally, the maker of a note either cannot or will not pay on the maturity date. In such a situation, the note is said to have been dishonored. This does not relieve the maker of the obligation and the institution should employ every legal means to obtain payment.

The balance of the notes receivable account should show only the amount of those that have not matured. A dishonored or past due note is always removed from the notes receivable account and the principal plus accrued interest is charged to the account receivable of its maker. For example, assume that the hospital holds a $4,000, 12 percent, 60-day note of C. Hill and that on the maturity date Hill dishonors the note. The following entry removes the debt from the note receivable account and charges the principal and interest to the Hill account:

Accounts Receivable—C. Hill	$4,082.85	
Notes Receivable		$4,000.00
Interest Income		82.85

In summary, transferring the dishonored note to the maker's account serves two purposes. First, the transfer removes the debt from the notes receivable account, so only those that have not matured remain in that account. Second, the entry assigns both interest and principal to the maker's account receivable and thereby retains it on the books of the institution until paid or recognized as a bad debt.

The reason for charging the interest and principal to the account receivable of C. Hill is that this individual owes both of those sums and that account should reflect the full amount due. The interest charges are recognized as revenue even though no cash is received.

7.3 FINANCING WITH NOTES RECEIVABLE

A note receivable is preferred to an open account because it may be discounted or sold to a bank. Discounting enables the institution to convert a note into cash without waiting for the debt to mature. To discount a note, the facility endorses and delivers it to a bank in exchange for cash. The maker of the note should be notified of the arrangement and the reasons for the arrangement, and instructed to make payments to the bank.

If the institution's credit is good, a bank usually is willing to accept and discount a note because the endorser agrees to pay it at maturity if it is dishonored. This means that when a note is discounted, the endorser assumes a contingent liability that hinges on the failure of the maker to honor the debt. If the maker honors the note, the endorser assumes no liability. On the other hand, if the maker dishonors the note, the contingent liability becomes a real liability. As a result, the contingent liability should appear in the books of the institution when a note is discounted.

7.3.1 Discounting a Noninterest-Bearing Note

For illustration, assume that on August 10, Hospital A accepts a noninterest-bearing 60-day, $900 note from P. Carson in granting an extension of time on an overdue account. The legal due date of this note is October 12. If the hospital discounts it on August 28, the bank must wait 45 days (until October 12) to collect the $900. The 45 days is called the discount period and is calculated as follows:

Number of Days in August	31
Date of Discount	28
Days Discounted in August	3
Days Discounted in September	30
Days Discounted in October (including 3 days' grace)	12
Days in Discount Period	45

Furthermore, if the bank's discount rate is 6 percent, it will deduct $6.66 ($900 × .06 × 45/365) from the maturity value of the note and the hospital will receive $893.34 ($900 − $6.66). The $893.34 is called the proceeds of the note and the $6.66 is an interest expense to the hospital. The transaction is recorded as follows:

Cash	$893.34	
Interest Expense	6.66	
Note Receivable Discounted		$900.00

Discounted the P. Carson note.

In that entry, the contingent liability of the hospital is recorded by the credit to notes receivable discounted. Assuming the hospital holds a $200 note from B. Jones as well as the one from Carson, the notes receivable and the notes receivable discounted accounts appear as follows after the entry is posted:

Notes Receivable			Notes Receivable Discounted	
Jones Note	$200		Carson Note	$900
Carson Note	900			

If a balance sheet is prepared before the maturity date of the note, the balance of these two accounts is presented thus:

Assets			
Cash		$8,000	
Notes Receivable	$1,100		
Less Notes Receivable Discounted	900	200	
Inventory		$7,500	
Net Accounts Receivable		4,000	
Total Current Assets			$19,700

Showing Notes Receivable Discounted as a reduction in notes receivable indicates the presence of a contingent liability to the knowledgeable balance sheet reader.

When a note is discounted, the bank takes possession of it in exchange for cash. If possible, the bank will attempt to collect on the note at the maturity date. In the example, if P. Carson honors the note at maturity, the hospital need only remove the contingent liability from the books by the following entry:

Notes Receivable Discounted	$900	
Notes Receivable		$900

To remove the contingent liability of P. Carson.

The effect of this entry is to eliminate the balance of the note receivable discounted account and to remove the amount of the debt from the notes receivable account:

Notes Receivable			Note Receivable Discounted			
Jones Note	$200	$900	Carson Note	$900	Carson Note	$900
Carson Note	900					

If the bank is unable to collect a discounted debt from the maker at maturity, it normally will protest the note and seek payment from the endorser. A notice of protest is prepared, attested to by a notary public, and mailed to the endorser. The cost of protesting a negotiable instrument is called a protest fee and the bank will seek payment of such fees as well as the principal from the one who discounted the dishonored note.

For example, suppose that instead of paying the $900 note above, P. Carson dishonors the debt. As soon as the note is not paid on the maturity date, the bank notifies the hospital by mailing a notice of protest and a letter asking for the payment of the maturity value and the protest fee. The hospital must pay both. If the protest fee is $7, the hospital will pay the bank $907 and charge the principal of the note as well as the protest fee to the account of P. Carson as follows:

Accounts Receivable—P. Carson	$907.00	
Cash—General		$907.00

The dishonoring of the note changes the contingent liability to a real liability. When the hospital pays the $907, both the real and contingent liabilities are liquidated. The entry above records the payment of the real liability while the following one eliminates the contingent liability and the value of the note from the books of the institution:

Notes Receivable Discounted	$900.00	
Notes Receivable		$900.00

When the bank receives the $907, the dishonored note is returned to the hospital, which then should make every effort to collect the maturity value as well as the protest fee and perhaps interest charges on both. However, in the event the hospital is unable to obtain payment, it will have to write off the account as a bad debt.

7.3.2 Discounting an Interest-Bearing Note

Discounting an interest-bearing note is somewhat different from a noninterest-bearing note. This is because when a bank discounts an interest-bearing note, it will collect from the maker *both* the note's principal and the interest on that sum. The principal plus interest is called the maturity value of the note. The bank bases the discount on the maturity value.

For example, suppose that on January 4, Hospital A discounts at 6 percent the $300, 90-day, 6 percent note, dated January 1, of Hospital K, which originally issued the instrument in exchange for laundry services provided by Hospital A. The maturity value of this note is $304.59, calculated as follows:

Principal of the Note	$300.00
Interest on $300 @ 6% for 93 days	4.59
Maturity Value of the Note	304.59

The discount period for the note is 89 days and is computed thus:

Number of Days in January	31
Date of Discount	4
Days Discounted in January	27
Days Discounted in February	28
Days Discounted in March	31
Days Discounted in April	3
Days in Discount Period	89

The bank then bases the discount of 6 percent on the maturity value of $304.59 for 89 days and will give the hospital $300.13 cash, computed as follows:

	Maturity Value of the Note	$304.59
Less	Interest on $304.59 @ 6% for 89 days	4.46
	Proceeds	$300.13

In this case, the proceeds exceed the principal of the note by $0.13. Consequently, the hospital records the transaction by the entry

Cash	$300.13	
Interest Income		$0.13
Notes Receivable Discounted		300.00

The hospital offsets the $4.46 interest expense by the $4.59 interest income that will be earned if the note is held to maturity, and records the net interest income of $0.13. If the discount exceeds the interest income that would have been earned at maturity, the hospital records the difference as an interest expense.

Suppose that Hospital K dishonors the note on the maturity date. As before, the bank will seek payment from Hospital A. In this case, however, the bank will demand not only the payment of the note's principal and protest fees but also the interest charges. Thus, assuming a protest fee of $5.50, the bank will demand $310.09 from Hospital A, computed as follows:

Maturity Value of the Note	
Principal	$300.00
Interest	4.59
	$304.59
Protest Fee	5.50
Total	310.09

The hospital must pay the bank $310.09. In recording the payment, it charges the amount to the account of Hospital K and cancels the contingent liability as well as the note receivable, as illustrated earlier.

When Hospital A receives the dishonored note from the bank, it should make every effort to collect its maturity value, the protest fee, and the interest on both from the date of maturity. For example, if Hospital K pays the value of the dishonored note, protest fees, and interest at 4 percent, 30 days after the legal due date, the total amount paid is calculated as follows:

Maturity Value	$304.59
Protest Fee	5.50
Interest on $310.09 @ 4% for 30 days	1.02
Total	311.11

This is recorded by Hospital A as follows:

Cash	$311.11	
Accounts Receivable—Hospital K		$310.09
Interest Income		1.02

The interest rate of 4 percent is assumed to have been one of the terms on which the note was accepted by Hospital A.

7.4 FINANCING WITH ACCOUNTS RECEIVABLE

Under a formal arrangement, the health care facility may pledge a portion or all of its accounts receivable in exchange for an immediate cash advance. The cash advance typically is less than 100 percent of the full value of the receivables and may be evidenced by an interest-bearing promissory note executed by the institution and issued to the bank. The hospital usually retains the credit risk and continues its normal collection efforts. The creditors of the institution generally are unaware of the arrangement and continue to make payments to the facility which, in turn, remits these amounts to the bank at the end of negotiated time intervals.

To illustrate, suppose that on April 1, the hospital exchanges $200,000 of its accounts receivable for a cash advance of $170,000 less a flat fee of 2 percent. The hospital also issues a $170,000 note that requires interest of 1 percent per month on the unpaid balance. The entry to record the April 1 entry is:

Assigned Accounts Receivable	$200,000	
Financing Expense (2% of $170,000)	3,400	
Cash ($170,000 − $3,400)	166,600	
Accounts Receivable		$200,000
Note Payable		170,000

During the month of April, assume the hospital collects $91,700 on these accounts and remits that amount to the bank. A summary entry for April is:

Cash—General	$91,700	
Assigned Accounts Receivable		$91,700

When payment is made to the bank on April 30 the entry is:

Note Payable	$90,000	
Interest Expense (1% × $170,000)	1,700	
Cash—General		$91,700

During May, the remaining amount owed to the bank is collected and the hospital remits the sum to the bank. The entries to terminate the agreement are as follows. The summary entry that records the cash received in May and reduces the assigned accounts receivable account is:

Cash—General	$93,000	
Assigned Accounts Receivable		$93,000

On May 31, the following entry eliminates the note payable and the payment of remaining interest charges:

Note Payable	$80,000	
Interest Expense (1% of $80,000)	800	
Cash—General		$80,800

At this point in the process of accounting for the cash advance, the assigned accounts receivable balance is $15,300:

Assigned Accounts Receivable	
$200,000	$91,700
	93,000

Debit Balance $15,300

To transfer the uncollected balance of this account to accounts receivable, the following entry is recorded:

Accounts Receivable	$15,300	
Assigned Accounts Receivable		$15,300

This entry permits the hospital to record payment on these accounts as illustrated earlier.

Questions for Discussion

1. Describe why it is important to report outstanding receivables in terms of their net realizable cash value.
2. Discuss the methods of estimating bad debts and other deductions in revenue.
3. Define the following terms:

    a. discount period
    b. maturity value of a note
    c. proceeds of a note
    d. promissory note

4. Describe how the institution can use notes receivable to finance temporary cash needs.
5. Explain how accounts receivable are used to finance a temporary cash need.
6. Discuss why a note receivable is preferred to an account receivable.

Problems for Solution

1. Suppose the following information is available on December 31, 198A:

    a. outstanding receivables generated during the period amount to $120,000
    b. previously, 5 percent of the outstanding receivables generated during a period resulted in bad debts
    c. the allowance for bad debt account has a current credit balance of $1,200

    Explain what adjusting entry is required to record the bad debts of the period.
2. Suppose the accounts receivable of the institution total $180,000 at the end of the accounting period. The probability of writing off one of these receivables as a deduction in revenue is as follows:

Bad Debt	.02
Charity Care	.01
Courtesy Discounts	.03
Contractual Agreements	.04

Explain the required adjusting entry and how these adjustments are reported in the financial statements.

3. Suppose the hospital accepts a $2,000, 60-day, 8 percent note from Henry Balk in settlement of a past due account. On day 20 the note is discounted at 6 percent. Subsequently, Henry dishonors the note, and the protest fees amount to $10. Later Henry pays the amounts due plus 6 percent interest for 30 days. Record all transactions regarding this note.
4. Suppose on day 30 a noninterest-bearing $1,000 90-day note is discounted at 8 percent. The note subsequently is dishonored and the protest fees are $25. Later, the maker of the note pays all amounts due plus interest charges of 6 percent for 20 days. Record all entries pertaining to this note, assuming it was received initially in settlement of a past due account.
5. Suppose the hospital accepts $500 and a $2,000 8 percent 60-day note from A. Klink in settlement of a past due account on August 1. On August 20, the hospital discounts the note at the bank, where the discount rate is 9 percent. Assuming that Klink dishonors the note and the protest fees are $10, record all entries pertaining to this note.
6. Suppose that on April 3 the hospital receives a $4,000 noninterest-bearing note that will run for 90 days. On May 2 the institution discounts the note at 6 percent. Suppose further that the note is dishonored on the maturity date and the protest fees are $5. If the maker of the note subsequently pays the hospital all amounts due 30 days after the maturity date plus 8 percent interest, record all entries pertaining to this note.
7. Suppose that on June 1 the institution assigns $200,000 of its accounts receivable to the bank. The hospital receives a 70 percent cash advance net of a flat finance charge of 2 percent on the advance. It makes the collections and remits them to the bank on a monthly basis. In addition, the hospital issues a $140,000 note that requires a 4 percent interest payment on the unpaid balance. Further, assume the following transactions completed:

   a. The hospital collects $75,600 in June.
   b. On June 30 the hospital remits the June collections to the bank.
   c. On July 31, the hospital pays the balance.

   Prepare all entries to record the foregoing transactions.
8. Suppose the hospital accepts $200 and a $400, 60-day, 6 percent note from I. Dink in settlement of a past due account. On day 15, the note is discounted at 8 percent at the bank. On the maturity date, Dink dishonors the note and the hospital pays the maturity value of the note plus protest fees of $10. Later, Dink pays the maturity value and the

protest fees plus 4 percent interest on both for 22 days. Record all transactions concerning this note.

9. Suppose that on January 1, the institution accepts a $10,000, 60-day, 10 percent note from A. Maur in granting an extension of time on an overdue account. On January 4, the note is discounted at 8 percent. On the maturity date, Maur dishonors the note and protest fees are $10. Record all transactions concerning this note.
10. Suppose the hospital accepts a $5,000, 90-day, 10 percent note from J. Dudd in settlement of a past due account. On day 30, it discounts the note at 7 percent. Later, Dudd dishonors the note and the protest fees are $20. Subsequently, Dudd pays all amounts due and 8 percent for 20 days. Record all transactions concerning this note.

Chapter 8

Accounting for Investments

Idle cash earns nothing for the health care facility and the purchasing power of cash declines during periods of rising prices. As a consequence, the well-managed institution invests all excess cash in securities that earn interest. Funds may be available for periods as short as 30 days or less, and temporary investments in short-term highly marketable instruments can be quite worthwhile. The major forms in which excess funds can be invested are Certificates of Deposit, Treasury bills, commercial bank savings accounts, high grade commercial paper such as 30-day notes of leading corporations, and bonds. Investments such as these earn income that would not have been produced if excess cash had remained idle in checking accounts.

The investment objectives of most health care administrators are to: (1) ensure the safety and the immediate availability of principal and (2) earn a reasonable income. Several potential alternatives are available, but of particular importance in evaluating these situations are the liquidity of the investment, safety of principal, and the extent to which the instrument is available in various maturities.

Liquidity may be defined as the ability to convert an investment into cash. If the demand for cash is underestimated, management may be forced to sell securities so it can meet unexpected financial requirements. From this perspective, a highly liquid security represents a more desirable investment than one that is less liquid.

An investment with several issues that mature at different times is a desirable choice for most health facilities. A wide range of maturity dates increases the flexibility required to permit the synchronization of future cash needs with the investments. Indeed, the effective use of cash funds and the maximization of investment income depends on such a synchronization.

These considerations suggest several guidelines for the investment of excess cash:

1. The investments should be readily marketable and characterized by stable prices.
2. Management, by limiting choices to highly liquid and marketable securities, can convert them into cash without a loss in principal; a relatively stable price tends to minimize risk.
3. Subject to the risk that management is willing to accept, the securities should yield a reasonable income.
4. The institution's portfolio should consist of securities that mature on different dates or in a relatively short period. This policy is desirable when viewed from the perspective of synchronizing maturity dates with the demand for cash.

8.1 BONDS

A bond is a promissory note to pay a definite sum of money to the owner or holder of record at a fixed future date. Similar to promissory notes discussed earlier, bonds bear interest. Unlike promissory notes, however, bonds do not name or identify the lender (holder) since these instruments may be owned and transferred by a number of people during the securities' lifetimes.

Since corporate lawyers and financiers have developed a wide variety of bonds, each with a slightly different set of characteristics, there is no single method of classifying these instruments. Rather, bonds may be classified according to the method of paying the principal and interest as well as the type of security pledged by the issuing institution.

When bonds are classified according to the method by which the principal is to be paid, they may be serial bonds or sinking fund bonds. As to the former, portions of the issue become due and are paid in installments over a period of years. For example, a $10,000,000 serial bond issue may provide that $1,000,000 becomes due and payable each year until the entire issue has been redeemed. As for sinking fund bonds, the issuing institution creates a sinking fund from which payments are made at maturity.

When classified according to the method of interest payment, they are either registered bonds or coupon bonds. Ownership of registered bonds is recorded with the issuing institution; this provides some protection against loss or theft. When ownership is transferred, the issuer records the transfer, and interest payments are made to the new registered owner. Coupon bonds, on the other hand, are characterized by interest coupons that are attached to each certificate. Each coupon calls for an interest payment on the date indicated on the bond to which it is attached. The coupons are detached as they become due and are deposited in a bank for collection. Frequently, the ownership of coupon bonds is not registered with the issuing institution, which implies that unregistered bonds are payable to the bearer. In that case, ownership is transferred by the act of delivering the bond from the previous holder to the new owner.

As noted, bonds may be classified by the type of security pledged by the issuing institution. They may be either secured or unsecured. Unsecured bonds are called debentures and depend on the general credit standing of the issuing institution for security. When bonds are secured, it normally is by mortgages or liens on the assets of the issuing institution. They are classified according to the type of asset pledged as security. For example, a real estate mortgage bond usually is secured by a mortgage on a portion or all of the land, plant, and equipment of the issuing institution, while collateral trust bonds are secured by stocks, bonds, and other negotiable instruments that are deposited with a trustee.

8.2 BONDS AS SHORT-TERM INVESTMENTS

When a bond is first issued, the transactions are between the institution and investors or between it and an underwriter who buys the issue and, in turn, sells it to the public. However, these transactions represent only a very small proportion of the total activity in the bond market on any given day. The vast majority of bond dealings involve buying and selling among investors through brokers who are paid commissions or fees.

Bonds normally are issued in $1,000 denominations but their price is quoted on a percentage basis. For example, a $1,000 bond quoted at 98½ sells at 98½ percent of $1,000, or $985. The $15 difference between the quoted price and the $1,000 par value is referred to as a discount. Similarly, a $1,000 bond quoted at 102⅛ sells for 102⅛ percent of $1,000, or $1,021.25. The $21.25 difference is called a premium. When bonds are held as a long-term investment, premiums or discounts must be amortized. These are considered in Section 8.3.

8.2.1 Acquisition of Bonds as Temporary Investments

Assume that a projection of the institution's cash position shows that approximately $10,000 will not be required for operating purposes during the next three months. Suppose further that on February 1, the facility purchases 10 Cable Co. 8 percent $1,000 bonds that pay interest semiannually on January 1 and July 1. At that time, suppose that the bonds are quoted at 96 and that the brokerage fees and other acquisition costs are $25. The following entry records the acquisition of these bonds:

Temporary Bond Investment	$9,625.00	
Accrued Interest Receivable	66.67	
Cash		$9,691.67

To record the purchase of 10 Cable Co. $1,000 bonds.

The values in this transaction are computed as follows:

Purchase Price (10 $1,000 bonds @ 96)	$9,600.00
Brokerage Fee	25.00
Book Value	9,625.00
Accrued Interest ($10,000 × 1/12 × .08)	66.67
Cash Disbursement	9,691.67

Several aspects of this transaction are worthy of note. First, the book value of these bonds is $9,625, which is the sum of the purchase price ($9,600) and any acquisition costs such as brokerage fees ($25). Any accrued interest must be recorded as a separate item. Since these bonds were purchased between interest payment dates, the seller is paid the interest that has accrued since January 1. In this case, the institution must pay the seller one month of accrued interest ($66.67), which will be recovered on July 1 when the next semiannual interest payment is received. On the other hand, should the hospital decide to sell these bonds before the next interest payment date, the $66.67 interest receivable plus any additional accrued interest will be recovered from the next buyer. Interest accrued between payment dates is paid by the buyer of the bond since it is not possible for the issuer to make these adjustments.

It will be noted that the Cable Co. bonds are purchased at a discount as indicated by the quoted price of 96. To complete the discussion of bond acquisitions as a temporary investment, assume that another $7,000 becomes available for a short period and, on March 1, the facility purchases 6 $1,000 bonds of Horse Co. that pay 6 percent interest on October 1 and April 1. Suppose also that on March 1 these bonds are quoted at 102 and the brokerage fees are $30. The acquisition of the Horse Co. bonds is recorded as follows:

Temporary Bond Investments	$6,150	
Accrued Interest Receivable	150	
Cash		$6,300

To record the purchase of 6 Horse Co. $1,000 bonds.

The values in this transaction are computed as follows:

Purchase Price (6 $1,000 bonds @ 102)	$6,120
Brokerage Fees	30
Book Value	6,150
Accrued Interest ($6,000 × .06 × 5/12)	150
Total Cash Disbursements	6,300

As before, the book value of these bonds is $6,150—the sum of the purchase price ($6,120) and all brokerage fees ($30). The institution also pays the interest ($150) that has accrued since the last interest payment date of October 1. As a consequence, the total cash disbursement for this acquisition is $6,300 ($6,150 + $150).

It will be noted that the Cable Co. bonds are purchased at a price below par value, the Horse Co. bonds above par. When such investments are purchased for short periods, amortization of the premium or discount generally is not necessary and their book value is given by the original cost.

8.2.2 Recording Interest

At the end of each month, an entry is required to record the interest income earned by the investment. The entry at the end of February to record the interest income that accrued from the Cable Co. bonds during the month is:

Accrued Interest Receivable	$66.67	
Investment Income		$66.67

To record the accrued interest income on Cable Co. Bonds.

The interest earned is given by:

$$(\$10{,}000 \times .08 \times 1/12) = \$66.67$$

as in Section 8.2.1. Similar entries should be recorded until the next interest payment period or until the bond matures.

On July 1, which is the next interest payment date, the following entry records the receipt of the semiannual interest on the bonds:

Cash	$400	
Accrued Interest Receivable		$400

The amount of the cash receipt and the corresponding accrued interest is given by $10,000 × .08 × 6/12 or $400.

The procedure outlined above is used to record interest on these bonds so long as the institution holds them. In the balance sheet, the bonds are reported at their original cost and any change in current market value may be indicated by a parenthetic comment. It generally is not appropriate to adjust temporary investments to reflect current market value.

8.2.3 Disposition of Bonds Held as Short-Term Investments

Suppose that on December 1, management realizes that it has estimated cash flows incorrectly and needs additional funds, so it is necessary to sell the Cable Co. bonds, which have a current book value of $9,625. Further, assume that the price of the bonds at the time of the sale is quoted at 99½ and that the brokerage fees are $30. If interest has been accrued properly, the entry to record the sale is given by:

Cash	$10,253.34	
Accrued Interest Receivable		$333.34
Temporary Bond Investment		9,625.00
Gain on Sale		295.00

To record the sale of 10 Cable Co. $1,000 bonds.

The values recorded in this entry are calculated as follows:

Sale Price (10 $1,000 bonds @ 99½)	$9,950.00
Less Brokerage Fees	30.00
Net Sale Price	9,920.00
Accrued Interest Receivable ($10,000 × .08 × 5/12)	333.34
Cash Proceeds	10,253.34
Net Sale Price (from above)	9,920.00
Less Book Value	9,625.00
Gain on Sale	295.00

In this transaction, it is important to note that the net sale price is the sale price less brokerage fees. Cash proceeds are derived by adding the accrued interest receivable to the net sale price. The difference between the net sale price and the book value of the Cable Co. bonds is recorded as a gain on sale and is treated as a nonoperating revenue when preparing the financial statements at the end of the period. Finally, the credit entry to the Temporary Bond Investment account eliminates the investment in Cable Co. bonds from the books of the institution.

To illustrate the method by which losses on sale are recorded, suppose that on November 1 additional funds are required to satisfy demands for cash and the institution is forced to sell the Horse Co. bonds, which have a book value of $6,150. On the date of the sale suppose that the bonds are quoted at 99½ and that the broker's fees are $70. If the interest receivable on this bond has been accrued properly, the entry required to record the sale is:

Cash	$5,930	
Loss on Sale	250	
Accrued Interest Receivable		$30
Temporary Bond Investment		6,150

To record the sale of Horse Co. bonds.

The values recorded in this transaction are computed as follows:

Sale Price (6 $1,000 Bonds @ 99½)	$5,970
Less Broker's Fees	70
Net Sale Price	5,900
Accrued Interest Receivable ($6,000 × .06 × 1/12)	30
Cash Proceeds	5,930
Net Sale Price (from above)	5,900
Less Book Value	6,150
Loss on Sale	250

As in the case of the Cable Co. bonds, the net sale price is the difference between the sale price of $5,970 and the broker's fees of $70, while the cash receipt is the sum of the net sale price and the interest that has accrued since the last interest payment date of October 1. Finally, since the book value of these bonds is $6,150 and the net sale price is $5,900, a net loss on sale of $250 is recorded.

8.3 LONG-TERM INVESTMENTS

As implied above, short-term investments are those that are readily marketable and that management intends to hold for a short time that generally does not exceed one year. The proceeds from short-term or temporary investments frequently are used to meet current or operating needs of the institution. In preparing the balance sheet, those that do not meet these criteria are classified as long-term investments.

Long-term investments may appear in any fund but are found most frequently in the Specific Purpose Fund, the Endowment Fund, or the Capital Fund. Long-term investments typically consist of corporate stocks and bonds, debt issues of various levels of government, and real estate held for future use or resale at an appreciated value. These assets are held to satisfy a need to use endowment and other restricted funds productively for a long period. Sometimes gifts are received in the form of stocks, bonds, and other noncash assets. In addition, the institution may invest cash set aside by the board to fund depreciation; this may result in the acquisition of long-term investments that are recorded in the Unrestricted Fund.

When long-term securities and other noncash assets are donated to the institution, they are recorded in the appropriate fund at their fair market value. Management may have to obtain an independent appraisal of that value. When stocks or bonds are purchased, their cost includes the purchase price, brokerage fees, and any other expenditure associated with the acquisition.

The income from long-term investments may be in the form of interest, dividends, rentals, royalties, and other similar items. This revenue must be recorded in accordance with sound accounting practice in the appropriate fund. Gains and losses are entered in the fund in which the asset is carried. It might be argued, however, that gains and losses realized when securities are sold should follow investment income rather than the principal. If the income generated by the investment of restricted funds is not restricted by the donor, gains or losses in disposing of such instruments might be similarly regarded as unrestricted. Depending on the legality of this argument, gains from the disposal of investments for which the income is not donor restricted may be recorded in the Unrestricted Fund and used to satisfy the operating needs of the institution rather than being assigned to the principal.

8.3.1 Acquiring Bonds As a Long-Term Investment

As noted earlier, the acquisition of bonds can involve a premium or a discount. As will be recalled, a discount is encountered whenever a bond is acquired at a price less than its face value. A bond is sold at a discount whenever the market rate of interest exceeds the nominal rate of interest or the rate quoted on the bond issue. For example, suppose the hospital purchases 10 6 percent 10-year $1,000 bonds of Teague Co. at 94 on November 1. Further assume that the bonds pay interest semiannually on April 1 and October 1 and will mature three years after the date of purchase. If the acquisition costs are $60, the entry to record the acquisition is:

Investment—Teague Co. Bonds	$9,460	
Accrued Interest Receivable	50	
Cash		$9,510

To record the acquisition of Teague Co. bonds.

The values recorded in this entry are computed as follows:

Price of Bonds ($10,000 @ 94)	$9,400
Acquisition Costs	60
Costs of Bonds	9,460
Accrued Interest (.06 × $10,000 × 1/12)	50
Cash Disbursement	9,510

Since the price is less than the face value of the bonds, the institution earns an annual interest income of $600 (.06 × $10,000), which exceeds a 6 percent yield on the investment of $9,400 ($564). Thus, when the market rate of interest exceeds the nominal rate, bonds sell at a discount to compensate for the disparity between the two rates.

Conversely, when the nominal or stated rate of interest exceeds the market rate of interest, bonds sell at a premium or at a price above face value. For example, suppose the institution purchases 20 of the 9 percent 10-year $1,000 bonds of Oak Co. at 107 on April 1. Assume also that these bonds pay interest semiannually on April 1 and October 1 and will mature 40 months after the date of purchase. Assuming further that the acquisition costs are $600, the entry to record the purchase is:

Investment—Oak Co. Bonds	$22,000	
Cash		$22,000

To record the acquisition of Oak Co. bonds.

The values in this entry are obtained as follows:

Price of Bonds ($20,000 @ 107)	$21,400
Acquisition Cost	600
Cost of Bonds	22,000

Since $21,400 is paid for these bonds, the annual interest of $1,800 (.09 × $20,000) yields an effective rate that is less than 9 percent.

8.3.2 Recording Interest Income on Long-Term Bonds

When bonds are acquired at a premium or a discount and will be held as short-term or temporary investments, no attempt is made to amortize the difference between the par and book values. However, when they are held as long-term investments, amortization of premiums and discounts is required.

Consider first the Teague Co. bonds described above as purchased at a discount. At the end of each month, the institution should record the interest income earned as well as the amortization of the discount:

Accrued Interest Receivable	$50	
Investment—Teague Co. Bonds	15	
Interest Income		$65

To record interest income and amortization of bond discount.

The values in this entry are calculated as follows:

Nominal Interest (.06 × $10,000 × 1/12)	$50
Discount Amortization:	
Maturity Value of Bonds	10,000
Cost of Bonds	9,460
Difference	540
Divide by Months to Maturity (3 × 12)	36
Monthly Amortization of Discount	15
Nominal Interest (above)	50
Monthly Interest Income	65

The difference between the maturity value and the acquisition cost of the bond is regarded as interest income over the 36 months between the acquisition and maturity dates. The credit to interest income is roughly the equivalent of the effective amount of interest earned on this investment.

The $15 amortization also is added to the book value of the Teague Co. bonds. On the maturity date, the bonds will have a book value of $10,000 ($9,460 + 36 months × $15/month) which, of course, is their maturity value. If the bonds are held until maturity, the entry on that date will be:

Cash	$10,000	
Investment Teague Co. Bonds		$10,000

To record the receipt of the maturity value of Teague Co. bonds.

The book value of long-term investments in bonds thus is given by the acquisition costs plus the amortization of the discount to date.

Consider next the Oak Co. bonds discussed earlier as acquired at a premium rather than at a discount. Just as the discount is amortized, the premium paid on the Oak Co. bonds also must be amortized through a series of monthly interest accruals. As a part of that accrual, the $2,000 bond premium is amortized as indicated by the following entry:

Accrued Interest Receivable	$150	
Investment—Oak Co. Bonds		$50
Interest Income		100

To record interest and the amortization of bond premium.

The values in this entry are computed as follows:

Nominal Interest (.09 × $20,000 × 1/12)		$150
Amortization:		
Cost of Bonds	$22,000	
Maturity Value	20,000	
Premium	2,000	
Divided by Months to Maturity	40	
Monthly Amortization		50
Monthly Interest Income		100

The amortization of the premium is recorded as a reduction in income during the 40 months that the bonds are held by the institution. The $100 credit to interest income is roughly the equivalent of the effective monthly yield on the investment. In addition, the $50 amortization of the premium reduces the book value. If the bonds are held to maturity, the book value of the investment on the maturity date will be $20,000 ($22,000 − 40 months × $50/month).

The receipt of semiannual interest on these bonds is recorded as indicated earlier. In the case of the Teague Co. bonds, the entry to record the interest payment is:

Cash	$300	
Accrued Interest Receivable		$300

To record interest on Teague Co. bonds (.06 × $10,000 × 1/2).

In the case of the Oak Co. bonds, the entry to record the receipt of the interest payment is:

Cash	$900	
Accrued Interest Receivable		$900

To record receipt of interest ($20,000 × .09 × 1/2).

These procedures also are applicable to bonds that have been received as an unrestricted gift. In such cases, the bonds should be recorded at fair market value in the Unrestricted Fund. If the fair market value is less than the maturity value, the accounting procedures outlined for the Teague Co. bonds should be applied. If the fair market value exceeds the maturity value, the accounting procedures applied to the Oak Co. bonds are appropriate.

8.3.3 Disposal of Bonds Held as Long-Term Investments

The entries to record the disposition of bonds that have been held to maturity have been illustrated. Consider now the disposition of bonds held as long-term investments and sold before their maturity date. Suppose that 10 months after the date of purchase, the institution disposes of the Teague Co. bonds at 102 plus 5 months' accrued interest. Also assume that the disposal costs are $50. The entry to record such a sale is:

Cash	$10,400	
Accrued Interest Receivable		$250
Gain on Sale		540
Investment—Teague Co. Bonds		9,610

To record the sale of Teague Co. bonds.

The values in this transaction are obtained by the following calculations:

Sale Price ($10,000 @ 102)		$10,200
Less Disposal Costs		50
Net Sale Price		10,150
Accrued Interest Receivable ($10,000 × .06 × 5/12)		250
Cash Proceeds		10,400
Net Sale Price (above)		10,150
Less Book Value Acquisition Cost	$9,460	
Add Amortization (10 Months × $15)	150	
Book Value on Sale Date		9,610
Gain on Sale		540

As before, the accrued interest is collected from the purchaser of these bonds. In computing the gain, the book value of the bonds on the date of sale includes not only the acquisition cost of $9,460 but also the $15 monthly amortization of the discount that has been recorded for ten months. As seen in the entry, the difference between the net sale price and the book value of the bonds as of the sale date is recorded as a gain.

Consider next the Oak Co. bonds that were purchased at a premium. Suppose that management decides to sell these bonds 20 months after their acquisition when they are quoted at 98. Also assume that the disposal costs are $60 and that interest for two months has been accrued. The entry to record the sale is:

Cash	$19,840	
Loss on Sale	1,460	
Accrued Interest Receivable		$300
Investment—Oak Co. Bonds		21,000

To record the sale of Oak Co. bonds.

The values in this entry are calculated as follows:

Sale Price ($20,000 @ 98)	$19,600
Less Disposal Cost	60
Net Sale Price	19,540
Accrued Interest Receivable ($20,000 × .09 × 2/12)	300
Cash Proceeds	19,840
Book Value	
Acquisition Cost	22,000
Less Premium Amortization to Date ($50 × 20 Months)	1,000
Book Value of Bonds	21,000
Less Net Sale Price (above)	19,540
Loss on Sale	1,460

As before, the accrued interest and disposal costs are incorporated in the calculation of the cash proceeds. In determining the loss, the book value of the bonds as of the sale date include both the acquisition costs and the amortization of the premium for the 20 months that the institution held the certificates as a long-term investment.

8.3.4 Endowment Fund Bond Investments

In general, the procedures outlined in the preceding discussion also apply to the bond investments of the Specific Purpose Fund, the Endowment Fund, and the Capital Fund, if the institution uses such a category. With the possible exception of income from endowments, the revenue generated by the investment of restricted funds should not be recorded as income in the Unrestricted Fund until the conditions specified by the donor have been satisfied. In those cases, the completion of such activities as the provision of charity care, the acquisition of plant and equipment, or the completion of a research project usually warrant the transfer of revenue to the Unrestricted Fund. As a result, no particular difficulty arises in accounting for the bond investments that are made possible by these funds.

However, application of the rules described above to the investment income from endowments gives rise to several complications because, while these instruments are recorded in the Endowment Fund, the income from them may be entered in another fund. As a result, special attention must be given to this interfund relationship.

By way of illustration, suppose that on December 1 the institution purchases 50 $1,000 10-year bonds of Himpty Dimpty Co. that pay 6 percent interest semiannually on April 1 and October 1. Further, assume that the acquisition is related to an endowment and that the bonds are purchased @ 102 plus two months' accrued interest. The acquisition costs are $200 and the bonds are acquired 50 months before their maturity date. The entry to record the acquisition is:

Endowment Fund

Investment—Himpty Dimpty Co. Bonds	$51,200	
Accrued Interest Receivable	500	
Cash		$51,700

To record the acquisition of Himpty Dimpty Co. bonds.

Similar to the earlier example, the values in the entry are calculated as follows:

Sale Price ($50,000 × 1.02)	$51,000
Acquisition Costs	200
Cost of Bonds	51,200
Accrued Interest (2/12 × .06 × $50,000)	500
Cash Disbursement	51,700

Suppose further that the use of the investment income is not restricted by the donor. In that case, the income from the investment is recorded in the Unrestricted Fund. Finally, assume that any gain or loss from the disposal of the bonds must be recorded in the Endowment Fund. The subsequent entries pertaining to this bond are summarized below. The monthly amortization and interest accrual is recorded by the entry:

Endowment Fund

Accrued Interest Receivable	$250	
Investment—Himpty Dimpty Co. Bonds		$24
Due to Unrestricted Fund		226

To record monthly interest accrual and amortization premium.

The values in this entry are calculated as follows:

Accrued Interest (.06 × 1/12 × \$50,000)		\$250
Premium Amortization:		
Cost of Bonds	\$51,200	
Maturity Value	50,000	
Premium	1,200	
Divide by Months to Maturity	50	
Monthly Amortization	24	

Since the revenue earned from the investment is unrestricted, the interest income is recorded in the Unrestricted Fund as follows:

Unrestricted Fund

Due from Endowment Fund	\$226	
Interest Income		\$226

The receipt of the semiannual interest payment is recorded by

Endowment Fund

Cash	\$1,500	
Accrued Interest Receivable		\$1,500

The transfer of semiannual interest to the Unrestricted Fund is accomplished by

Endowment Fund

Due to Unrestricted Fund	\$1,356	
Cash		\$1,356

To record payment of six months' interest (6 months × \$226/month).

Unrestricted Fund

Cash	\$1,356	
Due from Endowment Fund		\$1,356

Now suppose that management decides to dispose of these bonds 12 months after the date of purchase. At the time of the sale, the bonds are quoted at

103 and, if the disposal costs are $100, the entries pertaining to the disposal of these bonds are summarized as:

Endowment Fund

Cash	$51,900	
Accrued Interest Receivable		$500
Gain on Sale		488
Investment—Himpty Dimpty Co. Bonds		50,912

To record the sale of Himpty Dimpty Co. Bonds.

The values recorded in this transaction are calculated as follows:

Sale Price ($50,000 × 1.03)		$51,500
Less Disposal Costs		100
Net Sale Price		51,400
Accrued Interest Receivable (.06 × 2/12 × $50,000)		500
Cash Proceeds		51,900
Net Sale Price (above)		51,400
Book Value of Bonds:		
Acquisition Costs	$51,200	
Less Amortized Premium (12 months × $24)	288	
Book Value as of Sale Date		50,912
Gain on Sale		488

The transfer of cash from the Endowment Fund to the Unrestricted Fund is accomplished by the following entries:

Endowment Fund

Due to Unrestricted Fund	$452	
Cash		$452

To record the transfer of interest payment of previous two months to the Unrestricted Fund.

Unrestricted Fund

Cash	$452	
Due from Endowment Fund		$452

To record receipt of interest payment from the Endowment Fund.

If the hospital has a Capital Fund, and if the investment income is limited to the acquisition of plant and equipment, a similar set of entries is recorded. In this case, however, the transfers involve the Capital Fund rather than the Endowment Fund as assumed above.

8.4 STOCKS

When a person or institution invests in a corporation, a stock certificate is received as evidence of the shares purchased. An owner of stock may transfer part or all of the shares represented on the certificate. To do so, the holder simply completes the endorsement on the reverse side of the share and forwards it to a transfer agent, who cancels the old certificate and issues a new one that indicates the new ownership.

The earnings from stock holdings usually assume the form of dividend payments. A dividend, which is a distribution made by a corporation to stockholders, is declared by the board of directors, which generally is the final judge as to when a disbursement is to be made. Cash dividends are the most common and usually are stated in terms of a given number of dollars or cents per share. Dividends also may assume the form of other assets as well as the stock or stock rights of the corporation.

Since a corporation's stockholders usually change over time, dividends are paid to shareholders of record as of a specific date. In declaring a dividend, three dates are of significance. For example, on September 1 a board of directors may declare that dividends will be paid on October 7 to stockholders of record as of October 1. In this instance, September 1 is the date of declaration and October 1 the date of record. By specifying a date of record, new purchasers are given an opportunity to have ownership recorded in time to receive the dividend payment. Finally, October 7 is called the date of payment and represents the day on which dividends will be distributed.

Stockholders have no right to receive dividends until they are declared. Once declared, however, a cash dividend becomes a current liability of the corporation and must be paid. Furthermore, the stockholders have a right to sue and force the payment of a cash dividend once it has been declared.

In addition to the right to receive declared dividends, shareholders have other rights that depend on the type of stock they possess. If a company issues only one kind of share, it is known as common stock. When a person or institution acquires such stock, the shareholder has the right to:

1. vote at stockholders' meetings
2. sell or otherwise dispose of the stock
3. share pro rata with other common stockholders in any dividends declared
4. share in any assets remaining after creditors are paid if the corporation is liquidated

A corporation may issue more than one kind of stock. After common, the second prevalent type is called preferred stock. An owner of preferred stock is given preference in the payment of dividends. However, this preference does not give an absolute right to receive dividends but, if they are declared, preferred stock gives its owner the right to be paid before any disbursements to common stockholders.

Preferred stock dividends usually are limited to a fixed maximum amount that is stated as a percentage of par value (the dollar value originally assigned to a share). For example, a share of $100 par value 8 percent nonparticipating preferred stock would pay 8 percent of $100, or $8. In this example, the payout is limited to a fixed amount but dividends on common stock are constrained only by the earning power of the corporation and the judgment of the board of directors.

Some stocks have the right, under certain circumstances, to dividends in excess of the fixed percentage or amount. These are called participating preferred stocks. They may be either fully participating or partially participating—that is, participation may be limited to a predetermined amount.

For example, assume a company issues 6 percent $100 par value preferred stock that is fully participating. The owner of this stock has a right to 6 percent of $100 ($6 per share) in the years in which dividends are declared. Suppose the company issues $30 par value common stock. Each year, after the common stockholders have been paid a dividend of 6 percent ($1.80 per share), the preferred stockholders have a right to participate with common shareholders in any additional dividends declared by the board of directors. The participation usually is based on a percent of par value of each kind of stock. For example, if the common stockholders are paid an additional 7 percent of the $30 par value ($2.10 per share), the owners of fully participating preferred stock also will receive a dividend of $2.10 per share.

Preferred stockholders' participation in additional dividends may be limited. For example, a $100 par value 4 percent preferred stock may be issued with the right to participate in additional dividends up to 12 percent of its par value. Such a stock has the right to a dividend of $4 per share. In addition, after common stockholders receive a 4 percent dividend, owners of the preferred have the right to participate in additional dividends until 12 percent ($12 per share) has been received. The participation rights end at this point.

8.4.1 The Acquisition of Stock

Stock prices are quoted on the basis of dollars and one-eighth dollars per share. For example, a stock quoted at 73½ sells for $73.50 per share, and one quoted at 22⅛ for $22.125 per share. Similar to the accounting techniques used to enter bond acquisitions, the purchase of stocks is recorded at total cost that includes the quoted price and any brokerage fees. Unlike bonds, however, interest does not accrue on stocks, so accrued interest does not enter into the calculation of the cash disbursement associated with a stock acquisition.

For illustration, assume that a hospital decides to purchase 100 shares of Blitz Co. common stock as an investment at 26½ plus brokerage fees of $100. The entry to record the purchase is:

Blitz Co. Stock	$2,750	
Cash		$2,750

To record 100 shares of Blitz Co. common stock.

The book value of the stock and the related cash disbursement are calculated as follows:

100 Shares @ 26½	$2,650
Plus Broker's Fees	100
Book Value	2,750

When stock is acquired, it usually is not necessary to consider discounts or premiums. These are relevant only when stocks are issued originally and do not apply to transactions between investors.

8.4.2 Recording Dividend Income

Returning to the Blitz Co. stock, assume that on January 17 the board of directors declares a dividend of $0.50 per share payable on March 4 to stockholders of record as of March 1. If the dividends are unrestricted and are available for general use, the hospital records the following entry on the declaration date:

Dividend Receivable	$50	
Dividend Income		$50

When the dividend is paid and cash is received, the following entry records the cash receipt and eliminates the accrued dividend:

Cash	$50	
Dividend Receivable		$50

Although this treatment is theoretically superior, the entry for January 17 often is not recorded. Cash dividends usually are recorded when received and, as long as the end of the reporting period does not fall between the date of declaration and the date of payment, the practice is satisfactory.

8.4.3 Disposal of Stock

Investments in stock may be sold in response to a need for cash or to take advantage of temporary changes in their prices. When an investment in stock is sold, a gain or loss is recognized. When the amount received is greater than the original cost plus the commission on sale and other expenses, a gain is recognized. For example, assume that the hospital decides to sell the Blitz Co. stock, which has a book value of $2,750, at 42½ plus broker's fees and other costs of $20. The entry to record the sale is:

Cash	$4,230	
Blitz Co. Stock		$2,750
Gain on Sale		1,480

The values in this transaction are computed as follows:

Sale Price: 100 shares @ 42½	$4,250
Less Broker's Fees	20
Cash Proceeds	4,230
Less Book Value	2,750
Gain on Sale	1,480

The cash proceeds and the net sale price are equal to the difference between the sale price and broker's fees. In this case, the difference between the cash proceeds of $4,230 and the $2,750 book value of the stocks results in a gain of $1,480.

When stocks are sold at a price less than their book value plus sale costs, a loss in incurred. If the Blitz Co. stock in the previous example is sold at 17½ less disposal costs of $50, the transaction is recorded as:

Cash	$1,700	
Loss on Sale	1,050	
Blitz Co. Stock		$2,750

The values in this transaction are computed as follows:

Sale Price: 100 Shares @ 17½	$1,750
Less Broker's Fees	50
Cash Proceeds	1,700
Less Book Value	2,750
Loss on Sale	1,050

The gain or loss from the sale of a security carried in the Unrestricted Fund is reported as a nonoperating revenue in the income statement.

8.4.4 Additional Topics

Unless otherwise specified, assume that investment transactions in the following discussion pertain to the Unrestricted Fund. The primary purpose of the analysis is to consider the accounting procedures used when stocks are split and when stock dividends are declared by the issuing corporation.

8.4.4.1 Stock Splits

Assume the institution decides to purchase 100 shares of Funk Co. common stock for $7,000, which includes all acquisition costs, with money from the Unrestricted Fund. In accordance with the earlier discussion, the entry in the Unrestricted Fund is:

Investments—Funk Co. Stock	$7,000	
Cash		$7,000

A similar entry is recorded in any other fund. If the 100 shares of stock has been received as an endowment, however, the entry will involve a Restricted Gifts and Bequest account of the Endowment Fund and similar entry is required to record the receipt of any donor restricted gift. If these shares are received with no donor restrictions, the fair market value of the stock is recorded as a credit to an appropriate income account of the Unrestricted Fund.

A corporation also may split its stock in an effort to reduce the price per share and thereby make it more attractive to investors. For example, assume that Funk Co. subsequently splits its shares on a two-for-one basis at a time when the stock is quoted at $90. The institution then will own 200 shares (2 × 100) and the adjusted cost per share becomes $35 ($7,000/200 shares). The split will tend to reduce the market value of the stock since Funk Co. now has twice as many shares outstanding. It should be noted, however, that no revenue should be recognized at the time of the split. The only effect is to increase the number of shares held by the institution and to reduce the cost per share, even though the market value may be greater than before the split.

The adjusted cost per share is used in determining the cost of any portion of the stock that management may subsequently decide to sell. For example, suppose that the hospital sells 50 shares of the Funk Co. stock at 75. Also assume the acquisition costs are $40. The entry to record such a sale is:

Cash	$3,710	
Investment—Funk Co. Stock		$1,750
Gain on Sale		1,960

To record the sale of Funk Co. stock.

The values in this entry are computed as follows:

Sale Price (50 shares @ $75)	$3,750
Less Acquisition Costs	40

Net Proceeds	3,710
Less Cost of Stock (50 shares @ $35)	1,750
Gain on Sale	1,960

In computing the gain on sale, the cost of the stock given in exchange is valued at $35 (the adjusted cost per share) rather than $70 per share ($70,000/100 shares) that would have been the price in the absence of the split. In addition, the acquisition and disposal of shares as well as any splits or stock dividends are recorded in a subsidiary record. From the set of subsidiary records it should be clear that 150 (200 − 50) shares of Funk Co. common stock remain in the hospital's portfolio at a cost of $5,250 (150 shares × $35/share).

8.4.4.2 Stock Dividends

In addition to paying cash dividends, corporations frequently distribute stock dividends, which means that holders are given additional shares without charge. Assume, for example, that on May 1 the institution decides to use resources of the Endowment Fund to purchase 1,000 shares of H & K Co. common stock for $60,000, which includes all acquisition costs. The entry to record the acquisition is:

Endowment Fund

Investment—H & K Co. Stock	$60,000	
Cash		$60,000

Suppose that on June 1, the H & K Co. board of directors declares that stockholders of record on July 7 will receive a 25 percent common stock dividend payable on July 27. As a result, the institution will receive 250 (25% × 1,000) shares of the common stock. When the shares are received, an appropriate notation is made in the subsidiary record of investments.

However, no formal entry is required since stock dividends, as in the case of stock splits, do not give rise to income. These dividends and splits only increase the number of shares outstanding without any change in the assets of the issuing corporation. As a result, each shareholder has the same percent ownership in the resources of the corporation as before the stock split or dividend. In addition, revenue arises only from the sale of goods or services and no sale transaction is involved in a stock split or dividend. In this example, the effect of the stock dividend is to reduce the cost of the H & K common stock from $60 ($60,000/1,000 shares) to $48 ($60,000/1,250 shares) per share. When these shares are sold later, the adjusted cost per share of $48 is used as the basis for determining a loss or gain.

For example, assume that on August 27, management decides to sell 100 shares of the H & K stock. If the stock is quoted at $50 per share and the disposal costs are $40, the entry in the Endowment Fund is:

Cash	$4,960	
Investment—H & K Co. Stock		$4,800
Gain on Sale		160

To record the sale of H & K Co. stock.

The values in this entry are computed as follows:

Sale Price (100 shares × $50/share)	$5,000
Less Disposal Costs	40
Net Proceeds	4,960
Less Cost of Stock (100 shares @ $48/share)	4,800
Gain on Sale	160

Assuming that the income on this investment is not subject to donor restrictions and that the institution records this receipt as well as any gains or losses from the sale of such instruments in the Unrestricted Fund, the entries to record this sale are:

Endowment Fund

Cash	$4,960	
Investment—H & K Stock		$4,800
Due to Unrestricted Fund		160
Due to Unrestricted Fund	160	
Cash		160

Unrestricted Fund

Cash	$160	
Gain on Sale		$160

These entries (1) record the sale of the stock in the Endowment Fund where its acquisition was listed originally and (2) transfer the gain on sale to the Unrestricted Fund.

8.5 INVESTMENT POOLS

Many health care facilities have excess cash in both restricted and unrestricted funds that could be invested in revenue-generating instruments. This cash could, of course, be invested separately and individual records maintained to reflect the role of each fund. However, the cash in each fund, when considered separately, may be regarded as too little to warrant investment. On the other hand, if the excess cash in each fund is accumulated into a single fund, it may be large enough to invest profitably.

When investments are made by individual funds, a number of other important problems emerge:

1. The influence of good or poor investment decisions is likely to be concentrated in a single fund.
2. A large amount of cash may go uninvested.
3. A considerable amount of bookkeeping is required to maintain records on the investments of several funds.

These problems are overcome by accumulating these funds in a single investment pool through which the facility can spread the risk of both good and bad holdings among the participating funds. Thus, extremely good investments in one fund may be shared by all, and pooling provides greater assurance that the integrity of each fund will be maintained. Such a pooling also (1) provides for a greater diversification of investments, (2) produces a stable income for all funds, (3) eliminates the problem of investing small amounts of cash, and (4) eliminates excessive bookkeeping for each of the participating funds.

8.5.1 Creation of the Pool

Suppose the hospital creates an investment pool on January 1, 198A. Suppose also that the Unrestricted Fund (U.F.) contributes $100,000 in cash while Endowment Fund (E.F.) puts in securities that cost $400,000 but have a current market value of $600,000. A self-balancing set of accounts is established for the investment pool and the following entries are recorded:

Unrestricted Fund

Investment Pool Shares	$100,000	
Cash		$100,000

To record the purchase of 1,000 shares of $100 par value in investment pool.

Endowment Fund

Investment Pool Shares	$400,000	
Investments		$400,000

To record contribution of securities that cost $400,000 (current market value of $600,000) to investment pool in exchange for 6,000 shares at $100 par value.

Investment Pool

Cash	$100,000	
Investment	400,000	
U.F. Equity		$100,000
E.F. Equity		400,000

To record receipt of assets contributed by the Unrestricted Fund and the Endowment Fund and the issuance of shares at $100 par value as follows:

U.F. ($100,000/$100)	1,000
E.F. ($600,000/$100)	6,000
Total shares issued	7,000

It should be noted that the assets contributed to the investment fund are recorded at *cost* and that each of the participating funds enters the pool shares on the same basis. However, the investment pool distributes shares in accordance with the *fair market value* of the contributed assets. In addition, any subsequent purchases and redemptions are based on fair market values. On the other hand, fair market values are not recorded in the accounts; instead, the books are maintained on a cost basis. This is because no formal accounting recognition may be given to unrealized gains or losses except for declines in valuc that are likely to impair an investment permanently.

8.5.2 Operation of the Pool

During the first quarter of 198A, the investment pool engages in several investment transactions, the results of which are summarized by the following entries:

Investment Pool

Cash	$14,000	
Investment Income		$14,000

To record net investment income (i.e., gross investment income less expenses).

Cash	$370,000	
Investments		$300,000
Gain on Sale		70,000

To record net gain on sales of period.

Investments	$400,000	
Cash		$400,000

To record purchase of additional investments.

As a result, at the end of the period the pool has $84,000 in cash and investments recorded at a cost of $500,000. Assume that the investments have a current market value of $770,000.

8.5.3 Distribution of Gains, Losses, and Income

The net income as well as the net gain (or loss) for the first quarter of operation must now be allocated to the pool participants. The distribution is determined this way:

	Number of Shares	Market Value	Allocation Income	Net Gain	Total
Unrestricted Fund	1,000	$110,000	$2,000	$10,000	$12,000
Endowment Fund	6,000	660,000	12,000	60,000	72,000
	7,000	770,000	14,000	70,000	84,000
Per Share		110	2	10	12

The nature of the entries required in the investment pool and in each of the participating funds is:

Investment Pool

Allocations to U.F. and E.F.	$84,000	
Cash		$84,000

To record the transfer of investment income and gain as follows:

U.F.	$12,000
E.F.	72,000
	84,000

Unrestricted Fund

Cash	$12,000	
Investment Income from Pool		$2,000
Gain on Sale of Pool Investments		10,000

Endowment Fund

Cash	$72,000	
Investment Income from Pool		$12,000
Gain on Sale of Pool Investment		60,000

Under certain circumstances, it may be appropriate for the entire income earned by the pool to be recorded as income of the Unrestricted Fund. Conditions that must be satisfied are: (1) the investment income is not restricted by the donor and (2) gains on sale are recorded in the same fund in which the unrestricted income is entered.

8.5.4 Additional Fund Contributions and Withdrawals

The participants in an investment pool can increase its holdings by purchasing additional stock or redeem shares by withdrawing all or a portion of the investment. The purchase of additional stock or the redemption of shares usually is permitted only at the end of specified periods. When a fund increases or reduces its participation in the pool, the shares involved are valued at the current par. If withdrawals are permitted at any time, the shares may be valued at the price as determined at the end of the next accounting period.

In the following discussion, it is assumed that additional investments or withdrawals are permitted only at the end of the period. Suppose that at the end of the first accounting period the Unrestricted Fund increases its participation in the pool by purchasing an additional 2,000 shares and the Endowment Fund reduces its participation by redeeming 500 shares. These transactions are recorded at the current market value of $110 per pool share as computed above. The entries are summarized as follows:

Unrestricted Fund

Investment Pool Shares	$220,000	
Cash		$220,000

To record the purchase of an additional 2,000 shares @ $110/share.

Endowment Fund

Cash	$55,000	
Investment Pool Shares		$50,000
Gain on Redemption		5,000

To record the redemption of 500 shares.

The values in the entry to the Endowment Fund are calculated as follows:

Redemption Proceeds (500 × $110)	$55,000
Cost of Shares (500 × $100)	50,000
Gain on Redemption	5,000

The increased participation of the Unrestricted Fund is recorded in the investment pool as follows:

Investment Pool

Cash	$220,000	
Unrestricted Fund Equity		$220,000

To record the issuance of 2,000 additional shares to the Unrestricted Fund @ $110/share.

Similarly, the reduced participation of the Endowment Fund in the investment pool is recorded by the following entry:

Equity—Endowment Fund	$50,000	
Premium on Redemption of Shares	5,000	
Cash		$55,000

To record the redemption of 2,000 shares by the Endowment Fund.

After these transactions, the Endowment Fund has 5,500 shares, the Unrestricted Fund 3,000. If these shares are redeemed later, the value is entered on an average cost basis.

The Premium on Redemption of Shares account in the investment pool is not closed at the end of the fiscal year. Rather, it is a permanent account in which gains from the redemption of shares are accumulated. It also is used to preserve the self-balancing nature of the pool accounts. The redemption of shares by the Unrestricted Fund is recorded as a regular sale of stock that has been held as an investment. When the hospital's financial statements are prepared, gains from the redemption of pool shares are treated as if they are profits from the sale of investments to entities external to the institution.

Questions for Discussion

1. Define a bond. Discuss the various methods of classifying bonds.
2. Describe the types of stock available to the health facility and the advantages and disadvantages of each.
3. Define a bond premium, a bond discount. Discuss when a bond premium or bond discount should be amortized. Describe the objective of the amortization process.
4. Define a stock split, a stock dividend. Explain when each should be recognized by a formal accounting entry.
5. Identify what entry is required when a stock dividend is declared.
6. Define the following terms:

   a. declaration date
   b. date of record
   c. payment date

7. Describe an investment pool and its primary advantages.
8. Identify what rights are conferred on common stockholders, on preferred stockholders.

Problems for Solution

1. Suppose that on March 1 the institution decides to purchase 10 $1,000 bonds of Silver Co. These pay annual interest of 8 percent on January

1 and July 1. When the bonds are bought, the price is quoted at 102. Assuming the acquisition costs are $15 and that the bonds are a temporary investment, record their acquisition.

2. Suppose that on April 1 the hospital buys 5 $1,000 Gold Co. bonds that pay 10 percent annual interest on January 1 and July 1. At the time of purchase, the price is quoted at 103 and the acquisition costs are $25. On September 1 the bonds are sold at 97, with brokerage fees of $15. Record all transactions concerning these bonds.
3. Suppose that the Gold Co. bonds referred to in Problem 2 are quoted at 109 when sold on September 1. Record the disposition of these bonds.
4. Suppose the hospital purchases 100 shares of Brass Co. as an investment at 37½ with brokerage fees of $75. On January 6 the board of directors declares a dividend of $.75 per share payable on March 28 to stockholders of record as of February 28. Assume the investment income is unrestricted. On April 5, the institution sells the stock at 42, with brokerage fees of $10. Record all transactions concerning this stock.
5. Suppose the facility buys 200 shares of Iron Co. stock at 97⅛, with brokerage fees of $20. On January 1, the board of directors declares a 25 percent stock dividend payable on March 9 to holders of record of February 2. On May 2, the stock is sold at 65½, with brokerage fees of $15. Record all transactions concerning this stock.
6. Suppose the institution purchases 1,000 shares of Copper Co. for $85,000. On July 1, Copper Co. splits its stock on a two-for-one basis. On August 28, 500 shares are sold at 21¼, with brokerage fees of $50. Record all transactions concerning this stock.
7. Suppose that on June 1, 60 months prior to maturity, the institution purchases 10 of the 10 percent $1,000 bonds of Metal Co. as a long-term investment. Suppose further that the bonds are quoted at 107 and the costs of acquisition are $100. The bonds pay interest on April 1 and October 1. Record the acquisition of these bonds and the first two interest payments.
8. Suppose the bonds in Problem 7 are sold 40 months prior to maturity at 112 and that the costs of disposal are $60. Record the disposal of these bonds.
9. Suppose that on July 1, which is 100 months prior to maturity, 100 of the 14 percent $1,000 bonds of Mint Co. are bought as a long-term investment. These bonds pay interest on April 1 and October 1. At the time of acquisition, they are quoted at 95 and the broker's fees are $50. Record the acquisition of these bonds and the first two interest payments.

10. Suppose the institution sells the bonds of Mint. Co. in Problem 9 60 months prior to maturity at 90. If the broker's fees are $75, record the disposition of these bonds.
11. Suppose the institution creates an investment pool on January 1, 198A. Fund A contributes $200,000 in cash and Fund B contributes securities that cost $300,000 but have a market value of $800,000. If the pool shares are issued at a par value of $100, show the entries required to create the pool.
12. Suppose the activity of the pool in Problem 11 during the first quarter may be summarized as follows:

    a. investment income is $500
    b. investments totaling $40,000 are sold and a gain of $60,000 is realized
    c. additional investments of $210,000 are acquired

    If the pool investments have a fair market value of $1,070,000, show the entries to record these transactions as well as the distribution of pool income to the participating funds.
13. Suppose that, in Problems 11 and 12, at the end of the first quarter

    a. Fund A purchases an additional 100 shares
    b. Fund B redeems 50 shares

    Record the contribution of Fund A and the withdrawal of Fund B.
14. Suppose that on March 1, the hospital buys 10 Zinc Co. 12 percent, $1,000 bonds that pay interest on January 1 and July 1. At the time of acquisition the bonds are quoted at 95 and the brokerage fees are $40. On October 1, the bonds are sold at 106 with disposal costs of $35. Record the acquisition and disposal of the bonds as well as a representative entry at the end of the month and the first interest payment.
15. Suppose the facility purchases 500 shares of Blits Co. common stock at 52½. Assume further that the acquisition costs are $30. On January 1, the board declares a dividend of $1.50 per share payable on March 1 to stockholders of record February 1. On April 1, the stock is sold at 37½ and the brokerage fees are $40. Record all transactions concerning the stock.
16. Suppose the institution purchases 500 shares of Y Co. stock at 42½ and the broker's fees are $200. Also suppose that a dividend of $350 is declared and subsequently paid by Y Co. In addition, a subsequent dividend of 100 shares is received. Later, 200 shares are sold at 48¾,

with broker's fees of $170. Record all transactions concerning this stock.

17. Suppose that on April 1, the facility purchases, as a temporary investment, 10 $1,000, J Co., 6 percent 20-year bonds that pay interest on November 1 and May 1. The purchase price is 97½ and the commission $25. On December 1, the bonds are sold at 103 and the commission is $30. Record all transactions concerning this bond.
18. Suppose that the hospital buys, as a long-term investment, 10 F Co., $1,000, 8 percent bonds on the interest date five years before maturity. The purchase price is 98 and the commission fees are $30. On September 1, the annual interest on these bonds is received. Record these transactions in general journal form. Assume that two years after the purchase date, the bonds are sold at 102 and the commission is $40. Record the disposition of these bonds in general journal form.

Chapter 9

Accounting for Inventories and Prepaid Expenses

A considerable proportion of the resources appearing in the balance sheet of an unrestricted fund are reported as current assets; the majority of them are called quick assets. The so-called quick asset category includes cash, marketable securities, and accounts receivable. The accounting procedures pertaining to cash and the other assets that can be converted quickly to cash have been discussed in previous chapters. This chapter is devoted to the accounting procedures for inventories and prepaid expenses—the last of the current assets to be discussed. Since inventories usually are limited to the unrestricted fund grouping, the importance of supplies when viewed from a managerial perspective is considered first; then the techniques used in accounting for stock are considered.

9.1 THE IMPORTANCE OF INVENTORIES

The stochastic nature of the need for medical care and the resulting variability in the derived demand for supplies used in producing those services requires the health care facility to maintain adequate stocks of goods and consumable items. If the institution has too few supplies, the result may be pain, suffering, and even death. On the other hand, when too much inventory is maintained, cash is invested needlessly in inventories and the institution incurs opportunity costs in the form of foregone interest income. Thus, if inventories are to be maintained at a level consistent with the provision of required services while minimizing opportunity costs, a high order of inventory accounting is required.

Even though the inventory holdings at any moment in time may not be substantial in relation to other assets, it should be recognized that as much as 15 to 20 percent of overall hospital costs is attributable to supply expense. Only a fraction of the annual supply expense may be represented by inventories on hand at any given time, but the annual usage of articles from inventory results in substantial costs to the health facility.

Inventories thus are acquired, issued, and used continually in the normal course of day-to-day activity. Whenever an account is highly active, the possibility of error is magnified; these errors will have a direct impact on revenues and expenses. For example, if inventories are understated by $20,000, expenses will be overstated by $20,000, resulting in an understatement of net revenue in the same amount. The obverse is equally true. In either case, a misstatement of current assets occurs in the balance sheet.

Similar to cash and marketable securities, inventories are susceptible to theft and misappropriation. It is important to note that losses from theft and waste can be substantial. This means that every health care facility must have appropriate accounting procedures and internal control systems if it is to avoid these hazards.

These considerations suggest that, if management is to maintain a proper level of inventory and minimize the opportunity costs as well as the theft or waste losses, the accounting techniques must provide accurate information on inventory levels and the use of consumable supplies. Indeed, accurate accounting is essential to efficient inventory management.

What precisely is meant by inventory? The term may be defined as the total of the items of tangible property that are (1) held for sale in the course of ordinary business operations; (2) are in the process of production for sale; and/or (3) are to be consumed in the production of goods and services that will be made available for sale in an economic transaction.

The inventories of most health care facilities consist of a wide range of consumable items such as drugs and pharmaceuticals, food, trays, surgical packs, housekeeping supplies, blood, oxygen, sutures, and radiological film. Many of these items have extremely high unit prices while others have relatively low unit costs but may have high value from the perspective of their lifesaving properties. An obvious example of such an inventory item is blood, which is acquired at a relatively low unit cost but may be of critical importance in preventing pain, suffering, and death. Some of the inventory items are used continuously, others far less frequently. These considerations suggest the advisability of using different types of accounting practices for the various kinds of inventory items.

From a theoretical perspective, the cost of an inventory item should include all direct and indirect expenses incurred in acquiring, preparing, and placing it in use. From a practical perspective, however, it usually is not possible to allocate the costs of purchasing, handling, and storing to specific inventory items. In practice, then, theory is tempered by practical considerations and the cost of inventory acquisitions is represented by the sum of the list price and relevant freight charges less any discounts offered by vendors.

9.2 PERIODIC AND PERPETUAL INVENTORY SYSTEMS

A periodic inventory system is appropriate for some suppliers while the perpetual inventory system should be or, as in the case of drugs, must be used when accounting for other items. As a result, most health care facilities should and will employ the two basic inventory accounting systems concurrently. Supply items that should be accounted for on a perpetual or periodic inventory system should be stratified in accordance with unit prices, annual dollar usage, special storage requirements, the extent to which they are critical to the lifesaving function, and the extent to which they are subject to misappropriation.

Frequently, the ABC method of inventory stratification is used. The objective of this approach is to vary the extent to which inventories are controlled in accordance with potential savings or relative importance. When the ABC system of classification is employed, inventory items are grouped into three categories, A, B, and C, according to their relative importance. Items included in the A category require the use of precise control techniques while those in the C category need only general control methods. Finally, items contained in the B category should be subjected to procedures more stringent than general control techniques but less stringent than the most precise methods. A perpetual inventory system should be maintained for items that

1. have a high annual dollar usage, or
2. require special storage, or
3. are critical to lifesaving activities, or
4. are subject to misappropriation.

It should be noted, however, that the perpetual inventory system is expensive to maintain and should be used only for items requiring special attention.

To illustrate the perpetual and periodic inventory systems, suppose the following information is available for a given supply item:

April 1	Beginning Inventory	100 units @ $7/unit
April 15	Purchase	50 units @ $7/unit
April 25	Usage	80 units

On the basis of these assumptions, April begins with an inventory of $700. However, several questions arise. For example, what entry records the purchase on April 15, which one the usage of 80 items on April 25, and how is the value of the April 30 inventory determined? This last point is complicated if the items purchased on April 15 had been acquired at a price other than $7, but this is discussed later in the chapter.

9.2.1 The Periodic Inventory System

Under the periodic inventory system, no day to day entry is recorded when supplies are issued or used in providing service. As noted earlier, the acquisition of supplies may be charged to an inventory asset account or directly to a supply expense account. If it is assumed that the supplies purchased on April 15 are obtained on credit and that no cash discounts are available, the entry

Inventory	$350	
Accounts Payable		$350

records the supply acquisition. If the functional unit that will use the supplies is known at the time of the acquisition, the cost may be entered directly in the supply expense account of that unit. Otherwise, the debit entry should be recorded to an inventory asset account.

On April 25, no entry is made to record the issuance and usage of these items by the unit that requested them. Rather, periodic physical counts must be taken to ascertain the number of units remaining in inventory at the end of the period. Returning to the example, 150 units of the supply item (a beginning inventory of 100 units plus the acquisition of 50 units on April 15) are available for use during the period. In the absence of error or misappropriation, the physical inventory at the end of the period reveals that 70 units (the 150 units available less the issuance of 80 units on April 25) remain in inventory on April 30. Unit costs or prices are then assigned to the units still in inventory and to the units that were used during the period. This procedure constitutes the basis for adjusting the accounts as well as accurately reporting supply expenses and the ending inventory of the period.

If the April 15 purchase is recorded in an inventory asset account, the general ledger accounts discussed earlier will reflect the following balances as of April 30:

Inventory		*Supply Expense*	
Beginning Inventory $700 Purchase $350			

As noted above however, the physical count of supplies indicates that 70 units valued at $490 (70 units × $7/unit) remain unused at the end of the period. As a result, the following entry is required to reflect the supply expenses of the period and the ending inventory:

Supply Expense	$560	
Inventory		$560

This entry gives formal accounting recognition to the $560 supply expense for the period (80 units @ $7/unit) and reduces the inventory account in the general ledger from the preadjusted value of $1,050 to the correct ending inventory of $490 (70 units @ $7/unit):

Inventory		*Supply Expense*	
Beginning Inventory $700 Purchases $350	Adjustment $560	$560	

Without such an adjustment, the supply expense of the period will be understated and the ending inventory overstated. These misstatements also will result in an inaccurate fund balance.

Conversely, suppose that the department that required the supplies is known at the time of the acquisition and that on April 15 the purchase is recorded directly in an appropriate supply expense account. In this case the general ledger accounts will show the following balances as of April 30:

Inventory		*Supply Expense*	
$700		$350	

As before, a physical inventory at the end of the period should show that 70 units valued at $490 remain in inventory on April 30. Thus, the adjusting entry

Supply Expense	$210	
Inventory		$210

serves to increase supply expenses from $350 to $560 (which, of course, is the correct cost of the supplies used during the period) and to reduce the value of the inventory account from $700 to $490 (which is the correct value of the ending inventory). The effects of the adjusting entry on the general ledger accounts are:

Inventory		*Supply Expense*	
$700	$210	$350 $210	

In addition to its relative simplicity, the periodic inventory system is clerically inexpensive. On the other hand, because frequent counts of inventory items are impractical, the accounts will be distorted somewhat until a physical inventory is taken and the adjusting entry illustrated earlier is recorded in the books. These misstatements are not particularly important when interim reports are prepared and evaluated. However, to prepare annual financial statements, a physical inventory and appropriate adjusting entries are required if supply expenses and the ending inventory are to be reported accurately in the income statement and balance sheet, respectively.

The major disadvantage of the periodic inventory system is that it does not provide an adequate basis for the control of consumable supplies. As seen earlier, this system indicates the actual inventory only after a physical count. This implies that the system is incapable of indicating what the inventory *should* be at any given time and, as a result, significant shortages may go undetected by management. Germane to the latter observation is the notion that the periodic inventory system tends to magnify the problem of determining the point at which inventory should be reordered to avoid the depletion of stocks below acceptable levels.

9.2.2 Perpetual Inventory System

Under the perpetual accounting system, continuous records are maintained to reflect the quantity and value of supplies purchased, used, and available *at any moment in time.* The acquisition of supplies that are maintained in the perpetual inventory system must be debited to an inventory asset account. Referring to the earlier example, the entry to record the April 15 purchase under the perpetual inventory system is:

Inventory	$350	
Accounts Payable		$350

On the date the inventory is acquired, an entry also is made in subsidiary inventory records to reflect the purchase and to raise the inventory balance to 150 units.

As the supplies are issued from the stores section and used in the various units of the institution, journal entries are recorded to reduce the inventory asset account and to charge the appropriate supply expense accounts. Again referring to the example, the entry

Supply Expense	$560	
Inventory		$560

appropriately reduces inventory and increases supply expense in the amount of the April 25 usage. When the items are issued from the stores section, an additional entry is made in the subsidiary inventory records to reflect the 80 units issued and to lower the inventory balance to 70 units. The subsidiary records may be maintained in terms of quantities only or in terms of both quantities and costs. At least once a year, a physical inventory must be taken and perpetual inventory records adjusted, if necessary, to reflect the actual count. Recurring discrepancies between the physical and perpetual inventory records should be investigated since the latter method indicates the number of supply items that should be available.

As noted earlier, the choice of the inventory system depends on the characteristics of the supply item. If an item of stock is characterized by a high annual usage, is critical to the lifesaving function of the health facility, presents special storage requirements, or is subject to misappropriation, the perpetual inventory system probably is appropriate. As suggested, the perpetual inventory system provides continuous control over stocks since their level can be determined immediately at any moment. Even though the system is costly to operate, many of the items probably should be maintained by perpetual records. Careful studies should be conducted to determine the benefits and the costs of initiating and maintaining a perpetual inventory system.

9.3 METHODS OF INVENTORY VALUATION

Frequently, health care facilities purchase a particular supply item during a given period at different prices. The problem of assigning a value to the units of unused inventory available at the end of the period and a value to those used in providing care during the period is complicated by price changes during the period. Several methods are used to determine these values. The results of this process exert a direct impact on operating expenses for current and future periods as well as on the value of the inventories reported in the balance sheet. When selecting an inventory valuation method, the primary concern should be the cost of supplies used during the period so as to obtain a proper matching of revenues with expenses and thereby provide a proper determination of net income. The influence of any valuation technique on the inventory assets reported in the balance sheet is important but should be of secondary consideration.

It also is necessary to allocate supply expenses among the hospital's functional units. In this instance, it is assumed that inventory acquisitions are transferred from the receiving department to central supply where they are held until required by the functional units. Once a requisition has been initiated, the items are transferred from central supply to the floor stock of the unit, where they remain until used. After the items have been used in providing patient care, supply expenses are recognized and assigned to the functional unit.

To simplify the discussion, the focus here is on consumable supply CS_1, with the assumption that the information in Tables 9-1 and 9-2 is available.

Table 9-1 Acquisition and Issuance of Consumable Supply CS_1: Central Supply

Date	Transaction	Number of Units	Cost	
			Unit	*Total*
June 1	Inventory	50	$3.00	$150.00
June 6	Purchase	70	4.00	280.00
June 14	Issue	50		
June 22	Purchase	90	6.00	540.00
June 23	Issue	70		
June 25	Purchase	100	7.00	700.00
June 28	Issue	90		

This information depicts the relationship between central supply and functional units D_1 and D_2 that require the use of consumable supply CS_1 in operational activity. More specifically, the data in Table 9-1 portray the beginning inventory, the acquisition of the supply item during the month, and the issuance of the article to the functional units for the month of June. The data in Table 9-2 represent the floor stock of each unit at the beginning of the month, the quantity of the items received from central supply, and their use in the operational activity of the two units during the month.

The data in these tables are summarized in Table 9-3. The number of units issued from central supply (210) is just equal to the number received by the two functional entities (i.e., 70 + 140, or 210 units). Similarly, the ending inventory in the last column is calculated as follows:

Beginning Inventory		
Central Supply	50 units	
Unit D_1	40 units	
Unit D_2	80 units	
		170 units
Plus Purchases		260 units
Supplies Available		430 units
Less Usage:		
Unit D_1	70 units	
Unit D_2	180 units	
		250 units
Ending Inventory		180 units

As should be verified, the ending inventory of the institution is distributed as follows:

Central Supply	100 units
Unit D_1	40 units
Unit D_2	40 units
	180 units

Table 9-2 Receipt and Use of Consumable Supply CS_1 by Functional Units D_1 and D_2

Functional Unit D_1					Functional Unit D_2				
			Cost					Cost	
Date	Transaction	Number of Units	Unit	Total	Date	Transaction	Number of Units	Unit	Total
June 1	Inventory	40	$2.75	$110	June 1	Inventory	80	$2.75	$220
June 10	Use	20			June 7	Use	60		
June 14	Receipt	10			June 14	Receipt	40		
June 20	Use	25			June 18	Use	30		
June 23	Receipt	20			June 23	Receipt	50		
June 26	Use	15			June 25	Use	70		
June 28	Receipt	40			June 28	Receipt	50		
June 29	Use	10			June 29	Use	20		

Table 9-3 Summary of Inventory Operation

Organizational Unit	Beginning Inventory (in Units)	Purchases (in Units)	Issues (in Units)	Receipts (in Units)	Usage (in Units)	Ending Inventory (in Units)
Central Supply	50	260	210	—	—	100
Functional Unit D_1	40	—	—	70	70	40
Functional Unit D_2	80	—	—	140	180	40
Totals	170	260	210	210	250	180

In the following discussion, the objectives are to examine:

1. the accounting methods of determining the value assigned to the inventory items used by the two units in providing service
2. the accounting entries required to charge supply expenses to the two units
3. the accounting methods of determining the value of the units of inventory that remain unused at the end of the period

In addition, when considering the perpetual inventory system, it is necessary to examine

1. the accounting method of assigning a value to the supply items that are transferred from central supply to the functional unit
2. the accounting entries required to transfer supply items to the two functional units

More specifically, this section describes specific invoice prices, average weighted prices, FIFO cost evaluation, LIFO cost evaluation, and standard costs as methods that may be used in deriving reasonable solutions to these problems.

9.3.1 Specific Invoice Prices

When it is possible to identify each item with a specific purchase, the corresponding price or unit cost may be used to assign costs to the items remaining in inventory at the end of the period and to those used in producing service during the period. For example, suppose that the ending inventory is composed of:

1. 10 units acquired on June 6
2. 70 units acquired on June 22
3. 100 units acquired on June 25

The ending inventory is assigned a value of $1,160, which is calculated as follows:

Number of Units	*Unit Cost*	*Total Cost*
10	$4.00	$40
70	6.00	420
100	7.00	700
Total		1,160

With regard to the use of the supply item, suppose that

1. 40 units of the beginning floor stock,
2. 10 units of the beginning inventory assigned to central supply, and
3. 20 units that were acquired on June 6

are used by functional unit D_1 in providing service during the period. Similarly, assume that

1. 80 units of the beginning floor stock,
2. 40 units of the beginning inventory assigned to central supply,
3. 40 units that were acquired on June 6, and
4. 20 units that were acquired on June 22

are used by functional unit D_2 in providing service. As seen in Table 9-4, the supply expenses charged to units D_1 and D_2 are \$220 and \$620, respectively. Assuming that the purchases were assigned originally to an asset account, the entry

Supply Expense (classified by functional unit)	\$840	
Inventory		\$840

recognizes the expenses incurred in the two units and reduces the inventory holdings of the institution by \$840.

The major advantage of this approach is that it provides an accurate measure of the supplies actually used in providing care and the value of inventory items unused at the end of the period. The primary disadvantage is that it is difficult, if not impossible, to maintain records that accurately depict the physical flow of inventory items. As a result, it is necessary to use

---

Table 9-4 Assignment of Supply Expenses

Functional Unit D_1			*Functional Unit D_2*		
Number of Units	*Unit Cost*	*Total Cost*	*Number of Units*	*Unit Cost*	*Total Cost*
40	\$2.75	\$110	80	\$2.75	\$220
10	3.00	30	40	3.00	120
20	4.00	80	40	4.00	160
70		220	20	6.00	120
			180		620

an assumed flow of inventory items to determine the values of consumable supplies used in providing care and of the ending inventory.

9.3.2 Average Weighted Price

Many health facilities use the weighted average cost to determine the expense of supplies used during a given accounting period and the value of inventories on hand at the end. The basic assumption underlying the technique is that supply items are drawn more or less equally from the beginning inventory or floor stock and from each of the acquisitions of the period. Fortunately, it is not necessary for the actual flow of inventory to correspond to the assumed flow. As seen next, the average weighted cost method may be used in both periodic and perpetual inventory systems.

9.3.2.1 Average Weighted Cost and the Periodic System

The general formula for calculating the average weighted cost is given by

$$\overline{C} = \frac{\Sigma w_i p_i}{\Sigma w_i} \tag{9.1}$$

where

$\overline{C}$ = average weighted cost;

w_i = the quantity of the inventory item associated with acquisition *i*;

p_i = the unit cost or price associated with acquisition *i*.

Returning to Tables 9-1 and 9-2, assume for a moment that the periodic inventory system is used to record entries pertaining to the supply item referred to earlier. In this case, Equation 9.1 may be used to calculate an average weighted cost for the month of June, as follows:

Date		w_i	p_i	$w_i\ p_i$
June 1	Floor Stock	120	$2.75	$330
1	Inventory	50	3.00	150
6	Purchase	70	4.00	280
22	Purchase	90	6.00	540
25	Purchase	100	7.00	700
		430		2,000

Substituting $\Sigma w_i = 430$ and $\Sigma w_i\, p_i = 2{,}000$ into Equation 9.1, we obtain

$$\overline{C} = \frac{\$2{,}000}{430}$$

which indicates that the average weighted cost of these supply items is approximately $4.65116. The average weighted cost now may be used to calculate the ending inventory and the cost of the supply items used in the operational activity of the two functional units as follows:

$$\text{Ending Inventory} = 180 \text{ units} \times \$4.65116$$
$$\cong \$837.21$$

$$\text{Supply Expense Unit } D_1 = 70 \text{ units} \times \$4.65116$$
$$\cong \$325.58$$

$$\text{Supply Expense Unit } D_2 = 180 \text{ units} \times \$4.65116$$
$$\cong \$837.21$$

As before, if it is assumed that an inventory asset account is used to record the purchases, the adjusting entry

Supply Expense (Classified by functional unit)	$1,162.79	
Inventory		$1,162.79

recognizes the supply expenses incurred by the two units and reduces the balance of the inventory asset account from $2,000 to $837.21.

9.3.2.2 Average Weighted Cost and the Perpetual System

If the perpetual inventory system is used to record transactions involving the supply item and if expenses are recorded at the end of the month or at the end of other convenient intervals, the average weighted cost may be computed as above. On the other hand, it may be desirable to record the transfer of the item from central supply to the functional units and to enter expenses at the time supplies are used in operational activity. When this procedure is followed, a new weighted average must be computed whenever an inventory item is acquired at a unit cost that is different from the current weighted average. In other words, successive recalculations are required whenever inventory is acquired at prices different from the current weighted average cost.

As an example, consider Table 9-5, which is similar to the subsidiary inventory record that is maintained by the central supply unit of most facilities. For each of the inventory acquisitions, an average weighted cost is computed by dividing the current value of inventory held in central supply by the number of units available. For example, the acquisition of the supply item on June 6 increases inventory from 50 to 120 units; as a result, the inventory value grew from \$150 to \$430. Consequently, the average weighted cost of the 120 units is given by

$$\frac{\$430}{120} \cong \$3.5833$$

As should be verified, the other average unit costs in the table are calculated in a similar fashion.

Consider next the transfer of the item from central supply to the functional units of the organization. In Table 9-5, the value assigned to the 50 units of inventory that were transferred from central supply to functional units D_1 and D_2 on June 14 is given by

$$50 \text{ units} \times \$3.5833/\text{unit}$$

or \$179.16. The entry to record the transfer may be summarized in the form

Floor Stock (classified)	\$179.16	
Inventory		\$179.16

where the Floor Stock account represents an inventory asset of the institution. Consequently, the entry simply reflects the location of the supply item and does not alter total inventory holdings. Obviously, a similar entry is required for each of the other transfers during the month. A value of \$602.56 is assigned to the 100 units that remain in central supply at the end of the month.

As seen in Tables 9-6 and 9-7, the issuances from central supply are treated as a receipt of supplies when viewed from the perspective of the subsidiary records maintained for the functional unit. For example, consider the distribution of the \$179.16 worth of supplies to functional units D_1 and D_2. Table 9-6 shows that the value of the 10 units received by functional unit D_1 is given by

$$10 \text{ units} \times \$3.5833/\text{unit}$$

Table 9-5 Average Weighted Costs-Perpetual Inventory System Subsidiary Inventory Record: Central Supply

	Acquisitions			*Issues*			*Balance*		
		Cost			*Cost*			*Cost*	
Date	*Number of Units*	*Unit*	*Total*	*Number of Units*	*Unit*	*Total*	*Number of Units*	*Unit*	*Total*
June 1							50	$3.00	$150.00
6	70	$4.00	$280				120	3.5833	430.00
14				50	$3.5833	$179.16	70	3.5833	250.83
22	90	6.00	540				160	4.9427	790.83
23				70	4.9427	345.99	90	4.9427	444.84
25	100	7.00	700				190	6.0255	1,144.84
28				90	6.0255	542.29	100	6.0255	602.56

Table 9-6 Subsidiary Inventory Record of Functional Unit D_1

	Receipts			*Usage*			*Balance*		
		Cost			*Cost*			*Cost*	
Date	*Number of Units*	*Unit*	*Total*	*Number of Units*	*Unit*	*Total*	*Number of Units*	*Unit*	*Total*
June 1							40	$2.75	$110.00
10				20	$2.75	$55.00	20	2.75	55.00
14	10	$3.5833	$35.83				30	3.0277	90.83
20				25	3.0277	75.69	5	3.0277	15.14
23	20	4.9427	98.85				25	4.5596	113.99
26				15	4.5596	68.39	10	4.5596	45.60
28	40	6.0255	241.02				50	5.7324	286.62
29				10	5.7324	57.32	40	5.7324	229.30
						256.40			

Table 9-7 Subsidiary Inventory Record of Functional Unit D_2

Date	Receipts			Usage			Balance		
	Number of Units	Cost Unit	Cost Total	Number of Units	Cost Unit	Cost Total	Number of Units	Cost Unit	Cost Total
June 1							80	$2.75	$220.00
7				60	$2.75	$165.00	20	2.75	55.00
14	40	$3.5833	$143.33				60	3.3055	198.33
18				30	3.3055	99.17	30	3.3055	99.16
23	50	4.9427	247.14				80	4.3287	346.30
25				70	4.3287	303.01	10	4.3287	43.29
28	50	6.0255	301.27				60	5.7427	344.56
29				20	5.7427	114.85	40	5.7427	229.71
						682.03			

or approximately \$35.83, while Table 9-7 reveals that the value of the supplies received by functional unit D_2 is

$$40 \text{ units} \times \$3.5833/\text{unit}$$

or approximately \$143.33. The other transfers are treated in similar fashion.

Of particular importance at this point in the analysis is the calculation of the current average weighted costs in the subsidiary records of the functional unit. In functional unit D_1, the receipt of 10 units on June 14 increases the inventory holdings of this group to 30 from 20 units and the value of the floor stock of the unit grows to \$90.83 from \$55.00. Consequently, the average weighted cost of these 30 units is given by

$$\frac{\$90.83}{30} = \$3.0277$$

As should be verified, a similar technique is used to calculate a new average weighted cost on each occasion that the unit receives supplies.

Under a perpetual inventory system, expenses are recognized *at the time* supplies are used in operational activity. For example, the use of 20 units by functional unit D_1 on June 10 is recorded by the entry

Supply Expense (Classified)	\$55	
Floor Stock (Classified)		\$55

This entry recognizes the supply expense of \$55 and reduces the balance of the floor stock assigned to the unit from \$110 to \$55. Similarly, the entry

Supply Expense (Classified)	\$75.69	
Floor Stock (Classified)		\$75.69

recognizes the expenses incurred by using 25 units of supply on June 20 and reduces the value of the floor stock assigned to the unit to \$15.14 from \$90.83.

In summarizing Tables 9-5, 9-6, and 9-7, the inventory holdings of the institution at the end of the month may be calculated as follows:

	Ending Inventory
Central Supply	\$602.56
Functional Unit D_1	229.30
Functional Unit D_2	229.71
Total	1,061.57

Similarly, the supply expenses recognized during the period may be summarized:

	Supply Expense
Functional Unit D_1	\$256.40
Functional Unit D_2	682.03
Total	938.43

Finally, the use of average weighted costs in a perpetual inventory system results in expenses and an ending inventory that differ from the corresponding expenses and ending inventory in the periodic system.

9.3.3 First-In, First-Out (FIFO) Cost Evaluation

The first-in, first-out (FIFO) costing method is based on the assumption that goods are issued from inventory in the order they are received. In other words, under this method it is assumed that the oldest items are issued from inventory first. This, of course, means that inventory items remaining in stock are valued at the most recent costs or invoice prices. This method is intuitively appealing since some effort should be made to use the oldest stock first.

9.3.3.1 FIFO and the Periodic Inventory System

Under the assumption that a periodic inventory system and the FIFO method of evaluation are used to account for the inventory item described previously, the supply expenses charged to the functional units D_1 and D_2 are calculated as in Table 9-8.

Table 9-8 Charging Supplies to Functional Units

Functional Unit D_1			*Functional Unit D_2*		
Use (in Units)	*Unit Cost*	*Supply Expense*	*Use (in Units)*	*Unit Cost*	*Supply Expense*
40	\$2.75	\$110	80	\$2.75	\$220
10	3.00	30	40	3.00	120
20	4.00	80	50	4.00	200
70		220	10	6.00	60
			180		600

Similarly, the ending inventory is distributed thus:

	Number of Units	*Unit Cost*	*Ending Inventory*
Central Supply	100	$7.00	$700
Functional Unit D_1	40	6.00	240
Functional Unit D_2	40	6.00	240
	180		1,180

In this case, the value assigned to the items remaining in inventory at the end of the period is determined by the use of the most recent invoice prices. Similar to the earlier discussion, the entry

Supply Expense (Classified)	$820	
Inventory		$820

recognizes the supply expense incurred during the month and reduces the value of the inventory asset account to $1,180 from $2,000.

9.3.3.2 FIFO and the Perpetual Inventory System

Table 9-9 is an example of the subsidiary inventory record that central supply can maintain when a perpetual inventory system and the FIFO method of evaluation are used to account for the item. Purchases are recorded in the acquisition section and added to the inventory balance as before. In this case, the units of the item that are transferred from central supply to the functional units are assumed to have been selected from the oldest stock. For example, the units issued on June 14 are assumed to have been selected from the beginning inventory of central supply; the entry to record the transfer of these units is given by

Floor Stock (Classified)	$150	
Inventory		$150

This simply transfers items from central supply to the functional units and does not alter the value of the inventory holdings of the institution. After the items have been transferred, 70 units of inventory valued at $4.00 per unit remain in central supply. The other transfers in the subsidiary inventory record are treated in a similar fashion.

As before, the transfers recorded in central supply's subsidiary inventory ledger are regarded as a receipt when viewed from the perspective of the functional unit. For example, consider Tables 9-10 and 9-11, which represent the subsidiary records for functional units D_1 and D_2. In Table 9-10, the transfer of 10 units of the supply item to unit D_1 is recorded as a receipt and

Table 9-9 FIFO Evaluation and the Perpetual Inventory System: Central Supply

	Acquisitions			*Issues*			*Balance*		
		Cost			*Cost*			*Cost*	
Date	*Number of Units*	*Unit*	*Total*	*Number of Units*	*Unit*	*Total*	*Number of Units*	*Unit*	*Total*
June 1							50	$3.00	$150
6	70	$4.00	$280				50	3.00	150
							70	4.00	280
14				50	$3.00	$150	70	4.00	280
22	90	6.00	540				70	4.00	280
							90	6.00	540
23				70	4.00	280	90	6.00	540
25	100	7.00	700				90	6.00	540
							100	7.00	700
28				90	6.00	540	100	7.00	700

Arrows indicate flow of inventory.

Table 9-10 Subsidiary Inventory Record of Unit D_1: FIFO and Perpetual Inventory

Date	Receipts			Use			Balance		
	Number of Units	Cost: Unit	Cost: Total	Number of Units	Cost: Unit	Cost: Total	Number of Units	Cost: Unit	Cost: Total
June 1							40	$2.75	$110
10				20	$2.75	$55	20	2.75	55
14	10	$3.00	$30				20*	2.75	55
							10	3.00	30
20				20	2.75	55			
				5	3.00	15	5	3.00	15
23	20	4.00	80				5	3.00	15
							20	4.00	80
26				5	3.00	15	10	4.00	40
				10	4.00	40			
28	40	6.00	240				10	4.00	40
							40	6.00	280
29				10	4.00	40	40	6.00	240

* Arrows indicate flow of inventory.

Table 9-11 Subsidiary Inventory Record of Functional Unit D_2: FIFO and Perpetual Inventory

	Receipts			Use			Balance		
		Cost			Cost			Cost	
Date	Number of Units	Unit	Total	Number of Units	Unit	Total	Number of Units	Unit	Total
June 1							80	$2.75	$220
7				60	$2.75	$165	20	2.75	55
14	40	$3.00	$120				20	2.75	55
							40	3.00	120
18				20	2.75	55	30	3.00	90
				10	3.00	30			
23	50	4.00	200				30	3.00	90
							50	4.00	200
25				30	3.00	90	10	4.00	40
				40	4.00	160			
28	50	6.00	300				10	4.00	40
							50	6.00	300
29				10	4.00	40	40	6.00	240
				10	6.00	60			

Arrows indicate flow of inventory.

a unit cost of $3.00 is used to determine the value that is added to the balance of the floor stock maintained by the unit. A similar practice is employed in Table 9-11, where the subsidiary records pertaining to unit D_2 are summarized.

Consider next the use of the supply item in the operational activity of the functional unit. As seen in Table 9-10, the 25 units used on June 20 are composed of the remaining 20 units of the beginning floor stock and 5 units selected from the supplies received June 14. Recall that under the perpetual inventory system, supply expenses are recognized as stock is used in operational activity. As a result, the entry

Supply Expense (Classified)	$70	
Floor Stock (Classified)		$70

recognizes the expense of the use of supplies and reduces the floor stock.

At this point in the analysis, Tables 9-10 and 9-11 demonstrate that the supply expenses incurred during the month may be summarized as follows:

	Supply Expense
Unit D_1	$220
Unit D_2	600
Total	820

The value of the supply items that remain in inventory at the end of the period is distributed as follows:

	Ending Inventory
Central Supply	$700
Unit D_1	240
Unit D_2	240
Total	1,180

As can be verified, when the FIFO costing technique is used, the periodic and perpetual inventory systems yield identical results.

9.3.4 Last-In, First-Out (LIFO) Cost Evaluation

When the last-in, first-out (LIFO) method of evaluation is employed, it is assumed that supplies are issued and used from the most recently acquired stocks. As a result, the latest prices are assigned to units issued from central supply and used in operational activity. Consequently, the unit cost of the oldest stock is used when determining the value of the ending inventory.

9.3.4.1 LIFO and the Periodic Inventory System

Assume that the LIFO method of evaluation is used in conjunction with the periodic inventory system to account for the supply item referred to earlier. Since the ending inventory is assumed to consist of the oldest stock under the LIFO method, it can be verified easily that the value of the units of supply held by the institution at the end of the period may be determined by the following calculations:

	Number of Units	*Unit Cost*	*Ending Inventory*
	50	$3.00	$150
	10	4.00	40
Central Supply:			190
Functional Unit D_1:	40	2.75	110
Functional Unit D_2:	80	2.75	220
Totals	180		520

Thus, under the LIFO method, the unit cost of the oldest stock (i.e., beginning inventories and 10 units acquired on June 6) is used to determine the value of the ending inventory.

The supply expense of the period may be calculated thus:

Cost of Available Supplies	$2,000
Less Ending Inventory	520
Cost of Supplies Used	1,480

The cost of supplies used during the period also can be calculated as follows:

	Number of Units	*Unit Cost*	*Supply Expenses*
	60	$4.00	$240
	90	6.00	540
	100	7.00	700
Totals	250		1,480

In this case, the supply expense is determined by using the latest prices.

At this point in the analysis, it is necessary to allocate the supply expenses of the period to the functional units D_1 and D_2. It is assumed that the expenses are allocated in terms of the relative use of the supply item by the two units. Recall that

1. a total of 250 units are used during the period

2. functional unit D_1 uses 70 units of the supply item
3. functional unit D_2 uses 180 units of the supply item

As a result, 28 percent (i.e., $70/250 \times 100$) of the supply expenses are charged to unit D_1 and 72 percent ($180/250 \times 100$) to functional unit D_2. Consequently, the supply expense charged to unit D_1 is given by the product $.28 \times \$1,480$, or \$414.40 and that assigned to functional unit D_2 by $.72 \times \$1,480$, or \$1,065.60. Hence, the adjusting entry to record the expenses of the period is:

Supply Expense (Unit D_1)	\$414.40	
Supply Expense (Unit D_2)	1,065.60	
Inventory		\$1,480

9.3.4.2 LIFO and the Perpetual Inventory System

Assume that the LIFO method of evaluation and a perpetual inventory system are used. Table 9-12 is an example of the subsidiary inventory ledger that can be maintained by central supply. This shows that the items that are transferred to the functional units are assumed to have been selected from the most recently acquired stock. For example, the entry to transfer the 50 units on June 14 is given by

Floor Stock (Classified)	\$200	
Inventory		\$200

where the unit cost of the most recently acquired stock is used to determine the value of the items transferred to the functional entitics.

Consider next Tables 9-13 and 9-14, which present the subsidiary records maintained for functional units D_1 and D_2. Here, as in Tables 9-10 and 9-11, the transfer from central supply is regarded as a receipt that is added to the balance of the floor stock maintained on the unit. In accordance with the assumptions underlying the LIFO method, supply units used in operational activity are assumed to have been selected from the most recently acquired stock. For example, consider the use of the supply item by unit D_1 on June 20. In this case, it is assumed that the first 10 units are selected from the stock received June 14 and the remaining units from the beginning inventory. Consequently, the entry

Supply Expense	\$81.25	
Floor Stock		\$81.25

is recorded on June 20 to recognize supply expenses and to reduce the unit's floor stock.

Table 9-12 LIFO Evaluation and the Perpetual Inventory System: Central Supply

	Acquisitions			Issues			Balance		
		Cost			Cost			Cost	
Date	Number of Units	Unit	Total	Number of Units	Unit	Total	Number of Units	Unit	Total
June 1							50	$3.00	$150
6	70	$4.00	$280				50	3.00	150
							70	4.00	280
14				50	$4.00	$200	50	3.00	150
							20	4.00	80
22	90	6.00	540				50	3.00	150
							20	4.00	80
							90	6.00	540
23				70	6.00	420	50	3.00	150
							20	4.00	80
							20	6.00	120
25	100	7.00	700				50	3.00	150
							20	4.00	80
							20	6.00	120
							100	7.00	700
28				90	7.00	630	50	3.00	150
							20	4.00	80
							20	6.00	120
							10	7.00	70

Arrows indicate flow of inventory.

Table 9-13 Subsidiary Inventory Record of Unit D_1: LIFO and Perpetual Inventory

	Receipts			Use			Balance		
	Number	Cost		Number	Cost		Number	Cost	
Date	of Units	Unit	Total	of Units	Unit	Total	of Units	Unit	Total
June 1							40	$2.75	$110.00
10				20	$2.75	$55.00	20	2.75	55.00
14	10	$4.00	$40.00				20	2.75	55.00
							10	4.00	40.00
20				10	4.00	40.00	5	2.75	13.75
				15	2.75	41.25			
23	20	6.00	120.00				5	2.75	13.75
							20	6.00	120.00
26				15	6.00	90.00	5	2.75	13.75
							5	6.00	30.00
28	40	7.00	280.00				5	2.75	13.75
							5	6.00	30.00
							40	7.00	280.00
29				10	7.00	70.00	5	2.75	13.75
							5	6.00	30.00
							30	7.00	210.00

Arrows indicate flow of inventory.

Table 9-14 Subsidiary Inventory Record of Unit D_2: LIFO and Perpetual Inventory

	Receipts			Use			Balance		
		Cost			Cost			Cost	
Date	Number of Units	Unit	Total	Number of Units	Unit	Total	Number of Units	Unit	Total
June 1							80	$2.75	$220.00
7				60	$2.75	$165.00	20	2.75	55.00
14	40	$4.00	$160.00				20	2.75	55.00
							40	4.00	160.00
18				30	4.00	120.00	20	2.75	55.00
							10	4.00	40.00
23	50	6.00	300.00				20	2.75	55.00
							10	4.00	40.00
							50	6.00	300.00
25				50	6.00	300.00	10	2.75	27.50
				10	4.00	40.00			
				10	2.75	27.50			
28	50	7.00	350.00				10	2.75	27.50
							50	7.00	350.00
29				20	7.00	140.00	10	2.75	27.50
							30	7.00	210.00

Arrows indicate flow of inventory.

At this point in the analysis, it should be verified that the inventory of the institution at the end of the month is distributed as follows:

	Number of Units	*Unit Cost*	*Total Cost*	*Ending Inventory*
Central Supply:	50	$3.00	$150	
	20	4.00	80	
	20	6.00	120	
	10	7.00	70	
				$420.00
Unit D_1	5	2.75	13.75	
	5	6.00	30.00	
	30	7.00	210.00	
				253.75
Unit D_2	10	2.75	27.50	
	30	7.00	210.00	
				237.50
Totals	180			911.25

On the other hand, the total expenses charged to the functional units may be summarized as:

	Expense
Unit D_1	$296.25
Unit D_2	792.50
Total	1,088.75

As should be verified, the periodic and perpetual inventory systems do not normally yield equivalent results when the LIFO method of evaluation is used.

9.3.5 A Comparison of the Methods

Usually the health facility will use only one of the methods of evaluation, so it is necessary to evaluate the advantages and disadvantages associated with each approach. As a general guideline, management should select a method that will result in an accurate measure of the supply expenses during the period and a precise measure of the ending inventory. In addition, the method must be clerically feasible.

Table 9-15 summarizes the results when the three approaches are used in conjunction with the perpetual inventory system to account for the supply item. The three methods produce three different supply expenses for the

Table 9-15 Comparison of the Basic Methods of Evaluating Inventory

Method of Evaluation	*Cost of Available Supplies*	*Ending Inventory*	*Cost of Supplies Used*
FIFO	$2,000	$1,180.00	$820.00
Average Weighted Cost	2,000	1,061.57	938.43
LIFO	2,000	911.25	1,088.75

month and three different values for the ending inventory. All are acceptable methods of valuing ending inventory. The following attributes may be associated with the LIFO and FIFO methods that have differing effects during periods of price change.

During periods of price inflation, FIFO tends to result in smaller charges to expense, a larger net income, and a larger inventory for balance sheet presentation than does LIFO. Conversely, also during inflationary periods, LIFO tends to result in larger expenses, a lower net income, and a lower inventory asset in the balance sheet than does the FIFO method. These tendencies are of considerable importance when viewed from the perspective of increasing the amount of cost-based reimbursement from third parties. Since the amount of third party reimbursement of many institutions depends on cost, the accounting method that results in the highest cost also yields the highest reimbursement. Accordingly, the LIFO method is the more appropriate during inflationary periods; obviously, when prices are declining steadily, this tendency is reversed.

Whatever method is selected, it should be defensible, managerially useful, clerically feasible, and consistently applied from one period to another. The last observation is not intended to imply that management should not adopt a different method of inventory evaluation when conditions warrant. However, since complete freedom to abandon one method in favor of another permits the manipulation of expenses and net income in a more or less arbitrary fashion, changes in the method of valuing inventories and their effect on net income must be disclosed fully.

9.3.6 Standard Costs

Health administrators have expressed increased interest in using standard costs in connection with inventories. Suppose there is an inventory group or classification for which a standard price of $10 is established at the beginning of the year. That figure is based on anticipated or expected prices for the ensuing year and the purchasing policies that will prevail during the period. In other words, the use of standard costing techniques assumes efficiency in the purchasing function and the standard price represents what unit cost should prevail during the coming accounting period.

For example, assume the following data are germane to the inventory item during the year:

Date		*Units*	*Unit Cost*
1/1	Inventory	100	$10.00
1/3	Purchased	200	10.50
1/5	Used	150	
1/7	Used	100	
1/10	Purchased	200	9.40
1/11	Used	50	

Under standard cost techniques, inventory acquisitions are recorded by using the standard cost or price which, in the example, is $10. A purchase price variance account is used to record differences between the standard cost and actual expenses, while the issuance and use of inventory are recorded at standard cost. The entries for the year under this method are:

March 1	Inventory	$2,000	
	Price Variance	100	
	Accounts Payable		$2,100
May 1	Supply Expense	1,500	
	Inventory		1,500
July 1	Supply Expense	1,000	
	Inventory		1,000
October 1	Inventory	2,000	
	Accounts Payable		1,880
	Price Variance		120
November 1	Supply Expense	500	
	Inventory		500

The net purchase price variance for the year is $20 ($120 − $100); the supply expense is given by the product of the number of units used (150 + 100 + 50 = 300) and the standard cost of $10 per unit or $3,000; and the ending inventory is $2,000 (200 units @ $10/unit).

9.4 LOWER OF COST OR MARKET

Over the years, the traditional rule for reporting inventories in the balance sheet has been to price such assets at the lower of cost or replacement (market). This is a generally accepted practice because it reports the inventory holdings of the institution in the balance sheet at a conservative figure. The basic premise of the conservative approach is to anticipate no gains and to provide for all losses. In other words, if the inventory could be replaced at an amount that is less than its historical cost, the supply should be reduced to reflect the lower value. The amount of the reduction in inventory is treated as an expense of the period.

Suppose that the 180 units of the inventory item referred to in Section 9.3.5 could be replaced at a unit cost of $5.90 per unit or at a total cost of $1,062. No adjustment is required if the inventory is determined by the average weighted cost method or the LIFO method since these approaches result in inventory valuations of $1,061.57 and $911.25, respectively. Clearly, these values are less than the assumed replacement cost of $1,062. On the other hand, under the FIFO method, the value of the ending inventory is $1,180, which exceeds the replacement costs and, as a result, the inventory can be written down by $118.

The application of the lower of cost or replacement rule is not as simple as these comments might indicate. Several considerations in applying the rule should be noted: (1) replacement or market costs should not exceed the net realizable value that is the ordinary selling price less any reasonably predictable costs of completion and disposal; (2) replacement or market costs should not be less than the net realizable value reduced by an allowance for normal profit margins. These considerations suggest that there are upper and lower limits that should be considered in applying the rule. These and other complications are not considered in this text.

When inventory write-downs are required because of declines in prices, obsolescence, or damage, it may be desirable to credit the reduction in inventory to a contra inventory account rather than directly to the inventory asset account. This eliminates the necessity of adjusting subsidiary inventory records. Suppose that a $20,000 inventory is to be reduced by $4,000. The journal entry is

Loss on Inventory Reduction	$4,000	
Allowance for Inventory Reduction		$4,000

When such losses are material, they should appear as a separate entry in the income statement and the inventory asset in the balance sheet should be reported at the adjusted figure. When the inventory is sold or consumed in production during the subsequent period, the allowance account no longer is needed and is eliminated by:

Supply Expense	$63,000	
Allowance for Inventory Reduction	4,000	
Inventory		$67,000

9.5 ESTIMATION OF INVENTORIES

As indicated in Section 9.2.1, the periodic system does not provide the basis for determining what inventories should or ought to be. In preparing interim reports, supply items maintained under the periodic inventory system require a physical count to determine the supply expenses of the period and the inventory on hand at the end. The purpose of this section is to describe two basic methods that permit the estimation of the supply expenses of a given period and the inventory balances that are required when preparing interim reports. Since management requires interim reports on a frequent and timely basis, a physical inventory of items maintained on a periodic inventory system is not possible nor feasible each time these lists are prepared. In addition, by estimating what inventories should or ought to be, a comparison of actual and expected inventories provides the basis for controlling supply items maintained on a periodic inventory system.

9.5.1 Gross Margin Method

With respect to the periodic inventory system, it may be feasible to apply the gross margin method to estimate the amount that should be in inventory. Suppose that the following data are available on a supply item whose price is determined through a standard markup of 50 percent on cost:

Beginning Inventory	$20,000
Year ended December 31:	
Purchases	70,000
Billings	120,000

For these supply items, the price is determined by increasing costs by 50 percent. For example, an item costing $14 would be marked up to $21 and a $10 item to $15. In this case, $15 and $21 represent the price billed. Consequently, a 50 percent markup indicates that the price contains a one-third profit margin (33⅓ percent of the billed price). Assuming a 50 percent markup, the application of the gross margin method in estimating the December 31 inventory for the data assumed above is shown in Table 9-16. This shows that the total cost of supplies available during the period is determined by summing the beginning inventory ($20,000) and the purchases of the period ($70,000). The estimated costs of supplies billed (i.e., inventory withdrawals) is determined by subtracting the estimated gross margin (1/3 × $120,000) from the billings of $120,000, which are based on the price charged by the institution. The results of these operations are simply subtracted from the total cost of supplies available, yielding an estimate of the ending inventory ($10,000), which of course is valued at cost. This method provides reasonably good estimates of what the inventory should be and, when compared with actual inventory levels, offers the basis for detecting serious shortages. However, before concluding that theft or misappropriation has occurred, management should ensure that this method is reliable.

Table 9-16 Estimation of Inventory Gross Margin Method

Beginning Inventory	$20,000	
Purchases	70,000	
Total Cost of Supplies Available		$90,000
Billings	120,000	
Less Estimated Margin (33⅓% × 120,000)	40,000	
Estimated Cost of Supplies Billed		80,000
Estimated Inventory December 31		10,000
Less Physical Inventory (Assumed)		6,000
Inventory Shortage		4,000

The gross margin method of estimating inventories has other important uses when periodic inventory records are maintained:

1. When inventory has been destroyed by fire, the gross margin method may be used to determine the amount to be claimed for insurance purposes.
2. Insurance policies may require the institution to report approximate inventory levels at the end of each month. Since monthly inventories are impractical, the gross margin method provides a basis for determining such estimates and perhaps reducing insurance premiums.
3. The preparation of monthly financial statements requires the estimation of inventory levels and corresponding inventory expenses. The gross margin method can be employed for these purposes.

9.5.2 Retail Inventory Method

A variation on the gross margin method may be used in retail shops operated by the institution: the retail inventory method. Under this system, items that are placed in inventory are priced at retail using a uniform markup. The records also must reflect any additional price changes (markups or markdowns) that occur during the period.

By way of illustration, suppose the following data pertain to the activities of a retail shop operated by the hospital:

	Cost	*Retail*
Beginning Inventory	$14,000	$32,000
Purchases	10,000	15,000
Markdowns		7,000
Sales		20,000

The retail value of purchases is based on the prices at which the items were priced originally for sale. During the year, some unsold goods are marked down by $7,000. Table 9-17 presents the details of the retail inventory method of estimating ending inventories valued at cost. As the table shows, the inventory is determined on the basis of sales prices rather than costs. Now, assume that a physical inventory reveals that the value of the supply items held by the institution is $13,000. In this case, the inventory shortage is $7,000 ($20,000 − $13,000) when valued at retail or $4,200 ($7,000 × .6) when valued at cost. Both findings, of course, indicate a need to assess the system of controlling inventory.

9.6 PREPAID EXPENSES

As the name implies, a prepaid expense is one that has been paid in advance of its use. At the time of payment, an asset is acquired that will be used in operational activity. As it is consumed it becomes an expense. Typically an unrestricted fund will include prepayments for such items as insurance, rent, and interest. These prepayments represent rights to future services and it generally is assumed that these services will be used in the subsequent operating cycle.

Suppose, for example, that the institution pays a rental fee for the next three months and that the prepayment is $600. When the payment is made, the facility obtains the right to occupy space for three months; the entry to record the acquisition of the asset is:

Prepaid Rent	$600	
Cash		$600

With each passing day a portion of the prepaid expense expires and at the end of each month it is necessary to reduce the asset Prepaid Rent account

Table 9-17 Estimation of Inventories by Retail Inventory Method

	Cost	*Retail*
Beginning Inventory	$14,000	$32,000
Add Purchases	10,000	15,000
Less Markdowns		(7,000)
Total (Cost Percent = 24,000/40,000 = .6)	24,000	40,000
Less Sales		20,000
Ending Inventory at Retail		20,000
Cost Percent		.6
Ending Inventory at Cost		12,000

and to recognize the rent expense that has expired during the period by the entry

Rent Expense	$200	
Prepaid Rent		$200

Such an entry should continue to be made until the prepayment has been used up and the rental expense of each of the three-month periods has been recorded in the books of the institution.

Questions for Discussion

1. Distinguish between periodic and perpetual inventory systems. Describe conditions under which the facility should use a perpetual inventory system.
2. Describe briefly the following methods of valuing inventory:

   a. specific invoice method
   b. average weighted cost
   c. LIFO
   c. FIFO
   d. standard cost

3. Define a prepaid expense and give several examples.
4. Describe the retail inventory and gross margin methods of estimating inventory.
5. Explain what is meant by the lower of cost or market rule.

Problems for Solution

1. Suppose the following information pertains to a supply item that is used by the institution:

Central Supply

1/1	Inventory	400 units @	$7.00/unit
1/10	Issue	200 units	
1/14	Purchase	300 units @	$8.00/unit
1/21	Purchase	100 units @	$9.00/unit
1/28	Issue	300 units	

Functional Units

		D_1		D_2	
1/1	Floor Stock	100 units @	$6.00/unit	50 units @	$6.00/unit
1/9	Usage	60 units		10 units	
1/10	Receipt	150 units		50 units	
1/13	Usage	110 units		60 units	
1/28	Receipt	200 units		100 units	

If the institution uses a periodic inventory system, show all entries concerning this item, assuming that the

a. average weighted price
b. LIFO
c. FIFO

methods are used to value inventories.

2. Suppose the institution uses a perpetual inventory system to record transactions. Referring to the information in Problem 1, show all entries, assuming that

a. average weighted cost
b. LIFO
c. FIFO

methods of valuation are employed.

3. Suppose a standard cost system is used to record transactions concerning a given inventory item and that the following information is available:

2/1	Inventory	50 units @	$6.00/unit
2/10	Purchase	100 units @	$7.00/unit
2/14	Used	50 units	
2/21	Purchased	200 units @	$9.00/unit
2/28	Used	100 units	

Assuming a standard cost of $8.00/unit, record all transactions concerning this inventory item.

4. Suppose the following information is provided:

Inventory 1/1	$10,000
Purchases During the Year	60,000
Billings to Patients During the Year	90,000

Assuming that the institution uses a standard markup of 50 percent, estimate the inventory as of December 31.

5. Assume the following information is provided:

	Cost	*Retail*
Inventory 1/1	$9,000	$12,000
Purchases	12,000	16,000
Markups		6,000
Markdowns		8,000
Sales		15,000

Use these data to estimate the December 31 inventory at cost.

6. Suppose the following information pertains to an inventory item that is used in the institution's operations:

Beginning Inventory	200 units @	$5.50
Purchased	100 units @	6.00
Used	150 units	
Purchased	75 units @	10.00
Used	50 units	

Use the weighted average cost, LIFO, and FIFO methods of inventory evaluation to determine the costs of goods used and of goods remaining in inventory under the periodic inventory system.

7. Suppose the following information pertains to a supply item that is used by the institution:

Central Supply

1/1	Inventory	300 units @	$5.00/unit
1/10	Issue	100 units	
1/15	Purchase	400 units @	7.00/unit
1/20	Issue	200 units	
1/31	Purchase	100 units @	8.00/unit

	Functional Unit D_1			*Functional Unit D_2*	
1/1	Floor Stock	60 units @	$5.00	Floor Stock	40 units @ $5.00
1/3	Usage	20 units		Usage	10 units
1/10	Receipt	50 units		Receipt	50 units
1/12	Usage	10 units		Usage	20 units
1/20	Receipt	150 units		Receipt	50 units

Assume that:

a. all acquisitions are recorded as assets
b. the FIFO method of inventory valuation is used
c. the periodic inventory system is employed

Record all entries pertaining to the inventory item.

8. Assume on the basis of the information in Problem 7 that

a. the perpetual inventory system is used and
b. inventory is valued using the LIFO method

Excluding the acquisition of the supply article, record all transactions concerning the inventory item.

9. Assume that a standard costing system is used to record transactions concerning a given inventory item and that the following information is available:

1/1	Inventory	100 units @	$10.00
1/3	Purchase	200 units @	10.00
1/4	Used	150 units	
1/10	Purchased	100 units @	12.00
1/20	Used	150 units	
1/31	Purchased	20 units @	13.00

Assuming a standard cost of $12.00/unit, record all transactions concerning the inventory item.

10. Suppose the following information pertains to an inventory item used by the institution:

	Number of Units	*Unit Cost*
Inventory	10	$5.00
Purchased	20	10.00
Used	15	
Purchased	25	4.50
Used	20	

Using the periodic inventory method, record the transactions concerning this inventory item under the LIFO and FIFO methods of evaluation.

Chapter 10
Accounting for Current Liabilities

The liabilities of the health care facility represent economic obligations resulting from past transactions to pay cash, to remit other noncash assets, or to provide services at a future time. Given the credit-based economic environment in which the industry operates, the balance sheet frequently shows a wide variety of debt instruments representing goods and services purchased on account, borrowings from other institutions, payroll accruals, other payroll-related obligations, and deferred revenues (payments received in advance of providing service). As was seen earlier, almost all cash disbursements involve liabilities of one sort or another that were incurred previously.

The institution's financial obligations usually are classified in accordance with the general nature of their maturity. Some are shown as current liabilities, others as noncurrent or long-term liabilities. This distinction is important when evaluating the ability of the institution to meet maturing commitments to banks and other creditors as well as its financial position. This chapter deals only with the facility's current liabilities; the accounting treatment of long-term or noncurrent liabilities is the subject of Chapter 13.

10.1 THE NATURE OF CURRENT LIABILITIES

Current liabilities usually are defined as obligations that mature and will be paid within one year of the balance sheet date. Although this definition is simple and reasonably satisfactory in many situations, it fails to reflect the essential relationship between current assets and current liabilities. A strict one-year interpretation is much too narrow. A more useful definition designates current liabilities as those whose liquidation is reasonably expected to require the use of current assets or the issuance of other current liabilities. The latter part of this definition recognizes the potential for substituting one liability for another. For example, the institution might issue a note payable to a supplier in settling an account payable. In short, then, current liabilities are obligations that are expected to be liquidated within a short period of time, usually one year, by: (1) using resources classified as current assets or (2) the issuance of another short-term liability.

The current liability classification includes legally enforceable debts resulting from past transactions that will require future outlays in amounts that can be estimated or measured with reasonable accuracy. In certain circumstances, however, legal obligations may be so uncertain in amount that they cannot be measured with precision. As a result, they may not be formally recorded in the accounts but their existence should be disclosed by a parenthetic comment on the balance sheet. On the other hand, future outlays may arise from past transactions that are measurable and should be recorded as current liabilities even though they are not legally enforceable at present. These considerations suggest that an element of uncertainty is involved in the accounting treatment of some of the current liabilities of the health care facility. Most of the amounts associated with current obligations, however, are known with certainty and present little difficulty to the accountant.

In reporting current liabilities on the balance sheet, obligations are listed to reflect the best compromise between the value of the debt (largest to smallest) and the order of maturity dates. Both objectives seldom are satisfied and the amount of the debt usually takes precedence except when there are significant differences among maturity dates. The amount of detail presented will depend on the purposes for which the balance sheet is prepared. For general reporting purposes, it usually is sufficient to disclose broad totals by the major groups of liabilities discussed below: notes payable, accounts payable, liability accruals (payrolls, taxes), vouchers payable, deferred revenue, and current maturities of long-term debt.

10.2 NOTES PAYABLE

A note represents an unconditional promise to pay a definite sum of money on demand or at a fixed or determinable date. To the maker of a note, the document represents a liability. Notes are issued to vendors for supplies or other goods, to other organizations for the purchase of equipment, or to banks or other lending institutions in securing short-term loans. Unlike open accounts that generally fall due within one month, notes payable may be outstanding for longer periods, usually 30, 60, 90, or 180 days. When the maturity date of a note is beyond one year, it should be classified in the balance sheet as a long-term debt.

As seen earlier, liabilities in the form of notes payable may be secured by the pledge of certain assets such as accounts receivable or marketable securities. When such a security is pledged, its value should be disclosed in a footnote or by the accounting entries described earlier. In this way, the reader of the balance sheet is advised that the use or disposition of the proceeds from these assets is limited until the obligation has been satisfied.

10.2.1 Purchasing Capital Equipment

Notes payable are issued in purchasing capital assets that are characterized by a high purchase price or an excessively long credit period. Instead of buying the equipment on an open account, the institution may issue its note in exchange for the asset. For example, assume that a piece of equipment is acquired in exchange for a one-year $22,000 note with no reference to an explicit interest rate. If money is worth 10 percent per year (an assumed interest rate) the asset is recorded at its cash equivalent or the present value of the note. Thus, the entry to record the acquisition of the equipment is:

Equipment	$20,000	
Discount on Note Payable	2,000	
Note Payable		$22,000

To record the acquisition of equipment and liability at present value ($22,000/1.10).

The cost of the equipment for purposes of calculating depreciation is $20,000 and the discount is amortized to monthly interest expense through a series of accrual entries during the life of the note. For example, the monthly amortization of the discount involves the entry:

Interest Expense	$166.67	
Discount on Note Payable		$166.67

To amortize discount on note payable ($2,000/12).

In the balance sheet, any unamortized balance is deducted from the full value of the note and the interest expense is included in the income statement as is any other expenditure.

10.2.2 Obtaining an Extension of Time

A note also may be given to obtain an extension of time on an open account. For example, suppose the institution is unable to pay an account with M & F Supplies, which agrees to accept a 60-day, 6 percent, $400 note in settlement of the account. Clearly, M & F Supplies prefers the note to the open account since it represents written evidence of the debt and its amount. In this example, the note is recorded in the books of the institution by the following journal entry:

Accounts Payable—M & F Supplies	$400	
Note Payable		$400

To record the 60-day, 6 percent note in settlement or an open account.

The note does not liquidate the debt; rather, the entry simply changes the composition of the liability from an account payable to a note payable.

When the note becomes due, assume that the facility pays the principal plus the interest charges. The entry to record the payment is:

Note Payable	$400.00	
Interest Expense	4.14	
Cash		$404.14

To record payment of note and 63 days' interest.

10.2.3 Financing with Notes Payable

Finally, the institution may execute a note in obtaining a loan from a bank. In lending money, banks usually distinguish between a loan and a discount. In the case of a loan, the bank collects interest when it is repaid; for a discount, it deducts the interest when the loan is made. To illustrate the difference between loans and discounts, suppose that a hospital borrows $1,200 by issuing a 60-day, 7 percent note.

In lending the hospital the $1,200, the bank issues a loan in exchange for the note. The hospital records the transaction as follows:

Cash	$1,200.00	
Note Payable		$1,200.00

To record bank loan and issuance of related note.

When the note and interest are paid, the hospital records the following entry:

Note Payable	$1,200.00	
Interest Expense	14.50	
Cash		$1,214.50

To record payment of 60-day note and 63 days' interest.

In the case of a loan, interest expense is entered only when the note payable is extinguished.

If the bank is in the practice of deducting the interest at the time the loan is made, it discounts the hospital's note. If it does this, it deducts, from the face value of the note, 63 days' interest at 7 percent, which is $14.50 as above, and gives the hospital $1,185.50 ($1,200 − $14.50) that is called the proceeds of the note. The hospital then records the cash receipt and the related liability as follows:

Cash	$1,185.50	
Interest Expense	14.50	
Note Payable		$1,200.00

When the note matures, the hospital pays only the face value of the note and the payment is recorded by the entry:

Note Payable	$1,200.00	
Cash		$1,200.00

When the bank discounts the note, interest is deducted and recorded as an expense when the money is borrowed.

10.3 ACCOUNTS PAYABLE

Accounts payable usually emanate from the purchase of goods or services on account. As indicated in Chapter 6, the accounting procedures for this current liability must be systematized so that its existence, the amount due, the due date, and the entity to whom the institution is indebted may be discerned easily.

When the hospital uses the gross invoice method and it is expected that discounts will be taken in material amounts, these discounts should be anticipated. The entry required involves a debit to an Allowance for Purchase Discounts account and a credit to purchase discounts. The allowance account is then subtracted from the accounts payable in the balance sheet section reporting current liabilities. When the accounts are paid, the allowance account is eliminated by corresponding credits. If the net invoice cost method is used, however, such adjustments are unnecessary.

10.4 LIABILITY ACCRUALS

Accrued liabilities arise out of past transactions and operations that involve contractual commitments or tax legislation. In reporting accrued liabilities, it is common to report payroll liabilities and payroll-related accruals separate from other accruals such as rent, interest, etc., because of their materiality.

10.4.1 Accrued Payroll

Employees usually are paid periodically and the end of pay periods need not necessarily correspond to the end of an accounting period. As a result, it is not uncommon for the hospital's balance sheet to contain a current liability for unpaid wages and salaries. For example, if the institution pays its employees twice a month, a pay period can begin on Monday while the accounting period ends on Friday of the same week. Hence, the facility owes its employees for five days of work and the balance sheet therefore must include a liability for the unpaid salaries and wages earned during the five-day period.

In most cases, the accrual is made on a gross basis without recording the deductions mentioned earlier. The calculation of payroll accruals on an individual basis can be a tedious task that most institutions minimize by simply determining the average wage and salary cost per day and multiplying it by the number of days between the last pay date and the end of the accounting period. If, in the example above, the salary and wage cost for all employees is calculated to be $40,000 per day, the amount of unpaid salaries and wages earned at period's end is $200,000 ($40,000/day × 5 days). The entry to record the accrual is:

Salaries & Wages Expense	$200,000	
Salary & Wages Payable		$200,000

To record accrued salaries and wages.

At the beginning of the following period, the entry is reversed. In this way, the salary and wage expense is recorded in the period in which it is incurred, which means that a misstatement of net income has been avoided when evaluating periodic operating results.

10.4.2 Other Payroll Accruals

As mentioned earlier, the other major forms of payroll accruals include vacation pay, payroll withholdings, tax accruals, and deductions for health insurance premiums. As described in Chapter 4, these accruals must be recorded in accordance with sound accounting conventions if the information in the financial statements is to portray accurately the operating results of the period and the financial position of the institution at the end of the period.

10.5 VOUCHERS PAYABLE

In accounting, a voucher is a business paper on which a transaction is summarized and its correctness certified. A voucher system is developed to gain control over the accuracy of obligations as well as of the resulting cash disbursement. In a medium-to-large health facility, the individual signing the check is unable to be personally familiar with each transaction requiring a cash disbursement and thus cannot attest to the accuracy or validity of the cash outflow. In such a situation, the person signing the check must depend on an internal control system that indicates that a liability is a proper obligation and should be paid. The voucher constitutes the document upon which such a system is based.

The voucher also provides the basis for recording a liability and approving its payment. The voucher system gains control over cash disbursements by providing a routine that permits only certain departments or individuals to incur obligations requiring a cash disbursement. The system establishes the procedures for the verification, approval, and recording of obligations. In addition, the voucher system permits checks to be issued only in payment of properly verified, approved, and recorded obligations. Every liability is treated as a separate transaction and is recorded at the time it is incurred even though the institution may purchase supplies from the same vendor during a given operating cycle.

When a voucher system is in effect, control over cash outflows begins with obligations that will result in cash disbursements. As mentioned above, only certain individuals or departments are authorized to incur such obligations. Control is gained by establishing a more or less inflexible routine that must be followed for each kind of obligation and for evaluating as well as validating appropriate papers.

Consider, for example, the acquisition of supply items and recall the process by which they are obtained. If it is found that a particular item is required in the operation of a unit, the manager of the entity requests stock from central supply by completing a requisition slip. If the item is out of stock or the requisition will reduce the stock below acceptable levels, central supply will request the purchasing department to order more of the required item. That department issues a purchase order to the supplier, who ships the item and mails an invoice to the accounting department. The receiving department then examines the shipment and reports the results of the inspection to the accounting department in the form of a receiving report. The accounting department compares the requisition slip, the purchase order, the invoice, and the receiving report, thus providing the basis for approving the invoice for entry in the books and for ultimate payment. After the comparisons have been completed, a voucher is prepared that involves nothing more than summarizing the information in the invoice. After being approved by an independent crosscheck, the voucher is recorded and filed until its due date and cash is disbursed by a properly executed and authorized check.

When a voucher system is in use, an account called Vouchers Payable replaces the Accounts Payable one described in earlier chapters. As a result, when supply items are purchased, the voucher pertaining to the acquisition is recorded as a debit to inventory and a credit to Vouchers Payable. When the voucher is paid, payment is recorded by a debit to Vouchers Payable and a credit to Cash.

The substitution of the Voucher Payable Account for Accounts Payable is a small procedural change. However, the use of the account in recording expenses, such as wages and salaries, represents a somewhat greater change. To gain control over cash payments, *all* obligations resulting in a cash disbursement must be approved for payment and recorded as a liability (Vouchers Payable) when they are incurred. As a result, every expense of the institution must be verified and recorded as a voucher payable in the same way as a voucher is prepared and validated for an inventory acquisition. The basic difference, of course, is that the entry results in a debit to the appropriate expense category and a credit to Vouchers Payable.

Vouchers are recorded in a Voucher Register. Since they are prepared for the acquisition of all assets, goods, and services as well as the payment of all expenses, the Voucher Register represents an expansion of the Supply Acquisition Journal described earlier. As a result, the Voucher Register replaces the Supply Acquisition Journal.

The exact form of the Voucher Register may vary from institution to institution but in general it provides for the date, creditor's name, voucher number, and a record of voucher payments. There also is a column in which credits to the Voucher Payable account are recorded and several columns in which the corresponding debit associated with each transaction is shown. The columns may vary from facility to facility, but essentially two sets of debit columns should be provided: (1) pertaining to inventory acquisitions and (2) pertaining to the payment of all other expenses. The portions of the Voucher Register presented here are intended to be only illustrative in nature.

Table 10-1 is the portion of the Voucher Register involving the acquisition of inventory. The similarity between this and the Supply Acquisition Journal referred to earlier should be readily apparent. The basic difference in format involves the column provided for credit entries to Vouchers Payable (rather than an account payable, as in the Supply Acquisition Journal) and the column that indicates the date the voucher is paid. The table shows that the institution's inventory acquisitions are recorded in accordance with the accounting principles outlined in the preceding paragraph. Here, it is assumed that the institution engaged in the transactions summarized in Table 10-2. In each case in Table 10-1, the entry involves a credit to the Vouchers Payable account and a debit to the appropriate inventory account. As before, the acquisition of items maintained on a perpetual inventory basis is recorded immediately in the subsidiary inventory records. Information on the check numbers and payment dates are entered as each voucher is paid. The remaining information is listed as soon as each is validated and approved.

Table 10-1 Voucher Register: Inventory Acquisition

							Inventory			
Date	*Voucher No.*	*Payee*	*When Paid*	*Check No.*	*Vouchers Payable Credit*	*Freight In Debit*	*Surgical & Medical Debit*	*Food Supplies Debit*	*Drug Supplies Debit*	*General Supplies Debit*
1/1	1	M & F Co.	1/9	3	$10,000		$10,000			
1/7	3	Schaarf Co.	1/16	5	14,000					$14,000
1/10	5	Blue Co.	1/18	7	7,000			$7,000		
1/15	7	Sticks & Stones	1/19	9	12,000				$12,000	
1/20	9	A & B Food	1/25	11	16,000			16,000		
		Totals			59,000		10,000	23,000	12,000	14,000

Table 10-2 Listing of Transactions

Date	*Creditor*	*Payment Date*	*Ch. No.*	*Type of Supply*	*Cost*
1/1	M & F Co.	1/9	3	Surgical & Medical	$10,000
1/7	Schaarf Co.	1/16	5	General Supplies	14,000
1/10	Blue Co.	1/18	7	Food	7,000
1/15	Sticks & Stones	1/19	9	Drugs	12,000
1/20	A & B Food	1/25	11	Food	16,000

A portion of the voucher register for the expenses of the General Services Division of a hospital is shown in Table 10-3. The records involve a credit entry to the Vouchers Payable account and a debit entry to the appropriate expense category. The latter deserves further comment.

In Table 10-3, a primary three-digit code described earlier is entered in the Account Code column. The code identifies the expense center or unit incurring the expenditure. In addition, each transaction carries a secondary expense code that identifies the object of the expenditure. Consider, for example, the entry that records the voucher and payment of the facility's telephone bill. This entry results in a credit to the Vouchers Payable account and a debit entry to the expense account identified by the code 730.91. As discussed earlier, the first three digits (730) identify the expense center or department incurring the expense while the second two (91) refer to the type or object of the expenditure. Thus, in this case, the code 730.91 identifies the account to be credited as a telephone expense of the hospital's general administration. The remaining entries in this column identify the department incurring the expense and the object of the expenditure.

The use of code numbers to identify the expense center and object of expenditure facilitates the placement of expense accounts in subsidiary expense ledgers and the maintenance of accounts that control expenditures in the general ledger. When this practice is used, the usual technique is to post column totals to the control account of the general ledger and post individual accounts to the subsidiary expense ledgers.

When vouchers are used, some are paid as soon as recorded while others are filed according to their due date. This assists the institution in taking advantage of cash discounts since it automatically brings the voucher to the attention of management on its due date. In addition, the unpaid voucher file is a subsidiary record of creditors' accounts and, just as the Vouchers Payable account is substituted for the Accounts Payable account in the general ledger, the unpaid voucher file is substituted for the subsidiary Accounts Payable

Table 10-3 Voucher Register: General Services Division Expenses

						Expense Center—General Services Division									
						Administration		*Dietary*		*Laundry*		*Housekeeping*		*Plant Op.*	
Date	*Voucher No.*	*Payee*	*Ch. No.*	*When Paid*	*Voucher Payable Credit*	*Acct. Code*	*Amount Debit*	*Acct. Code*	*Amt. Debit*	*Acct. Code*	*Amt. Debit*	*Acct. Code*	*Amt. Debit*	*Acct. Code*	*Amt. Debit*
1/3	2	Frank Jones	4	1/3	$70	730.09	$70								
1/9	4	Betty Smith	6	1/9	100			755.09	$100						
1/11	6	Telephone Co.	8	1/11	110	730.91	110								
1/16	8	George Jay	10	1/16	300									770.09	$300
1/21	10	C. Finch	12	1/21	500					760.09	$500				
1/30	11	M. Clement	13	1/30	600							760.04	$600		
		Total			1,680		180		100		500		600		300

ledger. Consequently, after posting is complete, the balance of the Vouchers Payable account should equal the sum of the unpaid vouchers in the unpaid vouchers file as well as the sum of the vouchers listed as unpaid in the Voucher Register.

10.6 DEFERRED REVENUE

As mentioned earlier, when payment is received before service is provided, the institution incurs a liability that is called a deferred revenue. The accounting procedures for this category have been discussed; it will be recalled that prepayments of this sort must be recorded as a liability when received.

Many hospitals operate a formal education program under which students may pay tuition in advance. These receipts should be recorded as a deferred revenue. Tuition prepayments are earned and recognized as revenue as the program progresses through the school year or term. As revenue is earned, entries are recorded to transfer the deferred revenue to a tuition revenue account. This procedure gives proper accounting recognition to the facility's obligations and provides the basis for the appropriate matching of revenue and expenses.

It is possible to report all deferred revenue accounts in a separate balance sheet classification located between current and long-term liabilities. However, such a procedure fails to indicate whether the deferred revenue is a current or long-term liability and, as a consequence, serious misinterpretations of the financial position of the institution may result. This consideration indicates that the practice of reporting deferred revenues under a separate classification should be avoided.

10.7 CURRENT MATURITIES OF LONG-TERM LIABILITIES

Mortgages, bonds, and other long-term obligations of the institution should be reported as current liabilities to the extent they are to be paid within one year and involve current assets. In many cases, long-term debts mature in installments and a portion of the debt is reported as a current liability, with the remainder appearing as a long-term obligation. However, if the payment of the maturing portion does not involve current assets and will be paid from noncurrent assets such as a debt retirement fund, the obligation is listed as a long-term debt.

Questions for Discussion

1. Define the term current liability.

2. Describe a voucher and how a voucher system helps management gain control over cash disbursements.
3. Describe the use of a voucher register.
4. List conditions under which an obligation should be reported as a current liability. Explain why it is necessary to distinguish between current and long-term liabilities.
5. Define the term deferred revenue. Explain why deferred revenues are reported in the liability section of the balance sheet.

Problems for Solution

1. Suppose the institution issues a 90-day 10 percent $1,000 note to the bank. Assume further that the note is paid on day 93. Record all transactions concerning the note, assuming that

    a. the loan is obtained
    b. the bank discounts the note

2. Suppose that the note in Problem 1 is paid on day 65 rather than day 93. Record all transactions concerning the note.
3. Suppose that on January 1, the institution acquires a piece of equipment in exchange for a noninterest-bearing $11,400 note that is due in one year. If money is worth 14 percent per year, record the acquisition and the entries required on January 31.
4. Suppose the institution operates an educational program for which the annual tuition fees are $300 per student. Suppose further that the fees are collected on August 25 and that classes begin on September 1. If 1,200 students enroll, prepare the journal entries required on August 25 and September 30.
5. Suppose the following information pertains to the supply items acquired by the institution in January:

Date	*Vendor*	*Type of Supply*	*Amount*
1/1	J & G Co.	Drugs	$12,000
1/8	Binge Co.	Food	15,000
1/13	H & D Co.	Medical	20,000
1/20	Blimp Co.	Food	17,000
1/25	T & J Co.	General	6,000
1/28	S & C Co.	Surgical	7,000

Use a Voucher Register to record these acquisitions.

6. Suppose that on January 1 it is found that the institution requires $20,000. If the hospital issues a 90-day, 10 percent note, which is paid on day 60, record all transactions concerning this note, assuming that

   a. the bank issues a loan
   b. the bank discounts the note

7. Suppose the institution issues a 60-day, 12 percent, $3,000 note. Assume that the note is paid on day 45. Record all transactions concerning the note assuming that

   a. a loan is obtained
   b. the bank discounted the note

8. Suppose the institution issues a 90-day, 8 percent, $5,000 note to the bank and pays it off on day 62. Record the transactions concerning this note, assuming that:

   a. a loan is negotiated
   b. the bank discounts the note

9. Suppose the hospital exchanges a one-year $33,000 noninterest-bearing note for a piece of capital equipment. Assuming that money is worth 10 percent per year, record the acquisition. Indicate whether monthly entries are required and, if so, what they are.

Chapter 11

Accounting for Restricted Funds

Health facilities frequently receive donations, grants, and bequests from external donors who may restrict the use of these resources to specific purposes. The institution assumes a legal obligation to use or otherwise dispose of these resources in conformity with the donor's restrictions. From time to time, it must document its use of these funds and demonstrate that they have been used in a manner consistent with the donor's wishes. Fund accounting is the primary tool by which management controls these restricted assets and establishes accountability for them.

In accounting for restricted funds, procedures that must be considered are:

1. the receipt of funds during the period
2. the recording of income earned by the investment of these funds
3. the recording of expenditures or the disposition of special purpose funds
4. the maintenance of the record of equity
5. the closing entries for the restricted fund grouping(s)

This chapter discusses each of these elements. However, the recording of revenue earned by investing restricted funds receives only brief attention here because it was covered extensively in Chapter 8.

11.1 THE RECEIPT OF RESTRICTED FUNDS

Restricted funds may take the form either of an endowment or of another resource whose use is limited to specific purposes that are identified by the donor. The receipt of each type of restricted asset is discussed next.

11.1.1 Endowments

An endowment is a grant, donation, or bequest that may be used to earn investment income while maintaining the principal intact. The use of revenue thus earned may be either restricted to specific purposes or unrestricted and available for the institution's operating needs.

In either case, an endowment should receive accounting recognition when it is received. Assuming that the receipt of endowments is recorded on an accrual basis, the entry to record this involves a debit to a receivable account and a credit to a restricted fund income or equity account. Assume, for example, that on March 17 the institution becomes certain that it will receive an endowment of $100,000 from the estate of M. Rich. Further, suppose the investment income that will be earned on the bequest is unrestricted and the facility may use these revenues to meet current operating needs. The entry required in the Endowment Fund on March 17 is:

Bequests and Legacies Receivable	$100,000	
Bequests and Legacies—Endowment (Investment Income Unrestricted)		$100,000

To record the bequest of M. Rich.

Conversely, assume that this investment income is restricted by the terms of the Rich will. In that case, the receivable account is debited as above but the corresponding credit entry is to a different revenue account that indicates the restricted nature of the investment income that may be earned from the endowment. The entry to record an endowment for which investment income is restricted is:

Bequests and Legacies Receivable	$100,000	
Bequests and Legacies—Endowment (Investment Income Restricted)		$100,000

To record the bequest of M. Rich.

When the cash or noncash asset is received, the appropriate asset account of the Endowment Fund is debited while the Bequests and Legacies Receivable account is eliminated by the corresponding credit entry. In the case of M. Rich, assume that the endowment is in the form of cash. The entry in the Endowment Fund to record the cash receipt is:

Cash—Endowment Fund	$100,000	
Bequests and Legacies Receivable		$100,000

To record the cash receipt associated with the M. Rich endowment.

The recording of the receipt of the endowment is not sufficient in discharging the stewardship function and the associated fiduciary responsibilities. To provide detailed information on the receipt of restricted funds, any income or expenses associated with their investment, and, if the donor permits, their disposal, a set of subsidiary accounts is maintained to record such transactions. The methods for maintaining the records of equity are discussed briefly in Section 11.4.

11.1.2 Specific Purpose Funds

In addition to endowments, health facilities frequently receive grants, donations, or pledges that may be expended only on special projects specified by the donor. For example, suppose the hospital receives $75,000 from the Red Cross with the stipulation that this must be used to defray the costs of a particular research project. If the donation is recorded before the cash is received, the required entry involves a debit to an asset account and a credit entry to a revenue or to an appropriated equity account that indicates that the funds may be expended for special purposes only. As a result, the donation is recorded as follows:

Donations and Bequests Receivable	$75,000	
Appropriated Equity—Specific Purpose Fund		$75,000

To record the donation of the Red Cross.

When the cash is received, the entry

Cash—Specific Purpose Fund	$75,000	
Donations and Bequests Receivable		$75,000

records the cash receipt and reduces the donations and bequests receivable account by $75,000. As in the case of the receipt of an endowment, the acquisition of special purpose funds also should be recorded in a subsidiary record.

11.1.3 Capital Funds

As mentioned earlier, the receipt of funds that are restricted by donors and third party payers to the future acquisition of plant and equipment are recorded in the Capital Fund. Historically, the first entry pertaining to funds restricted to the future acquisition of capital was recorded at the time the cash or the noncash asset was received. However, to provide a more accurate portrayal of financial position, pledges, donations, and contributions should be recorded as an asset when it is certain that they will be received. When this practice is followed, capital grants and pledges should be recorded as debits to accounts such as Capital Donations Receivable or Capital Pledges

Receivable, depending on the type of funding. In addition, the receivable account may be modified to indicate the source of the capital funding. An offsetting credit entry is recorded in an appropriate equity account of the Capital Fund.

For illustration, assume that on May 28 the hospital is notified by a third party that a $10,000 capital donation that may be used only for the future acquisition of plant and equipment will be made available on June 3. Once it is certain that the institution will receive the donation, the corresponding receivable is recognized in the Capital Fund as follows:

Capital Donation Receivable	$10,000	
Capital Fund Equity		$10,000

The entry to record the cash receipt on June 3 is given by

Cash—Capital Fund	$10,000	
Capital Donation Receivable		$10,000

This entry increases the cash balance of the Capital Fund and eliminates the receivable that was recognized on May 28.

As noted, health care facilities occasionally acquire funds by issuing a debt instrument such as a bond, a note payable, or a loan payable. In such a situation, the cash receipt and the corresponding liability should be recorded in the Unrestricted Fund.

For example, suppose the hospital negotiates a 6 percent, 180-day, $70,000 note and the board of directors specifies that the proceeds must be used to acquire capital equipment. The transaction is recorded by the following entry:

Cash—Unrestricted Fund	$70,000	
Note Payable		$70,000

It also may be necessary to separate the funds that must be used for the future acquisition of capital equipment from the other Unrestricted Funds. In such a situation the hospital can use one of the board-designated accounts referred to earlier and record the following entry:

Cash—Board-Designated Capital Fund	$70,000	
Cash—Unrestricted Fund		$70,000

This procedure represents the accounting technique by which management ensures that the desires of the board are satisfied, at the same time gaining control over the portion of the Unrestricted Fund that is subject to board designation.

As has been mentioned, funds that are limited to capital acquisition are available for earning investment income until expended on the designated plant expansion or replacement. In that case, investment income is recorded on the accrual basis while gains or losses from the sale of investment instruments are entered on a cash basis. The fund into which investment income is recorded also must conform with the donor's desires.

11.2 THE EXPENDITURE OF RESTRICTED FUNDS

Expenditures associated with restricted funds are of two types:

1. Expenditures incurred in the process of earning investment income, including interest on a mortgage that may be related to property held as an endowment, and other expenses related to property such as taxes, occupancy expenses, manager's fees, etc.
2. Expenditures involving costs necessary to fulfill the purposes for which the funds were received.

It is important to note that the expenditures incurred in earning investment income should be recorded in the Specific Purpose Fund or the Endowment Fund if—and only if—the investment income is credited to a revenue account of the fund. On the other hand, if the investment income is entered in the Unrestricted Fund, the expenditures incurred in earning the revenue also must be recorded in that fund. These procedures represent an application of the accounting principle that requires a matching of expenses and the revenues they helped to produce so as to obtain a proper determination of net income. Thus, expenditures incurred in earning investment income must be recorded in the fund in which the revenue is recorded.

11.2.1 Accounting Procedures

The recording of expenditures incurred in carrying out special purposes designated by the donor usually involves the Unrestricted Fund and one of the Restricted Funds. First, an entry must be recorded in the Specific Purpose Fund or the Capital Fund to reduce the fund equity held for the designated purpose. Normally, cash is disbursed through the Unrestricted Fund where the normal operating accounts are maintained. As a result, it is necessary to transfer funds from the Specific Purpose Fund or the Capital Fund to the Unrestricted Fund. Funds are usually transferred to the operating fund where they will be used to offset or finance expenditures on the designated project. Assume for example that the hospital receives $175,000 to finance a research project that, during the current period, incurs costs of $100,000. Also assume that the original receipt of these funds is recorded in the Specific Purpose Fund as indicated earlier. To transfer these funds, two fund groups are affected, with the following entries:

Specific Purpose Fund

(1) Transfer to the Unrestricted Fund	$100,000	
Due to Unrestricted Fund		$100,000
(2) Due to Unrestricted Fund	100,000	
Cash		100,000

Unrestricted Fund

(3) Cash	$100,000	
Special Research Grant		$100,000

In entry (1) above, the Transfer to the Unrestricted Fund account represents a nominal account that, when closed at the end of the accounting period, reduces the equity of the Specific Purpose Fund. The second element of the transaction establishes the obligation of the Specific Purpose Fund to the Unrestricted Fund. Entries (2) and (3) effect the transfer of cash from the Specific Purpose Fund to the Unrestricted Fund. In entry (3), the debit to cash, which records the receipt of cash in the Unrestricted Fund, is offset by a credit entry to the Special Research Grants revenue account. Since the primary purpose for which these funds were received has been satisfied, the revenue is earned and recognized in the Unrestricted Fund where the expenditure is recorded as follows:

Expense—Research Project	$100,000	
Cash		$100,000

Since entry (3) results in a $100,000 debit to cash and a $100,000 credit to a revenue account, it can be seen that:

1. the two cash entries in the Unrestricted Fund are offsetting
2. the expenses incurred in conducting the research are offset exactly by the recognition of revenue that is earned after performing the research
3. other things held constant, the equity of the Unrestricted Fund is unchanged and the equity of the Specific Purpose Fund is reduced by the $100,000 cash outlay

The effects on the equity of the Unrestricted and Specific Purpose funds are recorded during the closing process, which is described in Section 11.3.

11.2.2 Encumbrance Accounting

The segregation of the assets of the Specific Purpose Fund and the Endowment Fund tends to preclude the possibility of expending resources on purposes other than those specified by the donor. However, there still is a need to ensure that funds are not spent on a project after resources available for the purpose have been exhausted. This implies that expenditures that are financed from the Specific Purpose Fund must be authorized. The expenditure should be compared with the balance of the fund to ensure that the balance is large enough to absorb the outlay. It also is necessary to ensure that authorization is not granted for two expenditures that individually do not exceed the balance but do so when considered jointly. For example, if a fund has a balance of $12,000 on January 15, and expenditures of $7,000 and $6,000 are authorized on January 16 and January 18, respectively, both might be authorized since each is less than the balance. However, when taken together, the authorization of the two will exceed the balance.

Unless the volume of restricted funds is very large, this problem may be resolved on an informal basis. However, in other cases it may be necessary to establish more formal controls in the form of encumbrances. Basically, encumbrance accounting is nothing more than establishing an amount available for expenditure as a credit balance. Each authorized expenditure is charged against the balance. As a result, the unencumbered credit balance represents the amount still available for the project. Thus, encumbrance accounting permits management to control funds restricted to specific purposes and thereby to avoid authorizing overspending.

For illustration, suppose the institution is given $20,000 that must be used to meet expenditures for a particular research project. To establish the amounts available for the project, the following entry is required:

Authorized Special Fund Expenditures	$20,000	
Available Special Funds		$20,000

Naturally, supplies are required during the course of the research and the required purchase orders are executed. At this point the special funds become committed and should be reduced to reflect the commitment. Assuming the supplies purchased are valued at $400, the entry

Available Special Funds	$400	
Encumbrances Outstanding		$400

reduces the special funds available from the original $20,000 to a balance of $19,600, which accurately reflects the sum that is uncommitted and available for future spending.

Once the supplies have been received, the outstanding encumbrances should be transformed into an account payable while preserving the balance of $19,600. This is accomplished by the entry:

Encumbrances Outstanding	$400	
Accounts Payable		$400

At the end of the accounting period, the original entry is reserved, as are any outstanding encumbrances. As a consequence, the balance available in the special fund account represents actual expenditures charged to the fund. In turn, the balance of the available special fund account is eliminated by the closing entries recorded at the end of the reporting period.

11.3 CLOSING ENTRIES

At the end of the year, or at more frequent intervals, the nominal accounts of the Specific Purpose Fund and the Capital Fund must be closed to the equity of the fund. As was seen in Chapter 2, there are two steps involved in the process by which the nominal accounts are closed to equity: (1) the revenue and expense accounts are closed to a revenue and expense summary; (2) the balance of the revenue and expense summary, which indicates the net addition to or the net reduction in the equity of the fund, is then closed to the fund balance. The process of closing the nominal accounts of the Restricted Fund group is similar to the closing entries discussed in Chapter 2.

11.4 MAINTAINING THE RECORD OF EQUITY

As mentioned earlier in this chapter, the maintenance of detailed information is required to discharge the fiduciary responsibility management assumes when it receives restricted funds. Thus, when expendable funds are received for more than one distinguishable purpose, it is necessary to establish subsidiary records to enter detailed information on the receipt of funds, restricted investment income earned, expenses, any other additions to equity, and the eventual disposal of the resource.

Such subsidiary records are controlled by the equity accounts of the relevant fund grouping. The accounting department or other persons who might be responsible for the approval of expenditures from the restricted funds also must have ready access to any documents that limit the use of donated resources.

Questions for Discussion

1. Explain the purposes for which the health care facility might receive restricted funds. Describe how restricted funds are reflected in the accounts of the institution.
2. Define conditions under which an endowment might become available to finance operating expenses.
3. Explain why restricted funds should be recorded on an accrual basis.
4. Describe the primary purpose of encumbrance accounting.
5. Describe the importance of the record of equity.
6. Describe the types of transactions that should be considered when accounting for restricted funds and the importance of each?

Problems for Solution

1. Suppose that on January 1 the institution receives $6,000 that must be used to defray the costs of providing care to indigent patients. During the year, the cost of charity care amounts to $4,500. Show the entries required to record these transactions.
2. Suppose that on April 1, the facility receives $60,000 that must be used to defray the costs of a specific research project. Also suppose that the following information is available:

   April 4 Ordered $500 of supplies
   April 8 Order of April 4 received
   April 13 Ordered supplies of $1,200
   April 20 Order of April 13 received
   April 25 Ordered supplies of $7,000

   Use encumbrance accounting to record these transactions. Explain what entry is required on April 30.
3. Suppose that on January 1 the hospital receives $1,000 from the estate of J. K. Will. These funds may be used to defray the costs of the health education program after April 1. If this bequest is used to finance expenses of $200 during the month of April, show the entries required to record:

   a. the receipt of the funds
   b. the transfer of the funds
   c. the expenditure of the funds

4. Suppose that on January 1 the facility receives $100,000 that must be used to acquire capital equipment. On March 1 these funds are used to

purchase $50,000 worth of equipment. Show the journal entries that record these transactions.

5. Assume the institution negotiates a 10 percent, 180-day $100,000 note and that the board specifies that the proceeds must be used to renovate the operating room. Show the journal entries required to record all aspects of the transaction.

Chapter 12
Accounting for Plant and Equipment

The term plant and equipment refers to physical assets that are of a relatively permanent nature and are not intended for resale. Capital assets are used repeatedly in the process by which patient care is provided. This category of assets includes land, land improvements, buildings, and several types of equipment. This chapter is concerned with the accounting problems associated with the health care facility's investment in these assets as well as the methods by which the depreciation on fixed or capital assets is computed and recorded, all of which are critical to sound management.

The health care sector has an extremely large investment in plant and equipment—for some institutions, as much as 60 percent of their assets. The substantial investment of resources in plant and equipment is a reflection of the rapid changes in medical technology and the increased importance of the health care facility in the system by which medical services are provided to the population at risk. Quite frequently, the funds for capital acquisition must be borrowed. Institutions must give careful consideration to their capability of financing the debt burden as well as to the terms of repaying these obligations. The nature of capital equipment implies that management's investment decisions exert long-term effects on the health delivery system and the care provided to the community.

For these and other reasons, sound investment decisions on the acquisition of plant and equipment are critical. Further, once acquired, the effective management of plant and equipment requires accurate plant asset and depreciation records.

12.1 TRANSFER OF PREVIOUSLY RESTRICTED FUNDS

Accounting procedures for recording the receipt of funds that are restricted to the acquisition of plant and equipment have been discussed in Chapter 11.

To transfer funds from the Capital Fund, where the receipt of restricted assets is recorded originally, to the Unrestricted Fund, where the resources are used to acquire capital assets, a series of transfer entries are required in those two funds. For example, if funds restricted to the future acquisition of capital are recorded originally in the Capital Fund, the entries:

Capital Fund

Transfer to Unrestricted Fund	$xx,xxx	
Cash		$xx,xxx

Unrestricted Fund

Cash	$xx,xxx	
Unrestricted Fund Appropriated Equity		$xx,xxx

serve to transfer cash assets from the Capital Fund to the Unrestricted Fund, where they will be used to purchase plant assets. The Transfer to the Unrestricted Fund account is treated as a temporary or nominal account of the Capital Fund; as such, this account is closed to the equity account at the end of the period.

As is noted in detail later, the cost of plant assets is recorded directly in an expense account or to an asset account that is subject to depreciation charges. In either case, the depreciation expense or the direct charge to a capital expense account are nominal accounts that are closed at the end of the period. Other things remaining constant, the equity account is reduced by the amount of the recorded expense when these accounts are closed.

12.2 ACQUISITION OF PLANT AND EQUIPMENT

When plant assets are purchased, records of the acquisition must be established and maintained. This requires a proper classification of capital assets and the proper determination of their cost. The acquisition also should be recorded in a subsidiary ledger and subjected to an internal control system that pertains to the facility's plant and equipment.

12.2.1 Classification

When recording transactions related to plant assets, it is convenient to use several major accounts. The following discussion identifies these accounts and describes the items of plant and equipment usually associated with each.

12.2.1.1 Land

This account reflects the cost of land owned by the institution and used in day-to-day operations. Items included are (1) purchase price; (2) buying costs such as commissions, legal fees, and title registration; (3) surveys, drilling, etc.; and (4) any accrued property taxes incurred by the institution. Land held for future expansion and not in use should be recorded as a long-term investment while land available for immediate resale should be shown as a current asset. Unlike buildings and equipment, land does not deteriorate and is not subject to depreciation.

12.2.1.2 Land Improvements

This category includes depreciable assets and reflects improvements in the usefulness of the land owned by the institution. Depreciation should be taken on land improvements such as on-site sewers, fences, sidewalks, parking lots, drainage systems, and lighting systems.

12.2.1.3 Buildings

The control account for buildings includes the cost or other valuations of structures owned by the institution, including those used in day-to-day activity, residences for personnel, storage areas, and utility structures. When buildings are purchased, the costs include the basic price, commissions, legal fees, title investigations, and renovation expenses if they are recognized as necessary.

12.2.1.4 Building Service or Fixed Equipment

This account includes the costs or other valuations of equipment that is affixed to and is a structural component of the building and is not usually subject to removal. Examples of building service equipment are elevators, generators, pumps, and other machines required to heat, light, or ventilate the facility and otherwise make it useful. Equipment of this sort has a relatively long life, but usually shorter than that of the building itself.

12.2.1.5 Major Movable Equipment

This category includes equipment items that have:

1. a relatively high unit cost
2. a more or less fixed location in the building, although such assets may be transferred from one location to another
3. an estimated life of more than five years

4. an economic value sufficiently large to justify the expense of controlling the item by means of a subsidiary record
5. an economic value great enough to justify the amortization of related costs throughout its useful life

In addition to these characteristics, items of major movable equipment possess an individuality that permits precise identification. Desks, cardiac synchronization systems, autopsy tables, and autoanalyzers are examples.

12.2.1.6 Minor Equipment

This classification includes equipment items that:

1. have a relatively small unit cost
2. have no fixed location in the facility and are small in size
3. are subject to requisition and use by various departments
4. are numerous in quantity and subject to storeroom control
5. have a maximum useful life of less than five years

Examples of minor equipment are wastebaskets, bedpans, sheets, glassware, basins, baskets, silverware, etc. In accounting for minor equipment, only the original cost is recorded as an asset and amortized by a series of charges to depreciation expense. The initial balance of the account should then be eliminated and all subsequent purchases of minor equipment recorded as expenses of the units requisitioning and using the items.

12.2.1.7 Accumulated Depreciation

A separate accumulated depreciation account should be maintained for each of the categories just described. The accounts should reflect the cumulative amount of the cost of the assets that has been charged to operations in the form of a depreciation expense. However, when preparing statements of financial position it is permissible to report all depreciation charges as a single entry in the balance sheet.

12.2.2 Determination of the Cost of Plant Assets

The value attributed to the acquisition of plant assets includes not only the cash outlay, which represents the cost or the price of such items, but also other incidental expenditures related to the purchase of a plant asset or to the preparation for its installation and use. Plant assets frequently are acquired in ways other than by cash purchase; in these cases, special accounting problems are encountered when determining the cost. Before discussing this, it is convenient to describe the difference between a capital expenditure and a revenue expenditure.

12.2.2.1 Capital vs. Revenue Expenditures

Expenditures for the acquisition and use of plant assets are incurred to obtain benefits or utility in the form of asset services. In recording such outlays, it is necessary first to differentiate between revenue and capital expenditures. When the outlay will benefit only the current period, it is regarded as a revenue expenditure. These are charged directly to an expense account that appears in the income statement and is deducted from the period's revenue in determining net income. If, on the other hand, management decides that the benefits will extend beyond the current period, the outlay is regarded as a capital expenditure and, rather than being charged to an expense account, the acquisition is recorded as an asset. An expenditure recorded in an asset account and subsequently reclassified as an expense through the depreciation process is said to have been capitalized.

Obviously, care must be exercised when distinguishing between capital and revenue expenditures when transactions are recorded since an erroneous distinction between the two can influence several accounting periods. For example, if an outlay is classified erroneously as a revenue expenditure, the expenses of the current period will be overstated and the net income of the period will be understated. Further, since a portion of the cost of the asset should be depreciated during the subsequent periods in which the resource contributes to operational activity, the depreciation expenses reported in future periods will be understated and, as a result, the net income of these periods will be overstated.

12.2.2.2 Cost of Cash Acquisitions

The cost of a plant asset that is acquired in a cash transaction includes the invoice or negotiated price as well as all incidental charges such as freight, sales taxes, installation, and any other expenses incurred in obtaining the item and preparing it for use. Plant assets should be recorded net of any discounts that are available to the institution; failure to take advantage of such discounts should be recorded as an expense. Expenditures incurred to repair or recondition a plant asset also should be included as a part of the cost of acquisition.

Special problems arise when land and a building constructed on it are purchased concurrently. Since land normally is nondepreciable, particular attention must be given to proper identification and separation of the land and building costs. Where land clearing is involved, it should be regarded as a land cost and the excavation expense as a building cost. The cost of a new building includes the expenditures for erecting temporary buildings on the site, architect's fees, permits, and insurance required during the construction period. Obviously, expenditures for material and labor must be included in the cost of buildings.

12.2.2.3 Acquisition of Plant Assets by Exchange

When one asset is traded for another, the cost of the new one should be recorded at the fair market value of the old item that is relinquished in the transaction. If a cash payment is required in addition to the trade-in, the new asset should be recorded at a figure that equals the total of the cash payment and the fair market value of the old one.

Since assets that are acquired in an exchange transaction are assigned a fair market value, the institution can realize a net gain or net loss. This gain or loss should be recognized at the time the new asset is obtained. An exception to this rule occurs when the fair market value of the acquired asset and/or the fair market value of the one given in exchange cannot be determined. In such a situation, the cost of the acquired asset is recorded at a value equal to the book value of the item given in exchange and no gains or losses are recognized.

12.2.2.4 Donated Plant Assets

When plant and equipment are donated to the institution, a fair market value, as determined by an independent appraisal, should be assigned to the asset. In this case, the institution's Plant and Equipment account should be increased by an appropriate debit entry. When recording the acquisition of donated equipment, a credit entry is recorded directly to the Unrestricted Fund balance rather than to a revenue account. If the donation or gift is contingent on conditions specified by the donor, the contingency should be disclosed in a special note in the balance sheet. In addition, the use of donated equipment should be reflected in the depreciation expenses that are reported in the income statement. In this regard, depreciation charges should be recorded before and after the institution acquires title to donated equipment so long as it is clear that management intends to comply with the restrictions or conditions specified by the donor.

12.3 NATURE OF DEPRECIATION

Most of the plant assets the health facility uses are depreciable resources. Associated with a plant asset is an amount of usefulness that will be employed in the provision of service throughout the life of the item. Furthermore, since the life of plant assets usually is limited, the amount of usefulness also is limited and is consumed over the life of the item. As the equipment is used each year, a portion of its service capability is consumed. Depreciation is nothing more than the expiration of a plant asset's usefulness, and depreciation accounting is a process of allocating and recording the cost of this asset as an expense during periods that benefit from its use. The use of an asset thus is an expired cost that is properly chargeable as an expense against the revenues that are directly or indirectly generated during its useful life.

Depreciation may be defined as

> an accounting procedure in which the cost or other recorded value of a fixed asset less estimated salvage (if any) is distributed over its estimated useful life in a systematic manner; it is a process of allocation, not valuation.

Clearly, then, the concept of depreciation must be sharply distinguished from the process by which plant assets are valued. More specifically, depreciation charges should not be regarded as a loss in market value, since depreciation accounting is simply a process by which the cost of a plant asset is allocated over its useful life.

Historically, depreciation expenses normally were not charged to functional units. However, Section 19 of Public Law 95-142 requires the hospital to charge depreciation expenses to the functional center that generates those costs. Unless otherwise specified, it is assumed here that depreciation expenses refer to items of plant and equipment that are used exclusively by a given functional unit.

12.4 FACTORS IN MEASURING DEPRECIATION

The measurement of periodic depreciation is dependent on three major factors: (1) the depreciation base, (2) the salvage value, and (3) the method of computing depreciation. Each is discussed next.

12.4.1 Depreciation Base

The depreciation base, also called depreciable cost, is simply the acquisition expense of a plant asset less the estimated salvage value. More specifically, the depreciation base is the portion of the asset's cost that should be charged to the revenue generated during the item's useful life. In equation form, the depreciation base is:

$$\text{Depreciation Base} = \text{Acquisition Cost} - \text{Salvage Value}$$

The problems in determining the acquisition cost were discussed in Section 12.2. As a practical matter, the acquisition expense is historical cost as measured by cash outlays or disbursements. When assets are acquired by other than cash, their cost is determined by the fair market value of the article received or the fair market value of the one relinquished.

The salvage value of a plant asset is the portion of its cost that management expects to recover at the end of its productive life. When the disposal of a plant asset requires dismantling or removal, the related costs should be deducted from the estimated salvage value. The institution may continue to use a plant asset until it is completely exhausted, so the salvage value will be quite nominal. On the other hand, certain types of plant assets may be replaced quite frequently and well before the end of their maximum useful life. In such a case, the salvage value may represent a substantial amount and a relatively high percentage of the acquisition cost.

This discussion suggests that there is no single formula for the determination of salvage value. Rather, the salvage value of a given asset is a matter of judgment that must be tempered by considerations such as the institution's asset retirement policy, past experience, and expected market conditions for used and scrapped equipment.

12.4.2 Productive Life of a Plant Asset

Plant assets, other than land, have a limited service life because of physical or functional factors and each of these should be considered in determining the items' useful service life. The physical factors include wear and tear from use in the productive process as well as deterioration caused by the action of natural elements. The functional factors of inadequacy and obsolescence also must be considered in determining service life. Rapid advances in medical technology and the embodiment of such advances in new equipment make older equipment obsolete just as changes in the scale of operations make some plant assets inadequate long before they are exhausted.

The useful life of an asset may be expressed in units of time (hours, weeks, or years) or in terms of units of output. In selecting an appropriate measure of service life, the physical and functional factors described above should be considered. Generally, functional factors have a greater impact on the useful or service life of medical equipment than do physical factors. On the other hand, physical factors are perhaps the most important determinants of the useful life of land improvements and buildings. As a matter of convenience, most institutions express the service life of plant assets in terms of time.

12.4.3 Depreciation Methods

Given the acquisition cost, the estimated salvage value, and the estimated service life, management must make a choice as to the method it will use in computing depreciation. The methods frequently used in the health industry are discussed in the next section.

12.5 METHODS OF DEPRECIATION

A number of methods by which depreciation may be computed are available for allocating the costs of a plant over is useful service life. For purposes of future illustration, assume the following data pertain to an item of new equipment that was purchased on January 1, 198A:

Acquisition Cost	$60,000
Less Salvage Value	15,000
Depreciation Base	45,000

Also suppose that the asset is estimated to have a five-year useful service life. The $45,000 depreciation base may be allocated over the five-year period by any of the methods described below. Whatever method is selected, it should (1) be systematic and rational and (2) result in a matching of revenue and expense to provide a proper determination of net income.

12.5.1 Straight-Line Method

The straight-line method of determining depreciation is a technique that charges an equal amount of depreciation to each year of the asset's useful life. The formula for the straight-line method is:

$$\frac{\text{Cost} - \text{Salvage Value}}{\text{Estimated Useful Life}} = \text{Annual Depreciation Expense}$$

In terms of the example, the annual depreciation expense is:

$$\frac{\$60{,}000 - \$15{,}000}{5} = \$9{,}000$$

Thus, in each year of the asset's useful life, $9,000 is charged as a depreciation expense for this item of equipment.

Since the financial statements should reflect all expenses, including depreciation charges, the following adjusting entry is required at the end of the year:

Depreciation Expense (Classified)	$9,000	
Accumulated Depreciation		$9,000

The entry is posted to the appropriate account in the general ledger.

Table 12-1 summarizes the results of the straight-line depreciation method for the five-year period. The basic advantage of the method is its simplicity. The effect of the method on expenses and the book value of asset is easily understood. Finally, to comply with P.L. 95-142, depreciation charges for plant assets used in operational activity must be reported as an expense of the Unrestricted Fund. The straight-line method also must be applied to all assets acquired after July 1970. As a result, hospitals cannot use other methods that are available and acceptable in terms of commonly accepted accounting principles.

12.5.2 Sum-of-Years'-Digits Method

Under the sum-of-years'-digits method, a declining portion of the depreciable cost is charged as a depreciation expense. This method often is referred to as an accelerated depreciation technique since it provides for writing off the depreciable cost at a more rapid rate than does the straight-line method. In computing depreciation by this method, a set of declining fractions is calculated in which the denominator is given by the sum of the years in the useful life of the asset. The numerator of the fractions is the number of years of life remaining at the beginning of the year.

Returning to the example, where it is assumed that the asset is expected to have a five-year service life, the denominator of the fraction is 15 (i.e., 5 + 4 + 3 + 2 + 1). The numerator of the fraction pertaining to the first year is 5 and as a result the proportion of the depreciable cost charged to depreciation is 5/15 or 1/3.

Table 12-2 summarizes the results obtained when the sum-of-the-years'-digits method is applied to the asset referred to earlier. As the table shows, the fractions for the second, third, fourth, and fifth years are 4/15, 3/15, 2/15, and 1/15, respectively. The declining fraction is applied to the depreciable cost of $45,000, resulting in a declining charge to depreciation expense. More specifically, during the first two years, the depreciation charges computed by the sum-of-the-years'-digits method exceed those calculated using the straight-line method. After the third year, however, the straight-line charges exceed those under the sum-of-the-years'-digits method. Also, as in the case of the straight-line method, the undepreciated cost at the end of the fifth year is $15,000, which is just equal to the estimated salvage value.

The sum-of-the-years'-digits method can be troublesome when an asset is acquired at a point other than the beginning of the year. For example, assume the plant asset is acquired on May 1 rather than January 1, 198A. The depreciation charges for 198A and 198B are calculated as follows:

For 198A:

$15,000 × 2/3 = $10,000

Table 12-1 Straight-Line Method of Calculating Depreciation

Year	*Depreciation Expense*	*Acquisition Cost*	*Accumulated Depreciation*	*Undepreciated Cost*
198A	$9,000	$60,000	$9,000	$51,000
198B	9,000	60,000	18,000	42,000
198C	9,000	60,000	27,000	33,000
198D	9,000	60,000	36,000	24,000
198E	9,000	60,000	45,000	15,000*

* Salvage value.

Table 12-2 Sum-of-Years'-Digits Method of Calculating Depreciation

Year	*Fraction*	*Depreciable Cost*	*Depreciation Expense*	*Accumulated Depreciation*	*Undepreciated Cost*
198A	5/15	$45,000	$15,000	$15,000	$45,000
198B	4/15	45,000	12,000	27,000	33,000
198C	3/15	45,000	9,000	36,000	24,000
198D	2/15	45,000	6,000	42,000	18,000
198E	1/15	45,000	3,000	45,000	15,000*

* Salvage value.

For 198B:

$15,000 × 1/3 =	$5,000	
12,000 × 2/3 =	8,000	
		13,000

A similar procedure is followed in subsequent years.

12.5.3 Declining Balance

The declining-balance method is another technique by which depreciation charges can be accelerated. Under this method a constant rate of depreciation is applied to a declining balance that represents the undepreciated cost of the asset that has *not* been reduced by the estimated salvage value. As a practical matter, the declining-balance rate is determined by multiplying 150 percent or 200 percent by the straight-line rate. In the example here, the straight-line rate of depreciation is 20 percent (1/5 or 9,000/45,000). When this rate is multiplied by 150 percent or 200 percent, the declining-balance rate of computing depreciation is 30 percent and 40 percent, respectively. Using the former rate, depreciation on the assumed asset is determined as in Table 12-3.

Table 12-3 Declining-Balance Method of Computing Depreciation

(Depreciation Rate = 150% × 20% = 30%)

Year	*Acquisition Cost*	*Undepreciated Cost at Beginning of the Period*	*Rate*	*Depreciation Expense*	*Accumulated Depreciation at End of the Period*
198A	$60,000	$60,000	.30	$18,000	$18,000
198B	60,000	42,000	.30	12,600	30,600
198C	60,000	29,400	.30	8,820	39,420
198D	60,000	20,580		5,580*	45,000

* $5,580 represents the remaining depreciable cost ($20,580 − $15,000) that results in a salvage value of $15,000, appearing as the undepreciated cost of the asset.

The salvage value is not considered in the declining-balance method until the last year of the schedule, when depreciation is taken in an amount that results in an equality between the salvage value and the undepreciated cost of the asset. No method of depreciation should reduce the book value of an asset below the salvage value. Under the declining-balance method, the salvage value need not be determined until late in the life of the asset, which may result in an improvement in the accuracy of the salvage estimate.

12.5.4 Units of Production Method

In the methods of determining depreciation discussed above, the usefulness of an asset is measured in terms of units of time. In certain instances, depreciation can be computed in terms of productivity as measured by hours of service or number of units produced. The use of such a method requires: (1) an estimate of the asset's life as expressed in terms of the number of hours of service or the number of units produced and (2) the maintenance of records on actual performance as measured in terms of capital use. Such a method may be costly from the standpoint of maintaining the required records but the additional cost may be offset somewhat since the productivity system produces charges that vary directly with the asset's use.

By way of illustration, assume that an asset has an estimated useful life of 120,000 units of service. The units may be expressed in terms of number of hours, number of services, number of films, etc. Also suppose that the acquisition costs are $30,000 and the estimated salvage value is $6,000. The depreciation charge per unit of output is computed by:

$$\text{Depreciation per Unit} = \frac{\text{Cost} - \text{Salvage Value}}{\text{Estimated Unit of Production}}$$

$$= \frac{\$30{,}000 - \$6{,}000}{120{,}000} = \$.20/\text{unit}$$

The results of the method along with the assumed production of the resource are presented in Table 12-4.

12.5.5 Composite Method

Thus far this analysis has examined the methods by which depreciation may be calculated for each individual plant asset used by the functional unit. Such a process is tedious and time consuming. As a result, many institutions may find it convenient to group depreciable assets and to compute composite depreciation expenses for groups of assets rather than to examine each item individually. This procedure is called the group or composite method of computing depreciation.

Under the composite depreciation procedure, a number of dissimilar assets may be depreciated as a single group. To illustrate, suppose that five items of equipment are acquired on January 1, 198A, with acquisition costs, salvage value, and useful lives as indicated in Table 12-5. Assume that the items of equipment will be used in one of the functional units of the institution. As seen at the bottom of Table 12-5, the composite life of these assets is ten years ($18,000/$1,800) and the composite rate of depreciation is .075 ($1,-800/$24,000). As a result, depreciation is recorded annually at 7.5 percent for ten years. At the end of the ten-year period the total accumulated depreciation is $18,000 ($1,800 × 10 years).

When an asset in the group is retired, the acquisition cost is eliminated from the books and the accumulated depreciation is debited for the amount of the salvage value indicated in the table. Moreover, when an asset is retired, no gain or loss is realized since the composite rate method assumes the plant asset is replaced with an item of equipment that has a similar cost and a similar useful life. If this assumption is violated, a new composite rate of depreciation must be computed.

12.5.6 Altering the Depreciation Rate

Because the institution is using a given method of computing depreciation does not mean that changes cannot be made in the rate or the method of calculating such charges. For example, material errors in judgment as to service life or salvage value may be recognized well before plant assets are fully depreciated. Furthermore, a depreciation method may be made inappropriate by changing conditions or operating methods. In such a situation it may be desirable to alter either the depreciation rate or the method of depreciation to correct earlier errors or to accommodate changing conditions.

For illustration, return to the $60,000 item that was purchased on January 1, 198A. The plant asset is assumed to have a useful life of five years and,

Table 12-4 Units of Production Method of Computing Depreciation

Year	*Units of Service*	*Rate*	*Depreciation Expense*	*Accumulated Depreciation*	*Undepreciated Cost*
198A	40,000	.20	$8,000	$8,000	$22,000
198B	20,000	.20	4,000	12,000	18,000
198C	25,000	.20	5,000	17,000	13,000
198D	35,000	.20	7,000	24,000	6,000*
	120,000				

* Salvage value.

Table 12-5 Composite Method of Computing Depreciation

Asset	*Acquisition Cost*	*Salvage Value*	*Depreciation Base*	*Useful Life*	*Annual Depreciation*
A	$1,000	$200	$800	8	$100
B	9,000	3,000	6,000	20	300
C	6,000	800	5,200	13	400
D	5,000	1,500	3,500	7	500
E	3,000	500	2,500	5	500
	24,000	6,000	18,000		1,800

Composite Rate of Depreciation: $1,800/$24,000 = .075.
Composite Life of Assets: $18,000/$1,800 = 10 years.

at the end of this period, is expected to have a salvage value of $15,000. Assuming that the asset has been depreciated on a straight-line basis for three years, the relevant balances in the general ledger on January 1, 198D are:

Equipment	$60,000
Accumulated Depreciation (3 Years × $9,000)	27,000

On this date, suppose it is decided that the useful life of the asset should have been established originally at nine years rather than five. In other words, on January 1, 198D, it is determined that the asset has six years of life remaining. In addition, suppose that it is determined that the salvage value should be reduced to $3,000.

To accommodate changes in management's expectations, it is necessary to revise the depreciation charges recorded during the asset's remaining years of service life. This is so even though the annual depreciation expense of $9,000 during the first three years of the asset's life is incorrect. No adjustment or restatement of previously recorded depreciation is required. Rather, the future rate of depreciation should be calculated thus:

Acquisition Cost	$60,000
Less Accumulated Depreciation January 1, 198D	27,000
Undepreciated Cost January 1, 198D	33,000
Less New Salvage Value	3,000
Depreciable Cost	30,000
Divide by Remaining Useful Life	6 Years
Revised Annual Depreciation	5,000

For each of the years remaining in the useful life of this asset, the following entry is made:

Depreciation Expense (Classified)	$5,000	
Accumulated Depreciation		$5,000

At the end of the asset's revised useful life, the equipment will carry a total accumulated depreciation of $57,000 and an undepreciated cost of $3,000, which of course is the revised salvage value.

In addition to changes in the expected salvage value and the estimated useful life, the depreciable cost of an asset can change during its service life. For example, suppose that the hospital purchases an item for $70,000 on January 1, 198A. The equipment is expected to have a useful life of five years and the salvage value is estimated at $10,000. Also assume that the straight-line method is used in computing depreciation and that on January 1, 198D, a capital expenditure of $20,000 is made on the equipment. If this capital expenditure does not prolong or extend the life of this asset, the entry to record the expenditure is:

Equipment	$20,000	
Cash		$20,000

The revised depreciation charge for 198D and 198E is calculated as follows:

$$\frac{\$70{,}000 - \$10{,}000}{5\text{ Years}} + \frac{\$20{,}000}{2\text{ Years}} = \$22{,}000/\text{Year}$$

↓	↓	↓
Annual Straight-Line Depreciation Rate	Additional Depreciation Due to Capital Expenditures	Depreciation Charge for 2 Years

Now assume that that $20,000 capital expenditure prolongs the service life of the asset by two additional years. The entry to record such a capital expenditure is:

Accumulated Depreciation	$20,000	
Cash		$20,000

To record capital expenditure that increases the service life of the asset by two additional years.

The new depreciation charge in each of the remaining four years is $11,000, which is computed as follows:

Acquisition Cost	$70,000
Less Accumulated Depreciation	36,000
Undepreciated Cost	34,000
Less Salvage Value	10,000
Balance	24,000
Add Capital Expenditure	20,000
Depreciation Base	44,000
Remaining Life	4 Years
Revised Annual Depreciation	11,000

It may be desirable to change the depreciation method. Before doing so, both the long-run and short-run effects must be considered from the standpoint of avoiding future changes in newly adopted methods. A further point involves the requirement that, when changes in the depreciation rate are implemented, the influence of the change on reported expenses and the determination of net income must be disclosed fully.

To illustrate the accounting procedures for changing the method of depreciation, return to the asset that is purchased for $60,000 and is expected to last five years. At the end of this period the asset is expected to have a salvage value of $15,000. Suppose that the sum-of-the-years'-digits method is employed in 198A and 198B in computing depreciation, as follows:

Depreciation:	198A	5/15	×	$45,000	=	$15,000
Depreciation:	198B	4/15	×	45,000	=	12,000
Accumulated Depreciation:	1/1/198C					27,000

If a change is made to straight-line depreciation in 198C, the cumulative influence on previously reported income must be estimated. Had the straight-line method been used at the end of 198A and 198B, the accumulated depreciation and total depreciation expense would have been $18,000 (2 years × $9,000/year). The retroactive and cumulative influence of the change, then, is the difference between the actual depreciation recognized under the sum-of-the-years'-digits and what would have been recorded if the straight-line method had been used during the first two years of the life of the asset. In this case, the net income for these years has been understated by $9,000 (i.e., $27,000 − $18,000). Consequently, the equity account also has been understated by $9,000.

To account for the change in the method by which depreciation is calculated it is necessary to reduce the balance of the accumulated depreciation account by $9,000. It also is necessary to increase the equity account of the Unrestricted Fund by the same amount. These adjustments are recorded by the following entry:

Accumulated Depreciation	$9,000	
Adjustment to Depreciation Expense		$9,000

The debit entry reduces the balance of the accumulated depreciation account. On the other hand, the Adjustment to Depreciation Expense account is a contra account that reduces the expenses of the period, which results in an increase of $9,000 in the net income of 198C. The increase in net income is transferred to the equity account of the Unrestricted Fund when the balances of the nominal accounts are eliminated by the closing entries. As a result, the balance of the equity account at the end of 198C reflects the net income that would have been reported in 198A and 198B assuming the straight-line method had been used to determine depreciation expenses for these two years.

The financial statements prepared for previous years need not be adjusted, although full disclosure is required in the financial statement of the period in which such changes occur. As seen, the depreciation charge for the year in which the change occurred and in subsequent years is $9,000 ($27,000/3 years).

12.5.7 A Comparison of Methods

Even though each of the methods described results in the same total accumulated depreciation in the long run, the amounts charged to depreciation in each year vary greatly among the various methods. As a result, a very real question emerges regarding which method should be used.

From a theoretical perspective, an enterprise should select the depreciation method that best approximates the use of plant assets in generating income; this, in turn, provides a proper matching of revenues and expenditures. As suggested earlier, the resulting balance sheet representation is of secondary importance. The process of selecting the method of determining depreciation in a given institution should focus on portraying operating results accurately.

In addition to theoretical concerns, practical considerations should play a role in the selection of the depreciation method. The practical concerns that must be considered are the simplicity of the method and the extent to which management understands it. Most would agree with the premise that the straight-line method is perhaps the simplest and the easiest to understand. It also needs a minimum of clerical effort and, when applied to a group of assets, may reduce accounting complications further.

Perhaps an even more important practical consideration involves the effect of the depreciation method on the institution's cash flows. As was suggested, plant assets should be capitalized and their costs charged to expense through the process of depreciation. In most cases, depreciation charges represent a cost that is recoverable from major third party payers. As a consequence, the selection of the depreciation method exerts a very real influence on the institution's cash flows.

For illustration, suppose that the hospital begins operations on January 1, 198A, with plant assets having a depreciable cost of $1,500 and an estimated useful life of five years. Assume that all hospital expenses, including depreciation, are reimbursable. Suppose also that the hospital has no liabilities and that all transactions occur on a cash basis. Finally, suppose that during the year the hospital's revenues amount to $1,100 and expenses, *excluding* depreciation, to $800.

If the straight-line method of computing depreciation is used, the depreciation expenses of the period will be $300 ($1,500/5 years). On the other hand, the sum-of-the-years'-digits method results in a declining charge to depreciation during the useful life of the plant assets. The results of the two methods are compared in Table 12-6.

If the straight-line method is used to calculate depreciation charges, revenues and expenses of $1,100 will be reported in the income statement of 198A. As a consequence, the hospital will have broken even for the year (i.e., no net income or net loss). At the end of the year, however, the cash balance will be $300, assuming that all transactions occur on a cash basis.

On the other hand, consider the results under the sum-of-the-years'-digits method. Revenues again are $1,100 but, under the sum-of-the-years'-digits method, expenses of $1,300 ($800 + $500) are reported. In this case, the hospital reports a net loss of $200 for the period. At the end of the year, however, it will have a $500 cash balance, which again assumes that all transactions occur on a cash basis. Thus, under the sum-of-the-years'-digits method, the cash inflow of the hospital is $200 greater than the corresponding cash receipts under the straight-line method.

Although this example is greatly simplified, it illustrates the basic fact that cash inflows are greatest during the early years of plant assets' useful life when the accelerated method of computing depreciation is employed. How-

Table 12-6 Comparison of Straight-Line and Sum-of-the-Years'-Digits Methods

	Depreciation Expense		
Year	*Straight-Line*	*Sum-of-the-Years'-Digits*	*Difference*
198A	$300	$500	$200
198B	300	400	100
198C	300	300	—
198D	300	200	(100)
198E	300	100	(200)

ever, the trend is reversed during the later years of the useful life of the assets. As can be seen in Table 12-6, the cash inflows during 198D and 198E under the straight-line method are greater than under the accelerated method. Thus, when an accelerated method is selected to improve current cash flows, the cash receipts in later periods are reduced. The use of accelerated methods implies that management in effect is borrowing from future cash flows. The wisdom of such a policy will depend on the use of these funds, anticipations of future economic conditions, and probable impact on the future replacement or expansion of plant assets.

12.5.8 Funding Depreciation

Many health facilities accumulate cash resources that may be used to finance the expansion or replacement of plant assets. When depreciation is funded, a portion of the revenue generated by operational activity is accumulated for the future replacement of plant and equipment. The accumulation of these resources is of importance for a number of reasons:

- One of the primary objectives of the institution is to maintain the plant and equipment required to provide care to the community. As mentioned earlier, the useful life of plant assets is limited by several factors and, to maintain productive capability, plant and equipment ultimately must be replaced.
- The costs of plant and equipment have increased dramatically in recent years and, to ensure that adequate funding is available, management should set aside resources that will be used for acquiring replacement capital. Moreover, by investing these resources in interest-earning securities, management can maintain the purchasing power of the designated funds.
- The importance of investing funded depreciation is enhanced further by the fact that the resulting income is not treated as offset revenue when calculating costs recoverable from major third party payers.

For illustration, suppose that the institution has implemented a policy of funding depreciation and that the depreciation charges for a given period are $65,000. The entry that records the depreciation expense of the period is:

Depreciation Expense (Classified)	$65,000	
Accumulated Depreciation		$65,000

This entry does not provide additional resources since the accumulated depreciation account contains no funds. Rather, it is only through adequate reimbursement that the facility will receive cash that it can use to offset the depreciation expenses of the period.

When the funding of depreciation is a voluntary action that the board may take, the annual entry to record a funding of 100 percent in the Unrestricted Fund is:

Cash—Board Designated (Capital Replacement)	$65,000	
Cash—General		$65,000

This entry simply changes the composition of the assets of the Unrestricted Fund from a general purpose cash account to a board-designated cash account and limits the use of these funds to the acquisition of replacement capital. Since the Restricted Fund grouping is used to record transactions involving resources that are subject to limitations imposed by outside parties, it is not proper to transfer the balance of the board-designated cash account to the Capital Fund.

12.6 DISPOSAL OF PLANT ASSETS

The health care facility may dispose of plant assets through the normal retirement process or through sale or exchange transactions. To show how the institution can dispose of plant and equipment, suppose the following information pertains to the asset in question:

Purchase Date:	January 1, 198A
Cost:	$160,000
Salvage Value:	$60,000
Service Life:	5 years
Depreciation Method:	Straight Line

12.6.1 Normal Retirement

If the useful life of the asset ends on December 31, 198E, as expected, and the salvage value of $60,000 is realized, the accounting entry for disposing of the asset is:

Cash	$60,000	
Accumulated Depreciation	100,000	
Equipment		$160,000

If the realized salvage value is greater than the estimated salvage value, a gain on retirement is recognized. Conversely, if the actual salvage value is less than the estimate, a loss on retirement is recognized. When an asset remains in use after being fully depreciated, no further depreciation is recorded and no adjustments to depreciation recorded previously are necessary.

12.6.2 Sale Transaction

An asset may be sold prior to the end of its estimated useful life. Assume, for example, that the piece of equipment just described is sold on July 1, 198C for $140,000. The entry to record such a sale is:

Cash	$140,000	
Accumulated Depreciation	50,000	
Equipment		$160,000
Gain on Sale		30,000

The values in this entry are calculated as follows:

Sale Proceeds			$140,000
Acquisition Cost		$160,000	
Accumulated Depreciation:			
198A	$20,000		
198B	$20,000		
198C			
($20,000 × 1/2)	10,000	50,000	
Less Book Value			110,000
Gain on Sale			30,000

If one of the accelerated methods of calculating depreciation had been used, the accumulated depreciation on this plant asset would have been greater than the $50,000 recorded under the straight-line method. The gain on sale would have been correspondingly greater than the $30,000 shown here. Accelerated depreciation, then, tends to increase gains recognized on the premature retirement of assets or to minimize or eliminate such losses.

12.6.3 Exchange of Plant Assets

Occasionally the institution will use an old asset as a trade-in on a new one. Suppose that the plant asset and $70,000 in cash are given in exchange for an asset with a cash price of $180,000 on July 1, 198C. The required entry is:

Equipment (New)	$180,000	
Accumulated Depreciation	50,000	
Equipment (Old)		$160,000
Cash		70,000

As mentioned earlier in this chapter, the basis for recording assets acquired in exchange is the fair market value of the item that is relinquished plus any cash disbursement or the fair market value of the one received, whichever is most clearly evidenced. If, for example, the asset has a cash price of $190,000, it is appropriate to recognize a gain of $10,000.

12.7 SUBSIDIARY RECORDS

As noted earlier in this chapter, it is desirable to maintain a set of subsidiary records for each of the plant assets used currently in operational activity. The subsidiary ledger contains information on the item pertaining to its acquisition cost, a description of it, where it is located in the facility, its estimated life, its salvage value, the amount of depreciation recorded monthly and annually, and details on its disposal. The balances appearing in the relevant control accounts of the general ledger also must balance with the sum of the entries on asset acquisitions, accumulated depreciation, and asset disposals in the subsidiary records.

Questions for Discussion

1. Describe the major categories into which plant and equipment are grouped.
2. Distinguish between capital and revenue expenditures.
3. Describe the mechanisms by which the facility can acquire plant and equipment. Discuss the methods of determining the value of capital acquisitions.
4. Define the term depreciation.
5. Define the term depreciation base. Identify what factors are considered when determining the depreciation base.
6. Name factors that influence the useful life of plant and equipment.

7. Describe the methods of calculating depreciation. Explain what influence accelerated methods exert on the cash flows of an institution that is reimbursed on a cost basis.
8. Define funding depreciation and describe its advantages and disadvantages.
9. Identify what procedure should be followed when depreciation has been estimated incorrectly in previous years.

Problems for Solution

1. Assume that the following information pertains to a piece of equipment that was purchased on January 1:

   Cost: $110,000
   Freight: $6,000
   Salvage Value: $16,000
   Useful Life: 4 Years

   What are the annual depreciation charges under:

   a. the straight-line method
   b. the sum-of-the-years'-digits method
   c. the double declining balance method

2. Describe what entries are required in Problem 1 to fully fund the depreciation in the first year under each of the methods.
3. Identify what entry is required in Problem 1 to write off the equipment at the end of the sixth year, assuming a salvage value of $14,000 was received.
4. Suppose that, in Problem 1, at the end of the third year it is decided that the useful life should have been six years rather than four years. In addition, suppose that the estimated salvage value is $10,000 rather than $16,000. If the straight-line method is used, describe the depreciation expenses for the remaining useful life.
5. Assume that the following information pertains to a piece of capital equipment that was purchased on January 1:

   Cost: $250,000
   Salvage Value: $10,000
   Useful Life: 10 Years

   Assume further that the equipment and $20,000 are given in exchange for a new capital asset at the end of the fifth year. If the straight-line method of calculating depreciation is used, describe what entry is required to record this transaction.

6. Assume the following information is available pertaining to a given piece of equipment:

Cost: $290,000
Salvage Value: $70,000
Useful Life: 100,000 Units of Service

Year	*Units of Service*
1	20,000
2	30,000
3	10,000
4	40,000

Record the depreciation charges using the productivity method for each of the four years.

7. Suppose the hospital acquires the following assets on January 1, 198A:

Asset	*Cost*	*Salvage Value*	*Useful Life*
A	$16,800	$800	8 years
B	20,500	500	4 years
C	3,750	750	5 years
D	40,800	800	10 years

Calculate the annual depreciation assuming that the assets are depreciated as follows:

Asset	*Method*
A and D	Straight Line
B	Sum-of-Year's-Digits
C	Double Declining Balance

Also calculate the composite rate of depreciation assuming that the straight-line method is used.

8. Suppose the hospital acquires a piece of equipment for $60,000 on January 1, 1980. The equipment has a useful life of five years and a salvage value of $15,000. The double declining balance is used to calculate depreciation during the first three years. However, on January 1, 1984, the straight-line method is used to calculate depreciation during the remainder of the asset's useful life. Calculate the depreciation charges during the remaining life of the asset.
9. Suppose the facility purchases a piece of equipment for $80,000 on January 1. Suppose further that the equipment is expected to have a salvage value of $20,000 and a useful life of 10 years. The straight-

line method of calculating depreciation is used. At the beginning of the fourth year, suppose the institution decides that the useful life of the machine is 15 years rather than 10 and that the salvage value is $10,000 rather than $20,000. Calculate the future rate of depreciation.

10. Suppose the institution buys a piece of capital equipment for $110,000 and that it is expected to have a salvage value of $10,000 and a useful life of 10 years. Two years later, a capital expenditure of $30,000 is made that prolongs the life of the equipment by five years. Under the straight-line method, describe what entry is required each year thereafter.
11. Suppose that the following information pertains to a piece of equipment used previously in the institution:

    Cost: $270,000
    Accumulated Depreciation: $162,000

    Assume that the equipment and $140,000 are given in exchange for a new piece of equipment. Record this transaction.
12. Assume that the facility purchases a machine that:

    a. costs $2,300
    b. has a salvage value of $200
    c. has an expected life of five years

    Use the straight-line, sum-of-year's-digits, and the declining balance methods to determine annual depreciation. Suppose further that this machine is sold at the end of the second year for $1,400. Record this sale for each method of calculating depreciation.
13. Suppose a piece of capital equipment is purchased for which the following information is available:

    Cost: $250,000
    Salvage Value: 50,000
    Estimated Use: 5 years

    Record the annual depreciation assuming that

    a. the straight-line
    b. the double declining balance
    c. the sum-of-the-year's-digits
    methods are used by the institution

14. Suppose the following information pertains to a group of units used in a functional unit of the institution:

Asset	*Cost*	*Salvage Value*	*Useful Life*
A	$18,750	$750	10 years
B	20,920	920	5 years
C	14,930	4,930	4 years
D	25,300	5,300	5 years

Calculate the annual depreciation changes, assuming that the assets are depreciated as follows:

Asset	*Depreciation Method*
A & B	Straight Line
C	Sum-of-the-Year's-digits
D	Declining Balance (150% × the Straight-Line Rate)

15. Use the composite depreciation method to calculate the following in reference to Problem 14:

 a. the composite life of the assets
 b. the composite rate of depreciation

16. Suppose the institution disposes of the Asset A item of equipment in Problem 14 at the end of the 11th year and realizes a salvage value of $1,000. If the straight-line method of depreciation is used, record the disposal of the equipment.
17. Suppose the following information pertains to a given piece of equipment:

Purchase Date	January 1, 1977
Cost	$20,000
Salvage Value	$4,000
Estimated Life	4 years
Depreciation Method	Straight Line

Suppose on January 1, 1980, this asset is exchanged for a new piece of equipment plus $40,000. Record this transaction.

Chapter 13
Accounting for Long-Term Debt

In addition to current liabilities, health care facilities incur obligations that will not be liquidated with the use of current assets. These obligations are referred to as long-term or noncurrent liabilities. Long-term liabilities frequently take the form of mortgages and bonds payable but also include notes, long-term leases, and certain deferred revenues. These accounts are found in the Unrestricted Fund but also may appear in one of the Restricted Funds. As mentioned earlier, a proper distinction between current and noncurrent obligations is important when evaluating the financial position of the institution and its ability to meet current obligations.

13.1 ACCOUNTING FOR BONDS PAYABLE

When the institution issues bonds, it contracts to pay: (1) the face or par value of the bonds at a specified maturity date and (2) interest, expressed as a percentage of the face value, at periodic intervals. The nominal rate of interest is predetermined on the basis of expectations concerning the rate of interest investors actually will demand at the time the bonds are issued. The market rate of interest varies according to the degree of risk, investors' preferences for liquidity, the terms of the bond, and general economic conditions. If the market rate of interest is equal to the nominal rate of interest, the bonds will sell at face value. If the market rate exceeds the nominal rate, the bonds will sell at a discount. Conversely, the bonds will sell at a premium if the nominal rate exceeds the market rate. As a result, differences between the nominal and market rates of interest are reflected in the prices investors are willing to pay for the bonds.

13.1.1 Issuance of Bonds at Discount

To illustrate the accounting procedures for bonds issued at discount, assume the hospital issues 500 $1,000 8 percent 20-year bonds at 96.7 on April

1, 197A. Also suppose that these bonds pay interest annually on April 1, and October 1 and will mature on April 1, 199A. Hence the hospital promises to pay $500,000 on the maturity date and $20,000 ($500,000 × .08 × 6/12) every six months for the next 20 years. Finally, suppose that bond issue costs—sales commissions, registration fees, appraisal costs, and printing expenses—amount to $24,000.

If all the bonds are sold on April 1, 197A, the following entries are recorded in the Unrestricted Fund:

Cash	$483,500	
Unamortized Bond Discount	16,500	
Bonds Payable		$500,000

As should be verified, the values in this entry are calculated as follows:

Par Value	$500,000
Price of bonds ($500,000 × .967)	483,500
Discount	16,500

The entry to record the costs of issuing the bonds is:

Unamortized Cost of Issuing Bond	$24,000	
Cash		$24,000

Technically, the unamortized cost of issuing the bonds should be reported as an asset in the balance sheet. However, the bond discount should be entered as a deduction from the face value of the bond:

8% Bonds Payable Due 199A	$500,000	
Less Unamortized Bond Discount	16,500	$483,500

When bonds are sold between interest dates, the seller collects accrued interest from the buyer. If, in the example above, the bonds are sold on July 1, 197A, the hospital will collect three months' accrued interest or $10,000 ($500,000 × .08 × 3/12) from the purchaser. The entry to record the sale is modified as follows:

Cash	$10,000	
Accrued Bond Interest Payable		$10,000

To record accrued bond interest on hand at date of issue.

This procedure permits the hospital to pay a full six months' interest to each bondholder regardless of the length of time the bonds have been held.

13.1.2 Issuance of Bonds at Premium

When the nominal rate of interest exceeds the market rate, the bonds will sell at a premium. For example, suppose that the hospital issues 500 $1,000 10 percent 20-year bonds @ 102.7 on April 1, 197A. These bonds pay interest annually on April 1 and October 1 and will mature April 1, 199A. Assume the issue costs are $7,600. The issue of the bonds is recorded in the Unrestricted Fund as follows:

Cash	$513,500	
Unamortized Bond Premium		$13,500
Bonds Payable		500,000

To record issue of 10 percent, $500,000 20-year bonds.

Unamortized Bond Issue Costs	$7,600	
Cash		$7,600

To record bond issue costs.

If a balance sheet is prepared immediately after issuance, the bonds appear as a long-term liability of the Unrestricted Fund:

10% Bonds Payable, Due 199A	$500,000	
Unamortized Bond Premium	13,500	$513,500

13.1.3 Bond Interest and Amortization

The bond interest expense is influenced by the bond premium or discount that is recorded when the certificates were issued. Amortization of a bond discount is regarded as an addition to periodic interest expense, while the amortization of the premium is regarded as a reduction in interest expenses. As a practical matter, bond discounts and premiums are amortized evenly throughout the life of the bond by the straight-line method.

Consider first the bonds issued at a discount of $16,500 that result in proceeds of $483,500. The $16,500 discount is amortized to interest expense over the 240-month life of the bond. Hence, the hospital receives $483,500 but must repay $500,000 on the maturity date. The $16,500 difference is an expense that is allocated to the 20-year period that is assumed to benefit from the resources provided by the bonds. The amortization of the bond discount, then, is simply an application of the matching concept introduced earlier.

If the bonds were issued on April 1, 197A, at the end of April and of each successive month in the 240-month period that the bonds are outstanding, the following entry is recorded in the Unrestricted Fund:

Bond Interest Expense	$3,402.08	
Unamortized Bond Discount		$68.75
Accrued Interest Payable		3,333.33

The values in this entry are calculated as follows:

Total Discount	$16,500.00
Monthly Amortization ($16,500/240)	68.75
Nominal Interest Expense ($500,000 × .08 × 1/12)	3,333.33
Monthly Interest Expense	3,402.08

In addition, a portion of the unamortized bond issue costs should be recognized as an expense:

Bond Issue Expense	$100	
Unamortized Bond Issue Costs		$100

To record monthly amortization of bond issue cost ($24,000/240).

In the first of these entries, the balance of the unamortized bond discount declines by $68.75 each month. As a result, the entire discount of $16,500 will have been charged to expenses by the time the bonds mature.

Consider next the example in which bonds are issued at a premium. As will be recalled, the $500,000 bond issue yields cash proceeds of $513,500. The premium of $13,500 should be amortized by credits to interest expense over the 240-month life of the bonds. Since the hospital receives $513,500 from the issue but must repay only $500,000, the $13,500 difference reduces the interest expense during the 20-year period.

If the assumption is maintained that all the bonds were issued on April 1, 197A, the following entries are recorded in the Unrestricted Fund at the end of each month of the 20-year period:

Bond Interest Expense	$4,110.40	
Unamortized Bond Premium	56.25	
Accrued Bond Interest Payable		$4,166.65

The values in this entry are obtained as follows:

Nominal Interest ($500,000 × .10 × 1/12)	$4,166.65
Amortization of Bond Premium ($13,500/240)	56.25
Bond Interest Expense	4,110.40

Thus the Unamortized Bond Premium is reduced by $56.25 each month until the balance of this account is reduced to zero by April 1, 199A.

13.1.4 Semiannual Interest Payment

In connection with the 10 percent bond issue described above, the semiannual interest payment is $25,000 ($500,000 × .10 × 6/12). On each April 1 and October 1 the following entry in the Unrestricted Fund records the interest payment:

Accrued Bond Interest Payable	$25,000	
Cash		$25,000

To record payment of semiannual interest on 10 percent $500,000 20-year bond.

In the case of the 8 percent bonds, the semiannual interest is $20,000 ($500,000 × .08 × 6/12) and, to record the interest payment, the entry

Accrued Bond Interest Payable	$20,000	
Cash		20,000

To record payment of semiannual interest on 8 percent $500,000 20-year bond.

is recorded in the Unrestricted Fund.

13.1.5 Bond Retirement

Three matters are considered in this section: (1) the retirement of term bonds at maturity, (2) the retirement of bonds prior to maturity, and (3) the redemption of serial bonds.

13.1.5.1 Bonds Retired at Maturity

In each of the examples above, the bonds have a maturity date of April 1, 199A. The entry recorded on that date is:

Bonds Payable	$500,000	
Cash		$500,000

The amortization process eliminates the premium or discount as well as the issue costs recorded at the time of the issue, so the retirement of these bonds requires the simple entry above.

13.1.5.2 Bonds Redeemed Before Maturity

The hospital may redeem its bonds before their maturity date if prices or other factors make such action desirable. For example, consider the bonds issued originally at a discount. Suppose the hospital redeems $200,000 of these bonds at 78 and accrued interest on August 1, 197D. Also assume the brokerage and other costs are $500. On the redemption date, the following balances will appear in the hospital's accounts:

Accrued Bond Interest Payable ($500,000 × .08 × 4/12)	$13,333.33 (cr.)
Bonds Payable	500,000.00 (cr.)
Unamortized Bond Discount ($16,500) − (40 months × 68.75)	13,750.00 (cr.)
Unamortized Bond Issue Costs ($24,000) − (40 × 100)	20,000.00 (cr.)

The entry to record the redemption usually requires a gain or loss when the amount paid for the bonds differs from the book value. The entry for recording the above redemption is:

Bonds Payable	$200,000.00	
Accrued Bond Interest Payable	5,333.33	
Unamortized Bond Discount		$5,500.00
Unamortized Bond Issue Cost		8,000.00
Cash		161,833.33
Gain on Redemption		30,000.00

The values in this entry are calculated as follows:

Bonds Payable (.40 × $500,000)		$200,000.00
Unamortized Bond Discount & Issue Costs (.4 × $13,750) + (.4 × $20,000)		13,500.00
Book Value of Redeemed Bonds		186,500.00
Price ($200,000 @ 78)	$156,000.00	
Brokerage Fees	500.00	
Total		156,500.00
Gain on Redemption		30,000.00
Redemption Cost (above)		156,500.00
Accrued Interest Payable ($200,000 × .08 × 4/12)		5,333.33
Cash Disbursement		161,833.33

After the redemption of the $200,000 in bonds, accounting for the balance continues until the maturity date. The monthly amount of interest expense, however, should be reduced to $2,041.25 (.6 × $3,402.08). In a similar fashion the monthly amortization of the bond issue costs would be 60 percent of $100, or $60.

13.1.5.3 Serial Bonds

Thus far this analysis has assumed that the bonds issued by the institution are term bonds (i.e., all bonds in the issue have a fixed single maturity date). Serial bonds, however, mature in periodic installments, which means that a portion of the original issue is retired annually. As a result, the retirement of serial bonds requires a slightly different treatment.

For illustration, suppose the hospital issues 500 $1,000 6 percent serial bonds on January 1, 1977, for $445,000 (net of issue costs). Assume the bonds mature at the rate of $50,000 per year beginning on January 1, 1978. A summary of the annual amortization and bond interest expense as computed by the "bonds outstanding" method is presented in Table 13-1. This system, rather than the straight-line method, is used for serial bonds. As in the sum-of-the-years'-digits method of calculating depreciation, the denominator of the fractions appearing in Column 3 is the sum of the years in the life of the bond (i.e., $10 + 9 + 8 + 7 + 6 + \ldots + 1$) while the numerator represents the number of years remaining in the life of the bond.

If interest is paid on January 1 of each year, and $50,000 of the bonds are retired as scheduled, the accounting entries are:

Cash	$445,000	
Unamortized Bond Discount	55,000	
Bonds Payable		$500,000

To record issuance of bond on January 1, 1977.

Bond Interest Expense	$40,000	
Unamortized Bond Discount		$10,000
Accrued Bond Interest Payable		30,000

To record discount amortization and interest payable on December 31, 1977.

Accrued Bond Interest Payable	$30,000	
Cash		$30,000

To record bond interest for 1977 on January 1, 1978.

Bond Payable	$50,000	
Cash		$50,000

To record retirement of bond on January 1, 1978.

13.1.6 Sinking Funds

When a bond issue does not mature in periodic installments but falls due in one lump sum at the maturity date, it is necessary to make provision for

Table 13-1 Summary of Bank Amortization and Interest Expense

Year (1)	Bonds Outstanding (2)	Fraction (3)	×	Bond Discount (4)	=	Discount Amortization (5)	+	6% Interest (6)	=	Interest Expense (7)
1977	$500,000	10/55		$55,000		$10,000		$ 30,000		$ 40,000
1978	450,000	9/55		55,000		9,000		27,000		36,000
1979	400,000	8/55		55,000		8,000		24,000		32,000
1980	350,000	7/55		55,000		7,000		21,000		28,000
1981	300,000	6/55		55,000		6,000		18,000		24,000
1982	250,000	5/55		55,000		5,000		15,000		20,000
1983	200,000	4/55		55,000		4,000		12,000		16,000
1984	150,000	3/55		55,000		3,000		9,000		12,000
1985	100,000	2/55		55,000		2,000		6,000		8,000
1986	50,000	1/55		55,000		1,000		3,000		4,000
						55,000		165,000		220,000

its payment over the life of the debt instrument. This is accomplished by a periodic deposit in a sinking fund. The deposits are made in amounts that, when combined with accrued interest, are sufficient to retire the bond issue.

The amount of the regular deposits depends on the interest that will be earned on sinking fund monies. The higher the rate of interest, the lower the required deposits. The annual rate of interest can only be estimated when the sinking fund is created. As the sinking fund approaches maturity, it may be necessary to adjust the contribution to correct for previous errors as well as to ensure that sufficient funds are available for retirement of the debt.

To compute the annual amount that must be contributed to the sinking fund, the concept of an ordinary annuity must be introduced first. An ordinary annuity is a series of equal cash flows that occur at the *end* of successive periods of equal length. For example, if the institution deposits $1.00 at the end of each year for three years in a savings account that will earn 6 percent interest compounded annually (i.e., the interest is computed on the principal *and* on any interest earned), the amount that will have accumulated in the account at the end of the third year is $3.1836:

Year	*Beginning Balance*	+	*Interest*	+	*1.00*	=	*Ending Balance*
1	$ 0		0		$1.00		$1.00
2	1.00		.06		1.00		2.06
3	2.06		.1236		1.00		3.1836

More generally, these calculations may be summarized in the form

$$V = \$1.00 + \$1.00(1.06) + \$1.00(1.06)^2$$
$$= \$3.1836 \quad \textbf{(13.1)}$$

where V represents the value of the annuity.

These results may be generalized further by assuming that A dollars are deposited at the end of each year for n years. Letting i represent the annual rate of interest, the result is that

$$V = A + A(1 + i) + A(1 + i)^2 + \ldots + A(1 + i)^{n-1} \quad \textbf{(13.2)}$$

Since V represents the sum of the first n terms of the geometric sequence having the common term A and $(1 + i)$, it can be shown that Equation 13.2 may be expressed in the form

$$V = \frac{A[(1 + i)^n - 1]}{(1 + i) - 1}$$

which indicates that

$$V = A\left[\frac{(1+i)^n - 1}{i}\right] \quad \textbf{(13.3)}$$

Referring to the earlier example, recall that $A = \$1.00$, $n = 3$ years, and $i = .06$. After substituting appropriately into Equation 13.3, we find that

$$V = \$1.00\left[\frac{(1+.06)^3 - 1}{(.06)}\right]$$
$$= \$1.00(3.1836)$$

or \$3.1836 which, of course, agrees with the earlier results.

Fortunately, it is not necessary to use the expression $\frac{(1+i)^n - 1}{i}$ to calculate factors similar to 3.1836 each time the value of an ordinary annuity is desired. Rather, the values of an ordinary annuity of \$1 associated with n periods and various interest rates have been computed using Equation 13.3 and are presented in Table A-2 of the Appendix at the end of this text.

The coefficients in Table A-2 also can be used to determine the amount that must be invested at the end of n periods so as to accumulate a desired balance. For example, suppose the interest rate is 10 percent and it is necessary to accumulate a balance of \$79,687 in 10 years. Using the coefficient 15.9374 obtained from Table A-2, we find that

$$\$79{,}687/15.9374$$

or \$5,000 must be invested at the end of each year to accumulate the desired balance.

The results of the foregoing discussion now may be used to calculate the annual contribution to a sinking fund from which a bond issue will be retired. Suppose that a bond issue requires the hospital to accumulate \$500,000 in a sinking fund by January 1, 1999, through a series of 25 equal annual deposits. If the sinking fund is expected to earn interest of 6 percent compounded annually, it can be verified that the annual contribution to the sinking fund is \$9,113.36 (\$500,000/54.8645).

The entry required in the Unrestricted Fund each year is indicated by

Bond Sinking Fund	\$9,113.36	
Cash—General		\$9,113.36

To record annual deposit.

and the income earned on the first deposit is recorded as follows:

Bond Sinking Fund	$546.80	
Income of Bond Sinking Fund		$546.80

To record earnings of bond sinking fund ($9113.36 × .06).

If the investment of bond sinking fund assets earn a return greater or less than 6 percent, the annual deposits are adjusted accordingly.

13.2 LONG-TERM LEASES

Hospitals and other health facilities are making increasing use of leases as alternatives to the outright ownership of plant assets. The use of the lease is a result of increased attempts to: (1) conserve existing capital, (2) avoid difficulties of long-term financing, and (3) obtain various economic advantages associated with leasing as opposed to purchasing capital assets. In fact, many leases provide the institution with the same rights and obligations as those of the owner of the capital asset.

13.2.1 Purchase and Operating Leases

Before considering the accounting techniques for lease contracts, it is necessary to distinguish between purchase and operating leases. In general, the difference involves the extent to which benefits are bestowed and risks are imposed on the lessee. Under a purchase lease, most of the benefits and risks of outright ownership of the asset are assumed by the lessee. Conversely, under an operating lease, these risks and benefits remain with the lessor and are not transferred to the lessee.

More specifically, Statement No. 13 of the Financial Accounting Standards Board identifies four criteria that may be used to distinguish a purchase or capital lease from an operating lease. Accordingly, if at its inception

a. the lease contract transfers ownership of the property to the lessee at the end of the lease term, or
b. the lease contains a bargain purchase clause, or
c. the term of the lease, excluding earlier years of use, is equal to or greater than 75 percent of the estimated economic life of the asset, or
d. the present value of the minimum lease payment, excluding executory costs such as insurance, maintenance, and taxes paid by the lessor, is equal to or greater than 90 percent of the excess of the fair value of the leased property over any related tax credits accruing to the lessor

the lease should be regarded as a purchase or capital lease by the lessee. On the other hand, unless the contract fails to satisfy one or more of these criteria, it should be regarded as an operating lease.

13.2.2 Accounting for Operating Leases

When accounting for operating leases, the property is not capitalized, so this type of contract exerts no influence on the facility's assets or liabilities. However, related rental payments should be recorded as expenses during the life of the lease contract and all relevant information concerning the operating lease must be disclosed in the financial statements. This procedure avoids the problem of presenting misleading information in the annual reports of the institution.

13.2.3 The Present Value of an Ordinary Annuity

Before describing the accounting procedures for purchase or capital leases, it is necessary to introduce the method of calculating the present value of an ordinary annuity. The present value of an annuity is the amount that, if invested today at interest rate *i*, would be sufficient to permit the withdrawal of equal rents or payments at the end of each of *n* periods. To develop this concept, let us first turn to the notion of present value. The present value formulation is analogous to the compound interest paid on a bank deposit. If $1 is invested in a savings account at a bank that pays 8 percent interest a year compounded annually, the amount in the account at the end of one year is given by

$$V_1 = \$1(1.08) = \$1.08$$

Accordingly the value (V_2) in the account at the end of the second year is

$$V_2 = \$1.08(1.08) = \$1(1 + .08)^2 = \$1.1664$$

and at the end of *n* years the value of the deposit is

$$V_n = \$1(1 + .08)^n$$

In the development of this section it is assumed for purposes of calculating present values that interest is compounded annually. If we now wish to determine the present value of V_n, we simply reverse the process outlined above and obtain

$$PV = \frac{1}{(1 + i)^n} \tag{13.4}$$

where i is the time value of money represented by the interest rate.

Suppose now that the institution considers the purchase of a noninterest-bearing instrument that promises to pay $1 at the end of each of three years and that a rate of return of 6 percent compounded annually is desired. A very real question regarding the amount that should be paid for such an instrument now emerges. To answer the question, the present value of the annuity must be calculated.

Using Equation 13.4, we may calculate the present value of the ordinary annuity, PV_A, as shown below:

	0	Year 1	Year 2	Year 3
Present Value of 1st Payment ($\$1/1.06$)	.943	$1.00		
Present Value of 2nd Payment ($\$1/(1.06)^2$)	.890		$1.00	
Present Value of 3rd Payment ($\$1/(1.06)^3$)	.840			$1.00
PV_A	2.673			

Hencc, the present value of the ordinary annuity is given by the sum of present values of each item. We may employ these results to accommodate n periods and obtain

$$PV_A = \frac{\$1}{1 + i} + \frac{\$1}{(1 + i)^2} + \frac{\$1}{(1 + i)^3} + \ldots + \frac{\$1}{(1 + i)^n} \tag{13.5}$$

Applying Equation 13.5 to the example yields

$$PV_A = \frac{\$1}{1 + .06} + \frac{\$1}{(1 + .06)^2} + \frac{\$1}{(1.06)^3} = \$2.673 \tag{13.6.1}$$

We may now manipulate Equation 13.6.1 to provide the basis for deriving a more general expression for calculating the present value of an ordinary annuity. Multiplying Equation 13.6.1 by 1/1.06, we obtain

$$PV_A \frac{1}{(1.06)} = \frac{1}{(1.06)^2} + \frac{1}{(1.06)^3} + \frac{1}{(1.06)^4} \tag{13.6.2}$$

Further, subtracting Equation 13.6.2 from Equation 13.6.1 yields

$$PV_A - PV_A \frac{1}{1.06} = \frac{1}{(1 + .06)} - \frac{1}{(1 + .06)^4}$$

which implies that

$$PV_A \left(1 - \frac{1}{1.06}\right) = \frac{1}{(1.06)} \left[1 - \frac{1}{(1 + .06)^3}\right]$$

or

$$PV_A \left(\frac{.06}{1.06}\right) = \frac{1}{1.06} \left[1 - \frac{1}{(1 + .06)^3}\right] \tag{13.6.3}$$

Dividing Equation 13.6.3 by .06/1.06, we obtain

$$\begin{aligned} PV_A &= \frac{1}{.06} \left[1 - \frac{1}{(1 + .06)^3}\right] \\ &= 2.6730 \end{aligned}$$

which agrees with our earlier results.

Thus, the general formula for the present value of an ordinary annuity of $1 can be expressed in the form

$$\boxed{PV_A = \frac{1}{i} \left[1 - \frac{1}{(1 + i)^n}\right] = \frac{1 - (1 + i)^{-n}}{i}} \tag{13.7}$$

This formula is the basis for calculating the coefficients appearing in Table A-3 of the Appendix, which presents the factors reflecting the present value of an ordinary annuity of $1 at the end of n periods for various rates of return.

13.2.4 Accounting for Purchase Leases

On the basis of this discussion, we now consider the accounting procedures that pertain to purchase or capital leases. When the institution acquires a purchase lease, the leased property is capitalized as an asset and the related obligation is recorded as a liability. The value assigned to the capitalized asset and the related liability should equal the lesser of

a. the fair market value of the leased property, or
b. the present value of the minimum lease payments anticipated during the life of the lease contract.

Moreover, the value of the capitalized asset should be depreciated over its useful life if the lessee is reasonably certain of acquiring ownership of it. On the other hand, if ownership is not assured, the value of the capitalized asset should be amortized during the life of the contract.

When accounting for purchase leases, the interest rate may be stated explicitly or may be implicit in the lease contract. Each of these situations is described next.

13.2.4.1 Explicit Interest Rate

Suppose the institution can either purchase a piece of equipment having a fair market value of \$36,048 or lease the equipment for a minimum payment of \$10,000 per year for five years. Suppose further that the estimated life of the equipment also is five years and that the institution is assured of acquiring outright ownership of the property. If the lease contract specifies an interest rate of 14 percent, we may use Equation 13.7 to compute the present value of the minimum lease payments. In this example, we find that

$$PV_{10,000} = \$10,000 \left[\frac{1 - (1 + .14)^{-5}}{.14} \right]$$

$$\cong \$10,000\ (3.433)$$

or approximately \$34,330. Since the present value of the minimum lease payments is less than the fair market value of the equipment, the entry to record the lease is:

Leased Property Rights	\$34,330	
Liability on Lease		\$34,330

The balance of the leased property rights account is reported as an asset of the Unrestricted Fund Balance and the balance of the Liability on Lease account as an obligation of the Unrestricted Fund.

The balance of the leased property rights should be amortized as an expense during each year of the five-year period. When calculating the depreciation charges associated with these rights, the $34,330 may be recognized as an expense using the declining balance, sum-of-the-years'-digits, or straight-line method. Using the straight-line method, depreciation expenses of $34,330/5 or $6,866 are recognized each year.

Consider next the cash disbursement associated with the first lease payment. Recall that the cash disbursement is accompanied by a reduction in the balance of the Liability on Lease account and a recognition of interest charges. Consequently, the entry to record the first payment is:

Liability on Lease	$5,193.80	
Interest Expense	4,806.20	
Cash		$10,000

The values in this entry are calculated as follows:

Rental Payment	$10,000.00
Interest Expense ($34,330 × .14)	4,806.20
Reduction in Liability	5,193.80

At this point in the analysis, it should be noted that the balance of the Liability on Lease account is $29,136.20 ($34,330.00 − $5,193.80), so the entry to record the second payment is:

Liability on Lease	$5,920.93	
Interest Expense	4,079.07	
Cash		$10,000

Similar to the earlier analysis, the values in this entry are calculated as follows:

Rental Payment	$10,000.00
Interest Expense ($29,136.20 × .14)	4,079.07
Reduction in Liability	5,920.93

The amount by which the balance of the Liability on Lease account is reduced increases each year while the annual interest expenses for the lease contract decline. To emphasize the latter point, it should be verified that the reduction in the balance of the Liability on Lease account in the third year is $6,749.86 and the interest expense recognized in that year is $3,250.14.

13.2.4.2 Implicit Interest Rate

Assume that the lease contract in the previous section fails to specify the interest rate explicitly. As before, we assume that the institution purchases the equipment for $36,048 or leases it for $10,000 per year for five years. Using Equation 13.7, we solve the expression

$$\$36{,}048 = \$10{,}000\left[\frac{1-(1+i)^{-5}}{i}\right]$$

uniquely for i and find that the implicit rate of interest is approximately 12 percent.

Since no interest is specified in the lease contract, the lessee and the lessor are essentially the same entity, so the institution should use the fair market value of $36,048 to capitalize the asset. Consequently, the entry

Leased Property Rights	$36,048	
Liability on Lease		$36,048

records the asset and related obligation under the assumption that the lease contract does not specify the interest rate explicitly. Similar to the discussion presented in the previous section, depreciation charges of $36,048/5 or $7,-209.60 should be recognized as an expense each year.

Consider next the cash disbursement for the first lease payment, which is recorded by the entry

Liability on Lease	$5,674.24	
Interest Expense	4,325.76	
Cash		$10,000

In this case the values are calculated as follows:

Rental Payment	$10,000.00
Interest Expense ($36,048 × .12)	4,325.76
Reduction in Liability	5,674.24

By analogy, the entry to record the cash disbursement for the second lease payment is:

Liability on Lease	$6,355.15	
Interest Expense	3,644.85	
Cash		$10,000.00

The values in the entry are calculated as:

Rental Payment	$10,000.00
Interest Expense ($30,373.76 × .12)	3,644.85
Reduction in Liability	6,355.15

Similar to the previous section, the balance of the Liability on Lease account is eliminated by a series of entries that are recorded during the remaining years in the life of the contract.

13.3 LONG-TERM LEASE CONTRACTS

As mentioned earlier, plant assets may be acquired under a deferred payment plan that requires a series of installment payments, with interest charges on the unpaid balances. The interest charges, whether explicit or implicit, must be deducted from the asset cost and recorded as expenses.

For example, suppose that equipment having a fair market value of $77,716.12 is purchased on January 1, 1979, under a contract calling for a down payment of $20,000 and 10 annual payments of $10,000 starting January 1, 1980. An interest rate of 15 percent per year is implicit in this contract, so the present value of the 10 annual payments of $10,000, each at a rate of 15 percent per year, is $57,716.20 (i.e., $10,000 × 5.0188* × 1.15). The acquisition of this equipment and the first annual payment are recorded as follows:

January 1, 1979

Equipment	$77,716.20	
Discount on Equipment Contract Payable	42,283.80	
Cash		$20,000
Equipment Contract Payable		100,000

To record purchase of equipment on installment notes contract.

December 31, 1979

Interest Expenses	$8,657.52	
Discount on Equipment Contract Payable		$8,657.52

To record 15 percent interest on $57,716.80 ($100,000 − $42,283.20).

* The value 5.0188 is obtained from Table A-3 of the Appendix.

January 1, 1980

Equipment Contract Payable	$10,000	
Cash		$10,000

This procedure provides a reasonable estimate of the cash equivalent price as well as an accurate measure of the related liability and the acquisition cost of the asset. The unamortized discount is reported in the balance sheet as a deduction from the Equipment Contract Payable account.

Questions for Discussion

1. Describe conditions under which a bond will sell at a premium; at a discount.
2. Describe the procedures followed when a bond is issued at a discount (premium).
3. Explain why it is necessary to amortize the bond premium or discount.
4. Define a sinking fund and the procedures to be followed when one is used.
5. Describe the problems associated with traditional lease-rental accounting procedures.
6. Explain the importance of the present value of an annuity to the problems of lease-purchase accounting.

Problems for Solution

1. Suppose the institution issues 10 $10,000 8 percent bonds at 100 and accrued interest on September 1, 1979. Issue costs are $120 and interest is payable on April 1 and October 1. The maturity date of these bonds is October 1, 1999. However, on March 1, 1980, 2 of the 10 bonds are redeemed at 96 and accrued interest. Record all transactions concerning this issue through March 1, 1980.
2. Assume the bonds in Problem 1 are issued at 93 and redeemed on March 1, 1980, at 91 plus accrued interest. Record this redemption.
3. Assume the bonds in Problem 1 are issued at 110 and redeemed on March 1 at 105. Record all transactions concerning this issue through March 1, 1980.
4. Suppose that on January 1, 1980, the hospital issues 100 $1,000 10 percent five-year serial bonds at 96. These bonds mature at a rate of $20,000 per year beginning January 1, 1981, and interest is payable on January 1. Show the amortization of the bond discount and the interest expense for the period.
5. Suppose the institution may either buy a piece of equipment for $144,720 or lease it for $20,000 for 10 years. In this case, the lessor

earns a rate of return of approximately 8 percent. If the rental payments are made at the beginning of each year, starting on January 1, 1980, prepare all entries for 1980, assuming that the equipment is leased.

6. Suppose that on January 1, 1979, the hospital purchases a piece of equipment for $100,000. Suppose further that it makes a down payment of $40,000 and agrees to pay the balance in six equal annual installments beginning January 1, 1980. Assuming an implicit interest rate of 10 percent, prepare the entries required on January 1, 1979, December 31, 1979, and January 1, 1980.

Part IV
Financial Statements

Chapter 14
Presentation of Financial Statements

One of the primary objectives of the accounting process is to provide information concerning the financial position and the operating activity of the health care facility. It is necessary to produce information that is required for the internal management of the institution and to prepare financial statements in a form specified by external authorities and third party payers. Fortunately, satisfying internal needs and providing information for external users are, in large part, mutually consistent goals that require little duplication of effort.

It is useful to consider first the criteria that should be used in evaluating reports generated for internal purposes. Obvious factors in evaluating the internal reporting system are the usefulness, timeliness, frequency, content, and form of periodic reports. Clearly, each report must serve some specified purpose and should be used by appropriate individuals. To be of maximum usefulness, reports must reach the recipients on a timely basis so that required information may be used in formulating and implementing managerial decisions. Consequently, reports must be provided at intervals that correspond to the managerial needs of the institution.

Although the number and type of reports will vary from institution to institution, the primary statements at most facilities include a balance sheet plus statements of revenues and expenses, of changes in fund balance, and of the sources and applications of funds. Supplementary schedules may be provided for certain users.

14.1 BALANCE SHEET

There are basically two different types of fund groupings—restricted and unrestricted. Accordingly, a balance sheet should be provided for each of those funds. It will be recalled that the restricted fund grouping usually consists of the Specific Purpose Fund, the Endowment Fund, and the Capital Fund.

The major function of the balance sheet is to provide users with information on the institution's assets, liabilities, and fund balance (equity). Of particular importance is the presentation of all material information concerning the institution's financial position that has been recorded in accordance with sound accounting practice. Clearly, any changes in accounting practice should be disclosed and their effects fully discussed in supplementary notes. As an example of the format used by many institutions, the balance sheet of a hypothetical hospital is presented in a somewhat condensed form in Table 14-1.

14.1.1 Fund Balances

This balance sheet shows a single fund balance that represents all unrestricted resources. As a result, there is no question as to the magnitude of the total unrestricted resources available to the hospital. On a less abbreviated balance sheet, the composition of the fund balance might be presented as follows:

Fund Balance	
Unappropriated	$500,000
Board-Designated Equipment Fund	300,000
Board-Designated Investment Fund	400,000
Board-Designated Specific Purpose	600,000
Total Fund Balance	1,800,000

Of primary importance is informing the user of the balance sheet as to the total of all unrestricted resources.

14.1.2 Assets

In a less abbreviated format, the composition of the current assets of the hospital might be presented as follows:

Current Assets		1980
Cash		$120,000
Accounts Receivable	$235,000	
Less Allowance	30,000	205,000
Short-Term Investments		700,000
Inventories		810,000
Prepaid Insurance		75,000
Prepaid Rent		90,000
Total Current Assets		2,000,000

Table 14-1 Typical Balance Sheet, Condensed

GENERAL HOSPITAL

Balance Sheet

(Condensed)

December 31, 1980

Unrestricted Funds

Assets		*Liabilities & Fund Balances*	
	1980		*1980*
Total Current Assets	$2,000,000	Total Current Liabilities	$13,000,000
Board-Designated Funds		Long-Term Liabilities	1,400,000
Cash	150,000	Fund Balance	1,800,000
Investment	50,000	Total	16,200,000
Property Plant & Equipment	15,000,000		
Less Depreciation	(1,000,000)		
	16,200,000		

Restricted Funds

Specific Purpose Fund

Assets		*Liabilities & Fund Balances*	
Cash	$100,000	Fund Balance	$125,000
Investment	25,000		
Total Assets	125,000		

Endowment Fund

Cash	$400,000	Permanent Endowments	$800,000
Investment	700,000	Term Endowments	300,000
Total Assets	1,100,000	Fund Balance	1,100,000

Capital Fund

Cash	$700,000	Fund Balance	$1,800,000
Investment	900,000		
Pledges	200,000		
	1,800,000		

The Unrestricted Fund of General Hospital consists of temporary or short-term investments of $700,000 (see the composition of current assets) and long-term investments of $50,000 (see Table 14-1). The latter appears as a board-designated asset, the former in the current asset section.

The basis of reporting investments in the balance sheet must be disclosed. As discussed earlier, short-term investments usually are carried at the lower of cost or market, long-term investments at cost. In the case of bonds, cost is adjusted to reflect the amortization of premiums or discounts.

14.1.2.1 Inventories

The presentation of information concerning inventories for external reporting purposes requires a disclosure of the method by which supplies are valued. Additional information on major categories of inventory, changes in supply sources, and other material matters should be disclosed through supplementary notes.

14.1.2.2 Prepaid Expenses

These assets usually arise from the prepayment of insurance, interest, rent, and other expense items. The accounting procedures for such assets were discussed earlier.

14.1.2.3 Receivables

As seen in the less abbreviated presentation of the current assets of the Unrestricted Fund (Section 14.1.2), General Hospital's receivables are reported at an amount reflecting their net realizable cash value. Details as to the composition of outstanding receivables are provided through a supplementary schedule. Details on the allowance for bad debt, contractual adjustments, courtesy discounts, and bad debt must also be disclosed fully.

14.1.2.4 Property Plant and Equipment

The Property Plant and Equipment account reflects the hospital's actual investment in plant assets it uses in day-to-day operations. These assets should not be reported in a restricted fund classification since this would imply restraints on their use or disposition. In addition, the basis of valuation, the method of depreciation, and the amounts invested in plant assets by major category should be disclosed through a supplementary schedule or footnote.

14.1.2.5 Board-Designated Assets

As noted earlier, the hospital's board may designate or earmark certain unrestricted resources for various purposes. These should not be reported as a part of the Restricted Fund but should be segregated in the Unrestricted Fund as seen in Table 14-1. The reason is that board-designated assets carry no legal restrictions imposed by external authority. Board decisions may be rescinded but donor restrictions can be changed only by the giver or by the court. As a result, board-designated assets should not be grouped with other restricted funds.

14.1.3 Liabilities

Most liabilities are reported in the Unrestricted Fund since they are satisfied by the use of unrestricted resources. These obligations are presented in two balance sheet categories: current liabilities and noncurrent or long-term liabilities. Only in unusual circumstances do liabilities in material amounts appear in restricted funds. Such amounts usually are related to interfund borrowing, which was discussed earlier.

The Restricted Funds are divided into three self-balancing groups. The Capital Fund does not contain the hospital's existing plant assets. Rather, this fund merely accumulates restricted resources until they are used for the actual acquisition of plant and equipment. As mentioned earlier, when resources are used in purchasing plant assets, the amount involved is transferred from the Capital Fund to the Unrestricted Fund, where such acquisitions are recorded.

14.2 INCOME STATEMENT

Table 14-2 is the income statement for the hypothetical hospital. As pointed out earlier, the income statement, or the Statement of Operations as it also is called, presents the results of operational activity in terms of the revenue earned and the expenses incurred during a specific period. Unlike the balance sheet, which provides a snapshot of the financial position of the institution at a given time, the income statement presents a series of events that influence the financial well-being of the facility.

In portraying the revenues and expenses during the accounting period, the income statement provides a measure of the extent to which management is successful in preserving the hospital's short-term financial viability. One of the major managerial responsibilities is to contain costs at a level that is commensurate with available revenues or, alternatively, to obtain revenues in amounts that are at least sufficient to avoid operating losses. The income statement, therefore, provides much of the information necessary for evaluating the extent to which management is successful in discharging these responsibilities.

Table 14-2 Example of an Income Statement

GENERAL HOSPITAL		
Income Statement		
For Year Ending December 31, 1980		
Income		
Inpatient Income	$3,000,000	
Outpatient Income	900,000	
Less Deductions from Patient Service Revenue	700,000	
Net Operating Patient Service Revenue		$3,200,000
Add Other Operating Revenues		20,000
Total Operating Revenue		3,220,000
Less Operating Expenses		
Patient Care Services	2,300,000	
Research	500,000	
Education	300,000	
General Service	100,000	
Depreciation	110,000	
Interest Expense	50,000	
Total Expenses		3,360,000
Net Operating Income (Loss)		(140,000)
Add Nonoperating Revenue		280,000
Net Income (Loss) for Year		140,000

As for the recognition of revenues and expenses, this occurs in accordance with the contribution and realization rules. Simply stated these rules are: (1) revenues should be recorded in the period in which they are earned, and (2) expenses should be recorded in the period in which they contribute to operations.

The income statement in Table 14-2 is easy to read and understand since it shows all the unrestricted income with a minimum of cumbersome or confusing detail. The income statement for General Hospital is presented in a multiple-step format in which the results of operations are reported through a series of intermediate subtotals or balances that depict patient service revenues, net operating patient revenues, other operating revenue, net operating revenue, and net income for the year. The multiple-step format emphasizes the deductions from patient service revenue and other adjustments as well as the net operating income before consideration of unrestricted gifts and other nonoperating revenues.

As indicated in Table 14-2, the income statement is presented in a condensed or abbreviated form that is relatively free of the mass of detail about the institution's operational results. The details supporting the totals should be provided in a series of supplementary schedules accompanying the financial statements. An indication of the type and nature of the supporting schedules is:

1. Patient Service Revenue Schedule: The details should be provided to indicate the source of revenues as well as the functional area of activity that earned the income. Such a schedule should be grouped in accordance with inpatient and outpatient categories as well as by type of service.
2. Deductions from Revenue: A supplementary schedule showing deductions by major type of deduction as well as by inpatient and outpatient categories should be attached to the income statement.
3. Other Operating Revenue Schedule: This supplementary schedule details the other operating revenues. As indicated, these revenues are derived from sales to persons or entities other than patients and from other activities that are related to the normal operations of the facility.
4. Operating Expense Schedule: This schedule reports the expenses incurred by the institution as classified by function and object of expenditure. Hence, the schedule should depict the direct costs over which management has effective control and primary responsibility. As a result, items such as employee benefits and depreciation should be apportioned among the departmental or functional areas.
5. Nonoperating Revenue Schedule: As indicated earlier, all unrestricted gifts and bequests must be included in this category in the year in which they are received, as should unrestricted investment income and other unrestricted contributions.

14.3 CHANGES IN FUND BALANCES

The third basic statement prepared by the institution reports the changes in balances for all fund groupings. The income statement (Table 14-2) represents only the change in the Unrestricted Fund balance that results from differences between the revenues and expenses of a given period. As will be recalled, a net income increases the fund balance and a net loss reduces it. However, factors other than a net income or a net loss may cause a change. Since the other factors are not reflected in the income statement as a revenue or an expense, it is necessary to provide an additional financial statement to report all changes in the balance of each fund grouping maintained by the hospital.

Tables 14-3, 14-4, 14-5, and 14-6 are the statements of changes in the fund balances for the Unrestricted Fund, the Specific Purpose Fund, the Endow-

Table 14-3 Statement of Changes in Fund Balances

Unrestricted Fund

	1980	*1979*
Fund Balance, January 1	$1,260,000	$1,060,000
Net Income for Year	140,000	60,000
Donated Medical Equipment	100,000	140,000
Transfer from Capital Fund	200,000	
Transfer from Specific Purpose Fund	100,000	
Fund Balance, December 31	1,800,000	1,260,000

Table 14-4 Statement of Changes in Specific Purpose Fund

	1980	*1979*
Fund Balance, January 1	$25,000	$10,000
Restricted Gifts	150,000	5,000
Research Grants	50,000	10,000
Transfer to Unrestricted Fund	(100,000)	
Fund Balance, December 31	125,000	25,000

Table 14-5 Statement of Changes in Endowment Fund

	1980	*1979*
Balance, January 1	$700,000	$500,000
Restricted Gifts & Bequests	200,000	100,000
Net Gain on Sale of Investments	50,000	40,000
Other Investment Income	150,000	60,000
Fund Balance, December 31	1,100,000	700,000

Table 14-6 Statement of Changes in the Fund Balance of the Capital Fund

	1980	*1979*
Fund Balance, January 1	$500,000	300,000
Restricted Gifts and Bequests	1,496,000	160,000
Investment Income	4,000	40,000
Transfer to Unrestricted Fund	(200,000)	
Fund Balance, December 31	1,800,000	500,000

ment Fund, and the Capital Fund of General Hospital, respectively. The following transactions apply to these fund groupings:

1. $100,000 is transferred from the Specific Purpose Fund to the Unrestricted Fund
2. $200,000 is transferred from the Capital Fund to the Unrestricted Fund
3. medical equipment with a fair market value of $100,000 is donated to the hospital
4. donations, bequests, and grants received by the hospital are reported in Tables 14-4 and 14-5
5. donor-restricted investment income is earned by resources of the Specific Purpose Fund, the Endowment Fund, and the Capital Fund.

Several comments concerning these transfers are warranted. The basic concept underlying the segregation of restricted from unrestricted funds is that these resources should be carried in the former until used for the purpose specified by the donor. At the time they are used for that purpose, the amount expended is transferred to the Unrestricted Fund. As a result, the transfer of $100,000 from the Specific Purpose Fund and of $200,000 from the Capital Fund to the Unrestricted Fund are used to finance the specified project and the acquisition of plant assets, respectively.

14.4 STATEMENT OF SOURCES AND APPLICATIONS

The income statement presents the results of operational activity in terms of revenues earned and expenses incurred during a given period. A balance sheet depicts the financial position of the institution in terms of assets, liabilities, and fund balances at a given moment. The statement of changes in fund balances provides a comprehensive survey of factors causing shifts in each of the fund groupings. These three financial statements provide essential information concerning the operating results and the hospital's financial position. However, changes in financial position as well as aspects of the financial and investment activities are not always disclosed by such statements. In the case of General Hospital, for example, a comparative balance sheet in which the previous year's assets, liabilities, and fund balances are reported in the financial statements reveals the following information:

	1979	*1978*
Property Plant & Equipment	$15,000,000	$14,000,000

On the basis of this information alone, it can be concluded that new assets costing $1,000,000 were acquired during the period. However, it is quite possible that new assets costing $2,000,000 were acquired while assets costing $1,000,000 were retired during the year. Offsetting activities such as these are not clearly discernible from the three tables.

The purpose of the Statement of Sources and Applications of Working Funds (see Table 14-7, later in this chapter) is to provide a summary of all operations and financial and investment activities of the institution. In this way, the statement accounts for all changes reported in successive balance sheets.

To illustrate the mechanics of the development of this statement, suppose that the following set of data pertains to Municipal Hospital:

	December 31		*Increase*
	198B	*198A*	*(Decrease)*
Current Assets	$4,150	$3,200	$950
Long-Term Investment	500	200	300
Plant & Equipment	9,760	8,500	1,260
Other Assets	50	70	(20)
Totals	14,460	11,970	2,490
Accumulated Depreciation	3,100	2,900	200
Current Liabilities	4,360	3,960	400
Mortgages Payable	2,000	2,410	(410)
Bonds Payable, Due 200B	2,000		2,000
Unrestricted Fund Balance	3,000	2,700	300
Totals	14,460	11,970	2,490

At this point in the analysis, net working capital is defined as the sum of the current assets of the institution less the sum of the current liabilities. Similarly, the change in working capital is defined as the change in current assets less the change in current liabilities. Algebraically, the change in working capital is given by the equation

$$\text{Change in Working Capital} = (CA_t - CA_{t-1}) - (CL_t - CL_{t-1}) \quad \textbf{(14.1)}$$

where CA represents the current assets, CL corresponds to the current liabilities, and the subscripts refer to the period in which the change occurred.

Referring to the example, an application of Equation 14.1 reveals that the change in the working capital of Municipal Hospital between December 31, 198A, and December 31, 198B, amounts to

$$(\$4{,}150 - \$3{,}200) - (\$4{,}360 - \$3{,}960)$$

Table 14-7 Statement of Sources and Applications of Working Funds

MUNICIPAL HOSPITAL

Year Ended December 31, 198B

Source of Funds		
Funds Generated by Operations		$530
Other Sources:		
Nonoperating Revenue (Not Including Gains and Losses on Sale of Assets)	$30	
Plant Expenditures Financed Through Capital Fund	30	
Issuance of Bonds	2,000	
Sale of Long-Term Investments	430	
Sale of Plant Assets	120	
Donated Equipment	120	
Decrease in Other Assets	20	
Total Other Sources of Revenue		2,750
Total Sources of Funds		3,280
Application of Funds		
Additions to Plant Assets	1,500	
Donation of Plant Asset	120	
Purchase of Long-Term Investments	700	
Retirement of Mortgage	410	
Total Applications of Funds		2,730
Increase in Working Capital		$550

or $550. As will be seen later, the details in Equation 14.1 are summarized by the data reported in the Statement of the Sources and Applications of Working Funds.

Before proceeding, it is necessary to be able to distinguish between sources and applications of funds. The basic accounting equation ($A = L + FB$) is expanded to:

$$CA + NCA = CL + NCL + FB \qquad \textbf{(14.2)}$$

where

NCA = noncurrent assets
NCL = noncurrent liabilities
FB = fund balance

Rearranging Equation 14.2 slightly yields

$$CA - CL = NCL + FB - NCA$$

where $CA - CL$ is the definition of the hospital's net working capital. From the rearranged formula, it can be seen that an increase in funds results from a gain in the value of the right-hand side of the equation. A decrease in funds occurs when the value of the right-hand side decreases. In summary, then:

1. Sources of funds are related to increases in the terms *NCL* and *FB* or decreases in the term *NCA*.
2. Applications of funds are related to decreases in the terms *NCL* and *FB* or increases in the term *NCA*.

An increase in the term *NCL* represents a source of funds since mortgages or bonds may be sold to obtain money. Similarly, a decrease in *NCA* (e.g., the sale of long-term investments) represents a source of funds to the hospital. On the other hand, a decrease in the term *NCL* (e.g., the repayment of mortgage notes) and an increase in *NCA* (e.g., purchase of long-term investments) represent an application of funds.

The following is a detailed analysis of the net increase or decrease in the noncurrent and fund balance accounts of Municipal Hospital so as to obtain the information necessary for the preparation of the Statement of Sources and Applications of Working Funds.

Long-Term Investments:

The $300 increase in the NCA account is given by	
Purchase of Additional Investments Costing	$700
Less: Sale of Investment for $430 That Cost	400
	300

Obviously, the purchase is an application of funds and the sale is source of funds.

Plant & Equipment:

The net increase of $1,260 in this NCA account results from:	
Expenditure for New Plant assets	$1,500
Donation of Plant Asset	120
	1,620
Less: Sale of Old Asset for $120 That Cost	360
	1,260

Other Assets:

The $20 decrease in other assets is treated as a miscellaneous source of funds.

Accumulated Depreciation:
This account shows a net increase of $200 that resulted from the following transactions:

Depreciation Expense for the Year	$500
Less: Write-off of Accumulated Depreciation on Plant Assets Sold During the Year	300
	200

Neither of these changes has any effect on funds provided or applied during the year. As will be seen, however, the depreciation expense of $500 must be added to net operating income of the period to determine the amount of funds provided by operations. This treatment is given to depreciation because it has been deducted in computing net income but does not require the use of funds.

Mortgage Payable:
The $410 decrease represents the payment of the annual installment of portions of the debt.

Bond Payable:
The $2,000 increase in this account reflects the 20-year $2,000 bonds issued by the hospital early in the year.

Unrestricted Fund Balance:
The $300 net increase in this account is calculated as follows:

Net Operating Income for 198B	$30
Nonoperating Income for 198B (includes $60 gain on sale of plant asset and $30 gain on sale of investments)	120
Plant Assets Donated in Kind	120
Transfer of Unrestricted Fund from Capital Fund for Financing of Plant Assets	30
	300

Funds are generated by the hospital's operations but the net operating income figure does not indicate the amount of funds generated from that source. This is because certain items that did not provide or require funds are added or subtracted from reported revenues when determining the net income of the period. The reported net income therefore must be adjusted for these items.

Table 14-7 is an example of the Statement of Sources and Applications of Working Funds for Municipal Hospital. The funds generated by operations in the amount of $530 are computed as follows:

	Net Operating Income	$30
Plus:	Items That Do Not Require the Use of Funds: Depreciation Expense	500
	Funds Generated by Operations	530

Recall that Municipal Hospital reported $500 in depreciation charges in 198B. When determining the net operating income of $30, however, these expenses are subtracted from the revenues reported in the income statement. Since the adjusting entry required to record depreciation does not involve a working capital account, the $500 should be added to the net operating income to determine the funds generated by operational activity. In addition to the Statement of Sources and Applications of Funds, a supplementary schedule showing the increase or decrease in each component of current assets (e.g., cash, marketable securities, etc.) and liabilities (accounts payable, accrued expenses payable, etc.) should be provided as an integral part of the financial statement.

As seen in Table 14-7, the total source of funds in 198B is $3,280. Most of these items are easily understood and are discussed first.

1. The resources transferred from the Capital Fund are recorded in the Unrestricted Fund as follows:

Cash	$30	
Unrestricted Fund Balance		$30

   This increases the working capital of the Unrestricted Fund and is a source of funds.

2. The bond issue results in a cash inflow that is recorded as:

Cash	$2,000	
Bonds Payable		$2,000

   This also represents a source of funds to the hospital since the bond issue increases its working capital.

3. The sale of long-term investments is recorded as follows:

Cash	$430	
Gain on Sale		$30
Investment		400

   Again, the $430 represents a source of funds to the hospital. The amount from this source is measured in terms of the proceeds and not in terms of the cost of the investment instrument.

4. The proceeds from the sale of plant assets is recorded in the Unrestricted Fund as follows:

Cash	$120	
Accumulated Depreciation	300	
Gain on Sale		$60
Equipment		360

   The sale of plant assets results in an increase in the cash balance and, as such, represents a source of funds.

Recall that the increase in the Unrestricted Fund balance is $300, including a nonoperating income of $120. The nonoperating income earned by the institution also includes the $30 gain realized from the sale of marketable securities as well as the $60 gain from selling plant assets. When preparing the income statements, the gains realized by selling securities and plant assets should be separated from the other nonoperating revenues. Consequently, nonoperating revenues of $30 (i.e., $120 − [$30 + $60]) should be reported in the income statement for 198B.

Consider next the second section of Table 14-7. The application of funds by Municipal Hospital is $2,730. In this case, the purchase of plant assets and long-term investments increases the noncurrent assets of the institution and, as a result, these transactions represent an application of funds. Similarly, the retirement of a portion of the outstanding mortgage payable reduces the noncurrent liabilities, so this transaction also represents an application of funds. Finally, the donated equipment is regarded as a source as well as an application of funds. As a consequence, the donated equipment exerts no effect on the funds statement.

Finally, Table 14-7 shows that the increase in working capital is given by the difference between the total source of funds ($3,280) and the total application of funds ($2,730), or $550. These results are identical to those obtained when Equation 14.1 is used to determine the change in the working capital of the institution.

Questions for Discussion

1. Identify and briefly describe the major financial statements prepared by most health care facilities.
2. Discuss the relationship between the Unrestricted Fund income statement and the Unrestricted Fund balance sheet.
3. Describe what factors other than the net income or loss of the period might influence the end-of-period fund balance.
4. Explain the primary purpose of the statement of sources and application of working funds.
5. Describe how working capital is increased; decreased.
6. Explain how board-designated funds are presented in the financial statements.

Problems for Solution

1. Suppose the following information appears in the general ledger accounts of Hill City Hospital on December 31, 198A:

Wages and Salaries	$10,100
Interest Expense	350

Supply Expense	$5,600
Inpatient Revenue	15,100
Outpatient Revenue	7,850
Depreciation Expense	2,100
Deductions from Revenues	900
Other Operating Revenue	1,300
Other Operating Expenses	780

Prepare an income statement for Hill City Hospital.

2. Assume that the following information appears in the general ledger of Mountain City Hospital on December 31, 198A:

Wages and Salaries	$21,700
Inpatient Revenue	26,499
Deductions in Revenue	1,750
Supply Expense	14,780
Outpatient Revenue	24,900
Depreciation Expense	4,500
Interest Expense	750
Rent Expense	900
Other Operating Revenue	7,300

Prepare an income statement for Mountain City Hospital.

3. Suppose the following information appears in the general ledger of the institution on December 31, 198A:

a. Fund Balances: January 1, 198A

Unrestricted Fund	$4,200
Specific Purpose Fund	580
Endowment Fund	3,600
Capital Fund	420

b. Donated Equipment	57
c. Net Income of the Period	720

d. Gifts and Bequests Received:

Specific Purpose Fund	400
Endowment Fund	300
Capital Fund	700

e. Restricted Income from Investments:

Specific Purpose Fund	207
Capital Fund	150
Endowment Fund	300

f. Transfers to Unrestricted Fund from

Specific Purpose Fund	200
Capital Fund	100

g. Transfer from Unrestricted Fund to

Capital Fund	75

h. Gains on Sales of Investments:

Specific Purpose Fund	10
Endowment Fund	20
Capital Fund	35

Prepare a statement of changes in fund balances for each of the fund groupings.

4. Assume the following information appears in the general ledger accounts of Bay City Hospital on December 31, 198A:

Cash (Undesignated)	$8,000
Accounts Payable	7,000
Mortgage Payable (Noncurrent)	8,000
Accounts Receivable	12,500
Mortgage Payable (Current)	700
Temporary Investments	15,100
Plant and Equipment	60,100
Accumulated Depreciation	3,100
Deferred Revenue (Current)	200
Inventory	7,100
Allowance for Uncollectable Accounts	3,100
Payroll Taxes Withheld	2,500
Prepaid Expenses	1,200
Accrued Expenses Payable	4,100
Other Current Liabilities	500

Prepare a balance sheet for Bay City Hospital.

5. Suppose the comparative balance sheet of Sick City Hospital is as follows:

	12/31/198B	12/31/198A
Current Assets	$900	$800
Long-Term Investments	360	400
Plant and Equipment	8,200	8,000
Accumulated Depreciation	(1,500)	(1,400)
	7,960	7,800

Current Liabilities	860	320
Mortgage Payable	3,500	4,000
Fund Balance	3,600	3,480
	7,960	7,800

Also suppose the following information is available:

a. Net income earned in 198B is $120.
b. Long-term investments that cost $240 are sold for $300.
c. Plant and equipment are sold for $100.
d. Depreciation expense for the period is $270.
e. Plant and equipment costing $730 are purchased.

Prepare a statement of sources and applications of working funds for Sick City Hospital.

Chapter 15
Introduction to the Analysis of Financial Statements

The primary focus of this text has been on the development of accounting information that is of value to the internal management of health care facilities. Management reaches important administrative and financial decisions that are based on the financial information generated by the accounting process.

In addition, the financial position and the results of operational activity are of interest to external agencies and entities. These groups also make extensive use of information provided by the accounting process. Also interested are creditors such as banks, suppliers and other lenders; planning agencies; investors; labor unions; and the general public. Some of these groups focus more on the institution's financial strength, others on the extent to which management has discharged its fiduciary responsibilities and complied with contractual agreements.

These entities frequently base their decisions on information in the institution's financial statements. The final chapter examines financial statements from the perspective of an external entity. It should be noted, however, that the techniques of evaluation and analysis also are important to the effective management of internal affairs.

15.1 BASIC METHODS OF ANALYSIS

Before financial statements are useful to the analyst, a basis for evaluating, measuring, and analyzing the information must be established. Analysts are not particularly interested in the absolute amount of current assets and current liabilities; rather, they are more concerned with the relationship between current assets and liabilities over time. As a result, financial analysis requires a set of comparative data. Comparative data make it clear that a set of financial statements represents a single point in a nexus that depicts the financial history of the institution as it evolves over time.

The reliance on the comparative approach means that the data in at least two successive years must be comparable. As noted in Chapter 14, all changes in accounting practices and their effect on financial information must be disclosed fully in annual reports. The reporting periods of course must be of equal length. Thus, accounting consistency and data comparability are critical to the analysis of financial statements.

15.1.1 Absolute and Relative Changes

Perhaps the most basic method of analyzing financial statements involves the development of data depicting the absolute and relative changes that have occurred over a period of time. Consider, for example, the comparative balance sheet of a hypothetical hospital in Table 15-1, where the absolute amount of change and the percentage change in each of the assets, liabilities, and the fund balance of the Unrestricted Fund are computed. The percentage change is calculated by dividing the absolute change by the base year (198A in this example) figure. Although not shown here, a similar set of calculations is required for the other financial statements of the hospital.

When more than two years of comparative data are available, trend percentages are used in analyzing the facility's financial history. Each figure in the base year (the earliest period for which data are available) is assigned the value of 100 percent; values in successive years are expressed as a percentage of the base figure. Trend percentages are useful in identifying unusual relationships that may not be detected by an examination of absolute changes over time.

15.1.2 Structural Ratios

Structural ratios are used in the analysis of relationships among data within each individual statement. For example, consider Table 15-2, which shows the balance sheet of the hospital reporting total assets of $3,235 and $2,830 at the end of 198B and 198A respectively. Accordingly, the value of each asset reported in the two years is expressed as a percentage of the total assets of the corresponding period. In Table 15-2, cash comprises 9.3 percent ($300/$3,235) of total assets in 198B and 8.8 percent ($250/$2,830) in 198A. A similar set of calculations permits an examination of the obligations and the fund balance of the institution. The ratios presented in the table are most useful in evaluating the balance sheet in terms of management's allocation of resources. Structural ratios also are helpful in analyzing the facility's capital structure.

Structural ratios also are useful in analyzing the income statement. Table 15-3 is an analysis of the hospital's condensed income statement. The first

Table 15-1 Example of a Comparative Balance Sheet

CIVIC HOSPITAL

Condensed Comparative Balance Sheet

Unrestricted Fund

December 31, 1979, and 1980

Assets	*December 31*		*Increase (Decrease)*	
	198B	*198A*	*Amount*	*Percent*
Current Assets				
Cash	$300	$250	$50	20.0
Temporary Investments	260	240	20	8.3
Receivables (Net)	400	420	(20)	(4.8)
Inventories	700	780	(80)	(10.2)
Prepaid Expenses	30	20	10	50.0
Total Current Assets	1,690	1,710	(20)	(1.2)
Board Designated Assets	500	100	400	400.0
Property, Plant, & Equipment (Net)	970	940	30	3.2
Other Assets	75	80	(5)	6.2
Total Assets	3,235	2,830	405	14.3
Liabilities and Fund Balance				
Current Liabilities				
Notes Payable	100	50	50	100.0
Accounts Payable	700	820	(120)	(14.6)
Accrued Expenses Payable	65	50	15	30.0
Other	200	190	10	5.3
Total Current Liabilities	1,065	1,110	(45)	(4.1)
Noncurrent Liabilities				
Long-Term Debt	1,400	1,200	200	16.7
Deferred Revenue	300	200	100	50.0
Total Noncurrent Liabilities	1,700	1,400	300	21.4
Total Liabilities	2,765	2,510	255	10.2
Unrestricted Fund Balance	470	320	150	46.9
Total Liabilities and Fund Balance	3,235	2,830	405	14.3

Table 15-2 Structural Ratio Analysis of Balance Sheet

CIVIC HOSPITAL

Condensed Balance Sheet—Unrestricted Fund

Structural Ratio Analysis

December 31, 1979, and 1980

Assets	*December 31, 198B*		*December 31, 198A*	
	Amount	*Percent*	*Amount*	*Percent*
Current Assets				
Cash	$300	9.3	$250	8.8
Temporary Investments	260	8.0	240	8.5
Receivables (Net)	400	12.4	420	14.8
Inventories	700	21.6	780	27.6
Prepaid Expenses	30	.9	20	.7
Total Current Assets	1,690	52.2	1,710	60.4
Board Designated Assets	500	15.5	100	3.5
Property, Plant, & Equipment	970	30.0	940	33.2
Other Assets	75	2.3	80	2.9
Total Assets	3,235	100.0	2,830	100.0
Liabilities and Fund Balances				
Current Liabilities				
Notes Payable	100	3.1	50	1.8
Accounts Payable	700	21.6	820	29.0
Accrued Expenses	65	2.0	50	1.8
Other	200	6.2	190	6.7
Total Current Liabilities	1,065	32.9	1,110	39.3
Noncurrent Liabilities				
Long-Term Debt	1,400	43.3	1,200	42.4
Deferred Revenue	300	9.3	200	7.0
Total Noncurrent Liabilities	1,700	52.5	1,400	49.4
Total Liabilities	2,765	85.5	2,510	88.7
Unrestricted Fund Balance	470	14.5	320	11.3
Total Liabilities and Fund Balance	3,235	100.0	2,830	100.0

Table 15-3 Structural Ratio Analysis of Income Statement

CIVIC HOSPITAL

Condensed Comparative Income Statements

Structural Ratio Analysis

Years Ended December 31, 198A and 198B

	198A		*198B*	
	Amount	*Percent*	*Amount*	*Percent*
Revenues				
Inpatient Revenue	$500	94.3	$400	94.1
Outpatient Revenue	30	5.7	25	5.9
Total Patient Service Revenue	530	100.0	425	100.0
Less Deductions from Patient Service Revenue	20	3.8	25	5.9
Net Patient Service Revenue	510	96.2	400	94.1
Net Patient Service Revenue (above)	510	92.7	400	93.0
Other Operating Revenue	40	7.3	30	7.0
Total Operating Revenue	550	100.0	430	100.0
Expenses				
Patient Service	350	63.6	290	67.4
Research	10	1.8	15	3.5
Education	20	3.7	10	2.3
General Services	70	12.7	65	15.2
Depreciation	30	5.4	40	9.3
Total Operating Expense	480	87.2	420	97.7
Net Operating Income	70	12.7	10	2.3
Nonoperating Income	20	3.6	30	7.0
Net Income (Loss) for the Year	90	16.3	40	9.3

two percentages pertaining to the years 198A and 198B indicate the relative contribution of inpatient and outpatient revenues to the total from that source in the two years examined. As indicated at the top of the table, the deductions from revenue are expressed as a percentage of gross patient service revenue. On the basis of these calculations, it can be concluded that, of each dollar of revenue generated, 3.8 cents results in a deduction in patient service revenue. The remaining percentages are computed by using total operating revenues as the base figure. For example, the expenses of providing patient services represent 63.6 percent of total operating revenue ($350/$550).

The Statement of Changes in Fund Balances and the Statement of the Sources and Applications of Funds may be examined by using structural ratios. It should be recognized, however, that in analyzing any of the financial statements, structural ratios must be supplemented with trends or observed changes over time to obtain an accurate portrayal of the various financial aspects of the institution.

15.2 RATIO ANALYSIS

The use of ratio analysis usually is limited to the examination of the financial position or balance sheet of a nonprofit hospital. This section also considers factors that influence the analysis of the operating results reported by the health care facility. It also examines this technique for evaluating the institution's current position.

15.2.1 Profitability Ratios

One of the primary objectives of the manager of a nonprofit institution is to ensure that the costs of operation are returned in the form of revenue. However, there is no clearcut criterion for judging the extent to which a "satisfactory" relationship between revenues and expenses has been obtained. On one hand, it can be argued that the hospital's financial objective should be to break even. On the other hand, given the pressures for improved service, the rapid advances in medical technology, and inflation, it can be argued that the institution should earn revenues in excess of expenses so it can meet the demands and pressures that confront it.

The most common measures of the excess of revenues over expenses are the net income ratio and the return on total assets. The first of these ratios is obtained by dividing net income by total operating revenues. The second, the return on total assets (ROA), is given by

$$ROA = \frac{\text{Net Income}}{\text{Total Tangible Assets}} \qquad \textbf{(15.1)}$$

To maximize the usefulness of these ratios, management should establish a desired relationship between net income and total operating revenue or between net income and total tangible assets. Such a relationship should be based, in part, on the need to replace or expand the capital complement of the institution. Once established, the desired relation between net income and tangible assets or total operating revenues should be regarded as a standard against which actual performance is compared.

Table 15-4 presents a set of ratios that can be used to evaluate the performance of a for-profit health facility. Since these ratios are self-explanatory, no further discussion seems necessary.

Table 15-4 Summary of Profitability Ratios

Profitability Ratio	*Definition*	*Comment*
Gross Profit Margin	$\frac{\text{Revenue} - \text{Expenses}}{\text{Revenue}}$	Shows that the higher the gross profit margin, the less susceptible the institution is to increases in costs.
Net Profit Margin	$\frac{\text{Net Profits After Taxes}}{\text{Patient Revenue}}$	Provides an indication of the institution's relative efficiency after taking into account all expenses and taxes.
Rate of Return on Common Stock Equity	$\frac{\text{Net Profits After Taxes} - \text{Preferred Stock Dividends}}{\text{Net Worth} - \text{Par Value of Preferred Stock}}$	Indicates the earning power of stockholder investment as stated in terms of book value.
Return on Assets	$\frac{\text{Net Profit After Taxes}}{\text{Total Tangible Assets}}$	Measures profitability in relation to investment.
Net Operating Rate of Return	$\frac{\text{Earnings Before Interest \& Taxes}}{\text{Total Tangible Assets}}$	Reflects profitability and is independent of the way the hospital is financed.

15.2.2 Activity Ratios

Closely involved with the measures of profitability is a set of ratios that relate operational performance to the asset holdings of the institution. Among the most important of these measures are: (1) the current asset turnover ratio, (2) the fixed asset turnover ratio, and (3) the total asset turnover ratio. Inventory turnover ratio and the number of days of inventory also are employed to measure the use of consumable supplies.

Consider first the set of ratios that relate the income generated during a given period to the assets of the institution. Normally, the total asset turnover ratio, TAT, is defined as

$$TAT = \frac{\text{Total Operating Revenues}}{\text{Total Tangible Assets}} \quad \textbf{(15.2)}$$

while

$$FAT = \frac{\text{Total Operating Revenues}}{\text{Fixed Assets}} \tag{15.3}$$

defines the fixed asset turnover ratio. Similarly, the current asset turnover ratio, *CAT*, is given by

$$CAT = \frac{\text{Total Operating Revenue}}{\text{Current Assets}} \tag{15.4}$$

These ratios measure the intensity with which the assets of the institution are used. It also is possible to substitute the working capital of the institution, as defined earlier, for current assets in Equation 15.4 and obtain a measure of the intensity of working capital use.

As mentioned previously, the information in the financial statements permits the analysis of the inventory the institution holds. In general, the health facility should maintain neither an excessive nor an insufficient quantity of consumable supplies. Consequently, management should maintain a reasonable relationship between inventory holdings and current assets as well as supply expenses. The relation between inventories and the total cost of supplies used may be evaluated by computing the inventory turnover ratio, *IT*, that is given by

$$IT = \frac{\text{Total Cost of Supplies Used}}{\text{Average Inventory}} \tag{15.5}$$

The ratio measures the number of times inventory is turned over during a given period. The value in the numerator usually is disclosed in the financial statements while the average inventory for the year is used in the denominator. An increase in *IT* (i.e., an increase in the number of times that inventory is turned over) is regarded as a favorable indication as to the efficiency of inventory management.

In addition to *IT*, the average number of days in supply, *NODS*, may be calculated:

$$NODS = \frac{\text{Number of Days in Year}}{IT} \tag{15.6}$$

In evaluating inventories, it should be recognized that they may be inadequate or excessive. Both of these situations can result in undesirable consequences.

For example, when excessive stocks are maintained, the institution incurs opportunity costs equal to the investment income that might have been earned on the funds spent on acquiring unnecessary supplies. Conversely, if inadequate supplies are maintained, the process of providing care could be interrupted, resulting in pain, suffering, and even death. It also should be noted that, when required data are available, management should compute both IT and $NODS$ by major categories of inventory so as to reflect the differing characteristics of the supplies used.

15.2.3 Liquidity Ratios

The analysis of the extent to which the health care facility is liquid closely parallels the examination of the current financial position of a commercial enterprise. However, the rules of thumb and ratio values regarded as acceptable in a commercial setting are not appropriate in the health care sector. Indeed, the best comparison available to management is one in which the institution's ratios are evaluated in terms of similar facilities in the same geographic area or in terms of ratio values that administration judges to be acceptable or desirable.

The hospital's current liquidity is of concern not only to financial managers but also to external groups such as bankers, creditors, governmental authorities, and third party payers. The ability to honor currently maturing obligations depends on the extent to which a sound financial position is maintained. In addition to assuring an adequate amount of working capital, management must be concerned with the liquidity of its current assets. That is, the institution should not invest in assets such as receivables or inventories that are not highly liquid. Some of the ratios used in obtaining impressions of the presence or absence of these conditions are discussed next.

15.2.3.1 Current Ratio

One of the most common measures of financial liquidity is the current ratio. This indicates the number of dollars of current assets for each dollar of current liabilities. In other words, the current ratio indicates the number of times the current assets of the institution will pay its current liabilities. Using the notation developed earlier, the current ratio, CR, is defined as:

$$CR = \frac{CA}{CL} \qquad \textbf{(15.7)}$$

A popular rule of thumb is that the current ratio should be 2:1 or higher. However, no one value for the current ratio applies to all health facilities. A ratio of 1.5:1 may be quite acceptable for one institution while a 2.5:1 ratio may be quite low for another. If the institution can pay its current obligations promptly and without undue hardship, the current ratio, whatever it is, must be adequate. Again it may be necessary for management to determine internally that the value of the current ratio is to be regarded as adequate.

15.2.3.2 Quick Ratio

Too much emphasis should not be placed on the current ratio as a measure of the facility's ability to meet its current obligations promptly. Clearly, some of the current assets (e.g., inventories) are not highly liquid and cannot be converted into cash immediately to satisfy maturing obligations. Further, the current ratio does not reflect the composition of current assets nor of current liabilities. For these reasons, the quick ratio, which sometimes is called the acid test, also is computed. The quick ratio is a more severe test of the ability of the facility to meet currently maturing obligations. Accordingly, the quick ratio, *QR*, is defined as

$$QR = \frac{\text{Cash} + \text{Temporary Investments} + \text{Net Receivables}}{CL} \qquad \textbf{(15.8)}$$

where the less liquid current assets have been excluded in the numerator.

15.2.3.3 Analysis of Receivables

As mentioned earlier, receivables are generated through the provision of patient care and the sale of goods or services (recoveries) to entities other than patients. The amount of receivables from patient services and from recoveries should not exceed a reasonable proportion of patient billings and charges to external agencies, respectively. This relationship may be quantified by computing the accounts receivable turnover ratio, *ART*. The accounts receivable turnover pertaining to patient accounts is defined as:

$$ART = \frac{\text{Net Patient Service Revenue}}{\text{Patient Receivables}} \qquad \textbf{(15.9)}$$

The numerator of *ART* should exclude revenues that are offset by a debit to cash and are not recorded as an account receivable. This ratio indicates the number of times during the year that the receivables are collected or turned over. An increase in this ratio usually is regarded as a favorable sign.

Another ratio used frequently in the analysis of receivables is the number of days charges in receivables, *NODCIR*. In general, *NODCIR* indicates the average time required to transform an outstanding receivable into cash. This measure is defined for patient service receivables and is calculated as follows:

$$NODCIR = \frac{\text{Number of Days in Year}}{ART} \qquad \textbf{(15.10)}$$

Unlike *ART*, a reduction in the *NODCIR* value indicates that the rate at which the receivables of the institution are transformed into cash has been accelerated.

ART and *NODCIR* are of value from the perspective of managing the institution's financial affairs. For example, whenever *ART* is low and *NODCIR* is high, the hospital forgoes income it could have earned by investing the amounts owed to it in an interest-earning security. To avoid such opportunity costs, management should carefully evaluate outstanding receivables. In such an evaluation, however, it is important to note that the resulting ratios are only averages that may fail to reflect the age distribution of the receivables adequately.

15.2.4 Capital Structure Ratios

Thus far, the analysis has considered neither the institution's level of debt nor its ability to support the debt burden. Obviously, both factors are of importance when assessing the long-run financial position of the health facility.

The capital structure of the institution is evaluated by constructing the debt ratio, the equity ratio, or the debt-to-equity ratio. More specifically, the debt ratio, *DR*, is given by

$$DR = \frac{\text{Total Debt}}{\text{Total Debt} + \text{Equity}} \qquad \textbf{(15.11)}$$

and indicates the proportion of all assets that is financed by liabilities as opposed to noncredit sources of funding. Since total assets must equal the sum of the total liabilities and the equity of the institution, the complement of the debt ratio is given by

$$ER = \frac{\text{Equity}}{\text{Total Assets}} \qquad \textbf{(15.12)}$$

which is called the equity ratio. In addition, the debt ratio may be combined with the equity ratio to obtain the debt-to-equity ratio. Letting D/E represent the debt to equity ratio, DR may be divided by ER to obtain

$$D/E = \frac{\dfrac{\text{Total Debt}}{\text{Total Debt + Equity}}}{\dfrac{\text{Equity}}{\text{Total Assets}}}$$

which means that

$$D/E = \frac{\text{Total Debt}}{\text{Equity}} \qquad \textbf{(15.13)}$$

Similar to the equity and debt ratios, the debt-to-equity ratio measures the extent to which assets are financed by noncredit sources of funding.

As noted, the ratios in this section may be used to evaluate the facility's capital structure. As a general rule, a reduction in the reliance on credit sources of funding (i.e., lowering DR and D/E or increasing ER) tends to improve the health care facility's long-run financial position. For example, a high debt ratio coupled with a series of periods during which operating results are unfavorable may impair the ability of management to honor currently maturing obligations. Moreover, if the institution is forced to seek a long-term loan, potential creditors may view a high debt ratio unfavorably and reject an application for funding.

On the other hand, a high debt ratio may be desirable during periods of inflation or when the institution uses equity as financial leverage. Concerning the latter possibility, an institution with a high debt ratio is said to be *trading on equity*. When trading on equity, the objective of management is to earn a percentage return on borrowed funds that is greater than the interest rates charged by the lender for the use of that money. As to the first of the two situations, suppose that the interest rate charged on long-term indebtedness is less than the rate of inflation. In that case, debtors repay long-term loans with dollars having a lower purchasing power than those borrowed initially. Even though such gains are not formally recognized in the accounting records, the advantages of repaying debts during periods of rapidly rising prices can be substantial.

Consider next the problem of evaluating the ability of the institution to support a given level of indebtedness. In addition to the ratios discussed earlier, potential creditors frequently use the times interest earned ratio to evaluate the safety of their investments. The times interest earned ratio, TIE, expresses the number of times interest charges are earned in the form of net income and is calculated as follows:

$$TIE = \frac{\text{Annual Net Income} + \text{Annual Interest Expense}}{\text{Annual Interest Expense}} \quad \textbf{(15.14)}$$

Obviously, the institution's ability to support a debt burden improves as the value of the *TIE* ratio increases. Moreover, it should be noted that no single value of the *TIE* ratio is regarded as satisfactory for all health facilities. Rather, the acceptability of the ratio depends not only on the stability of past earnings but also on the projected performance of the institution.

15.3 SUMMARY

In conclusion, the information in the financial statements of the health care facility can be of considerable value in evaluating its performance and financial position. However, managers must be cautioned against placing too much emphasis on the information in financial statements while ignoring the vital role performed by the institution. Rather, the data in the financial statements must be supplemented with many other factors when evaluating the institution's role as a community resource.

Questions for Discussion

1. Discuss the role of structural ratios in the analysis of financial statements.
2. Define and briefly describe the usefulness of the following ratios

   a. current ratio
   b. quick ratio
   c. *ART*
   d. *NODCIR*
   e. *IT*
   f. *NODS*

3. Explain the limitations of the financial statements in evaluating the performance of the health facility.
4. Describe the primary advantage of reporting comparative data in financial statements.
5. Define conditions under which data are comparable.
6. Explain the advantages and disadvantages of using ratios and percentages in the analysis of financial statements.

Problems for Solution

1. Suppose that Jamestown Hospital provides the following information:

	December 31	
	198B	*198A*
Cash	$600	$300
Investments (Current)	400	350
Accounts Receivable (Net)	1,000	1,200
Prepaid Expenses	500	470
Inventory	700	900
Plant and Equipment (Net)	9,100	9,000
Total Assets	12,300	12,220
Notes Payable (Current)	$200	$300
Accounts Payable	900	200
Accrued Expenses	100	400
Long-Term Debt	4,000	4,500
Deferred Revenue (Noncurrent)	1,000	200
Fund Balance	6,100	6,620
Liabilities and Fund Balance	12,300	12,220

Using these data, construct structural ratios and analyze the balance sheet of Jamestown Hospital.

2. Suppose that the following data also are provided by Jamestown Hospital:

	198B	*198A*
Revenues		
Inpatient	$4,000	$4,500
Outpatient	2,000	1,900
Deductions from Revenue	1,200	900
Other Operating Revenue	700	400
Expenses		
Supplies	2,850	3,100
Wages and Salaries	8,500	9,000
Depreciation	1,100	890
Interest Expense	50	45
Other Expenses	2,500	3,000

Use these data to construct structural ratios and analyze the operational performance of the hospital.

3. Construct the following ratios for 198A an 198B, using the information in Problems 1 and 2:

   a. Current Ratio
   b. Quick Ratio

c. *ART*
d. *NODCIR*
e. *IT*
f. *NODS*

On the basis of these calculations, describe conclusions that might be reached.

4. Calculate the debt ratio, the equity ratio, and the debt-to-equity ratio, using the information in Problem 1. Discuss conclusions that might be reached on the basis of these calculations.
5. Suppose the following information is available:

	198B	*198A*
Net Income	$150,000	$100,000
Interest Expense	20,000	25,000

Calculate the times interest earned ratio for these two years. Discuss the conclusions these calculations suggest.

Appendix

Table A-1 Present Value of $1.00

$$P = \frac{S}{(1 + r)^n}$$

Periods	4%	6%	8%	10%	12%	14%	16%	18%	20%	22%	24%	26%	28%	30%	40%
1	0.962	0.943	0.926	0.909	0.893	0.877	0.862	0.847	0.833	0.820	0.806	0.794	0.781	0.769	0.714
2	0.925	0.890	0.857	0.926	0.797	0.769	0.743	0.718	0.694	0.072	0.650	0.630	0.610	0.592	0.510
3	0.889	0.840	0.794	0.751	0.712	0.075	0.641	0.609	0.579	0.551	0.524	0.500	0.477	0.455	0.364
4	0.855	0.792	0.735	0.683	0.636	0.592	0.552	0.516	0.482	0.451	0.423	0.397	0.373	0.350	0.200
5	0.822	0.747	0.681	0.621	0.567	0.519	0.476	0.437	0.402	0.370	0.341	0.315	0.291	0.260	0.186
6	0.790	0.705	0.830	0.564	0.507	0.450	0.410	0.370	0.335	0.303	0.275	0.250	0.227	0.207	0.133
7	0.760	0.605	0.583	0.513	0.452	0.400	0.354	0.314	0.279	0.249	0.222	0.198	0.178	0.159	0.095
8	0.731	0.027	0.540	0.467	0.404	0.351	0.305	0.266	0.233	0.204	0.179	0.157	0.139	0.123	0.068
9	0.703	0.592	0.500	0.424	0.361	0.308	0.263	0.225	0.194	0.167	0.144	0.125	0.108	0.094	0.048
10	0.676	0.558	0.463	0.386	0.322	0.270	0.227	0.191	0.162	0.137	0.116	0.099	0.085	0.073	0.035
11	0.650	0.527	0.429	0.350	0.287	0.237	0.195	0.162	0.135	0.112	0.094	0.079	0.066	0.056	0.025
12	0.625	0.497	0.397	0.319	0.257	0.208	0.168	0.137	0.112	0.092	0.076	0.062	0.052	0.043	0.018
13	0.601	0.469	0.368	0.290	0.229	0.182	0.145	0.116	0.093	0.076	0.061	0.050	0.040	0.033	0.013
14	0.577	0.442	0.340	0.263	0.205	0.160	0.125	0.099	0.078	0.062	0.049	0.039	0.032	0.025	0.009
15	0.555	0.417	0.315	0.239	0.183	0.140	0.108	0.084	0.065	0.051	0.040	0.031	0.025	0.020	0.006
16	0.534	0.394	0.292	0.218	0.163	0.123	0.093	0.071	0.054	0.042	0.032	0.025	0.019	0.015	0.005
17	0.513	0.371	0.270	0.198	0.146	0.108	0.080	0.060	0.045	0.034	0.026	0.020	0.015	0.012	0.003
18	0.494	0.350	0.250	0.180	0.130	0.095	0.069	0.051	0.038	0.028	0.021	0.016	0.012	0.009	0.002
19	0.475	0.331	0.232	0.164	0.116	0.083	0.060	0.043	0.031	0.023	0.017	0.012	0.009	0.007	0.002
20	0.456	0.312	0.215	0.149	0.104	0.073	0.051	0.037	0.020	0.019	0.014	0.010	0.007	0.005	0.001
21	0.439	0.294	0.199	0.135	0.093	0.064	0.044	0.031	0.022	0.015	0.011	0.008	0.006	0.004	0.001
22	0.422	0.278	0.184	0.123	0.083	0.056	0.038	0.026	0.018	0.013	0.009	0.006	0.004	0.003	0.001
23	0.406	0.262	0.170	0.112	0.074	0.049	0.033	0.022	0.015	0.010	0.007	0.005	0.003	0.002	
24	0.390	0.247	0.158	0.102	0.066	0.043	0.028	0.019	0.013	0.008	0.006	0.004	0.003	0.002	
25	0.375	0.233	0.140	0.092	0.059	0.038	0.024	0.010	0.010	0.007	0.005	0.003	0.002	0.001	
26	0.361	0.220	0.135	0.084	0.053	0.033	0.021	0.014	0.009	0.006	0.004	0.002	0.002	0.001	
27	0.347	0.207	0.125	0.078	0.047	0.029	0.018	0.011	0.007	0.005	0.003	0.002	0.001	0.001	
28	0.333	0.196	0.118	0.089	0.042	0.026	0.016	0.010	0.006	0.004	0.002	0.002	0.001	0.001	
29	0.321	0.185	0.107	0.053	0.037	0.022	0.014	0.003	0.005	0.003	0.002	0.001	0.001	0.001	
30	0.368	0.174	0.099	0.057	0.033	0.020	0.012	0.007	0.004	0.003	0.002	0.001	0.001		
40	0.208	0.097	0.045	0.022	0.011	0.005	0.003	0.001	0.001						

Source: Reprinted from *Cost Accounting: A Managerial Emphasis* (3rd ed.) by Charles T. Horngren by permission of Prentice-Hall, Inc., © 1970.

Table A-2 Amount of an Ordinary Annuity

Amount of an Ordinary Annuity of $1 = $Ao\,\overline{n}\backslash\, i$

	Rate of interest, %							Rate of interest, %			
n	.5	1.0	1.5	2.0	2.5	3.0	4.0	5.0	6.0	8.0	10.0
1	1.0000	1.0000	1.0000	1.0000	1.0000	1.0000	1.0000	1.0000	1.0000	1.0000	1.0000
2	2.0050	2.0100	2.0150	2.0200	2.0250	2.0300	2.0400	2.0500	2.0600	2.0800	2.1000
3	3.0150	3.0301	3.0452	3.0604	3.0756	3.0909	3.1216	3.1525	3.1836	3.2464	3.3100
4	4.0301	4.0604	4.0909	4.1216	4.1525	4.1836	4.2465	4.3101	4.3746	4.5061	4.6410
5	5.0503	5.1010	5.1523	5.2040	5.2563	5.3091	5.4163	5.5256	5.6371	5.8666	6.1051
6	6.0755	6.1520	6.2296	6.3081	6.3877	6.4684	6.6330	6.8019	6.9753	7.3359	7.7156
7	7.1059	7.2135	7.3230	7.4343	7.5474	7.6625	7.8983	8.1420	8.3938	8.9228	9.4872
8	8.1414	8.2857	8.4328	8.5830	8.7361	8.8923	9.2142	9.5491	9.8975	10.6366	11.4359
9	9.1821	9.3685	9.5593	9.7546	9.9545	10.1591	10.5828	11.0266	11.4913	12.4876	13.5795
10	10.2280	10.4622	10.7027	10.9497	11.2034	11.4639	12.0061	12.5779	13.1808	14.4866	15.9374
11	11.2792	11.5668	11.8633	12.1687	12.4835	12.8078	13.4864	14.2068	14.9716	16.6455	18.5312
12	12.3356	12.6825	13.0412	13.4121	13.7956	14.1920	15.0258	15.9171	16.8699	18.9771	21.3843
13	13.3972	13.8093	14.2368	14.6803	15.1404	15.6178	16.6268	17.7130	18.8821	21.4953	24.5227
14	14.4642	14.9474	15.4504	15.9739	16.5190	17.0863	18.2919	19.5986	21.0151	24.2149	27.9750
15	15.5365	16.0969	16.6821	17.2934	17.9319	18.5989	20.0236	21.5786	23.2760	27.1521	31.7725
16	16.6142	17.2579	17.9324	18.6393	19.3802	20.1569	21.8245	23.6575	25.6725	30.3243	35.9497
17	17.6973	18.4304	19.2014	20.0121	20.8647	21.7616	23.6975	25.8404	28.2129	33.7502	40.5447
18	18.7858	19.6147	20.4894	21.4123	22.3863	23.4144	25.6454	28.1324	30.9057	37.4502	45.5992
19	19.8797	20.8109	21.7967	22.8406	23.9460	25.1169	27.6712	30.5390	33.7600	41.4463	51.1591
20	20.9791	22.0190	23.1237	24.2974	25.5447	26.8704	29.7781	33.0660	36.7856	45.7620	57.2750
21	22.0840	23.2392	24.4705	25.7833	27.1833	28.6765	31.9692	35.7193	39.9927	50.4229	64.0025
22	23.1944	24.4716	25.8376	27.2990	28.8629	30.5368	34.2480	38.5052	43.3923	55.4568	71.4027
23	24.3104	25.7163	27.2251	28.8450	30.5844	32.4529	36.6179	41.4305	46.9958	60.8933	79.5430
24	25.4320	26.9735	28.6335	30.4219	32.3490	34.4265	39.0826	44.5020	50.8156	66.7648	88.4973
25	26.5591	28.2432	30.0630	32.0303	34.1578	36.4593	41.6459	47.7271	54.8645	73.1059	98.3471
26	27.6919	29.5256	31.5140	33.6709	36.0117	38.5530	44.3117	51.1135	59.1564	79.9544	109.1818
27	28.8304	30.8209	32.9867	35.3443	37.9120	40.7096	47.0842	54.6691	63.7058	87.3508	121.0999
28	29.9745	32.1291	34.4815	37.0512	39.8598	42.9309	49.9676	58.4026	68.5281	95.3388	134.2099
29	31.1244	33.4504	35.9987	38.7922	41.8563	45.2189	52.9663	62.3227	73.6398	103.9659	148.6309
30	32.2800	34.7849	37.5387	40.5681	43.9027	47.5754	56.0849	66.4388	79.0582	113.2832	164.4940
35	38.1454	41.6603	45.5921	49.9945	54.9282	60.4621	73.6522	90.3203	111.4348	172.3168	271.0244
40	44.1588	48.8864	54.2679	60.4020	67.4026	75.4013	95.0255	120.7998	154.7620	259.0565	442.5926
45	50.3242	56.4811	63.6142	71.8927	81.5161	92.7199	121.0294	159.7002	212.7435	386.5056	718.9048
50	56.6459	64.4632	73.6828	84.5794	97.4843	112.7969	152.6671	209.3480	290.3359	573.7702	1163.9085

Source: Reprinted from *Hospital Financial Accounting: Theory and Practice* by L. Vann Seawell by permission of the Hospital Financial Management Association, © 1975.

Table A-3 Present Value of an Ordinary Annuity

Present Value of an Ordinary Annuity of $1 = $P_{o\,\overline{n}|\,i}$

n	Rate of interest, % .5	1.0	1.5	2.0	2.5	3.0	4.0	5.0	6.0	Rate of interest, % 8.0	10.0	15.0	20.0	25.0
1	.9950	.9901	.9852	.9804	.9756	.9709	.9615	.9524	.9434	.9259	.9091	.8696	.8333	.8000
2	1.9851	1.9704	1.9559	1.9416	1.9274	1.9135	1.8861	1.8594	1.8334	1.7833	1.7355	1.6257	1.5278	1.4400
3	2.9702	2.9410	2.9122	2.8839	2.8560	2.8286	2.7751	2.7232	2.6730	2.5771	2.4869	2.2832	2.1065	1.9520
4	3.9505	3.9020	3.8544	3.8077	3.7620	3.7171	3.6299	3.5460	3.4651	3.3121	3.1699	2.8550	2.5887	2.3616
5	4.9259	4.8534	4.7826	4.7135	4.6458	4.5797	4.4518	4.3295	4.2124	3.9927	3.7908	3.3522	2.9906	2.6893
6	5.8964	5.7955	5.6972	5.6014	5.5081	5.4172	5.2421	5.0757	4.9173	4.6229	4.3553	3.7845	3.3255	2.9514
7	6.8621	6.7282	6.5982	6.4720	6.3494	6.2303	6.0021	5.7864	5.5824	5.2064	4.8684	4.1604	3.6046	3.1611
8	7.8230	7.6517	7.4859	7.3255	7.1701	7.0197	6.7327	6.4632	6.2098	5.7466	5.3349	4.4873	3.8372	3.3289
9	8.7791	8.5660	8.3605	8.1622	7.9709	7.7861	7.4353	7.1078	6.8017	6.2469	5.7590	4.7716	4.0310	3.4631
10	9.7304	9.4713	9.2222	8.9826	8.7521	8.5302	8.1109	7.7217	7.3601	6.7101	6.1446	5.0188	4.1925	3.5705
11	10.6770	10.3676	10.0711	9.7868	9.5142	9.2526	8.7605	8.3064	7.8869	7.1390	6.4951	5.2337	4.3271	3.6564
12	11.6189	11.2551	10.9075	10.5753	10.2578	9.9540	9.3851	8.8633	8.3838	7.5361	6.8137	5.4206	4.4392	3.7251
13	12.5562	12.1337	11.7315	11.3484	10.9832	10.6350	9.9856	9.3936	8.8527	7.9038	7.1034	5.5831	4.5327	3.7801
14	13.4887	13.0037	12.5434	12.1062	11.6909	11.2961	10.5631	9.8986	9.2950	8.2442	7.3667	5.7245	4.6106	3.8241
15	14.4166	13.8651	13.3432	12.8493	12.3814	11.9379	11.1184	10.3797	9.7122	8.5595	7.6061	5.8474	4.6755	3.8593
16	15.3399	14.7179	14.1313	13.5777	13.0550	12.5611	11.6523	10.8378	10.1059	8.8514	7.8237	5.9542	4.7296	3.8874
17	16.2586	15.5623	14.9076	14.2919	13.7122	13.1661	12.1657	11.2741	10.4773	9.1216	8.0216	6.0472	4.7746	3.9099
18	17.1728	16.3983	15.6726	14.9920	14.3534	13.7535	12.6593	11.6896	10.8276	9.3719	8.2014	6.1280	4.8122	3.9279
19	18.0824	17.2260	16.4262	15.6785	14.9789	14.3238	13.1339	12.0853	11.1581	9.6036	8.3649	6.1982	4.8435	3.9424
20	18.9874	18.0456	17.1686	16.3514	15.5892	14.8775	13.5903	12.4622	11.4699	9.8181	8.5136	6.2593	4.8696	3.9539
21	19.8880	18.8570	17.9001	17.0112	16.1845	15.4150	14.0292	12.8212	11.7641	10.0168	8.6487	6.3125	4.8913	3.9631
22	20.7841	19.6604	18.6208	17.6580	16.7654	15.9369	14.4511	13.1630	12.0416	10.2007	8.7715	6.3587	4.9094	3.9705
23	21.6757	20.4558	19.3309	18.2922	17.3321	16.4436	14.8568	13.4886	12.3034	10.3711	8.8832	6.3988	4.9245	3.9764
24	22.5629	21.2434	20.0304	18.9139	17.8850	16.9355	15.2470	13.7986	12.5504	10.5288	8.9847	6.4338	4.9371	3.9811
25	23.4456	22.0232	20.7196	19.5235	18.4244	17.4131	15.6221	14.0939	12.7834	10.6748	9.0770	6.4641	4.9476	3.9849
26	24.3240	22.7952	21.3986	20.1210	18.9506	17.8768	15.9828	14.3752	13.0032	10.8100	9.1609	6.4906	4.9563	3.9879
27	25.1980	23.5596	22.0676	20.7069	19.4640	18.3270	16.3296	14.6430	13.2105	10.9352	9.2372	6.5135	4.9636	3.9903
28	26.0677	24.3164	22.7267	21.2813	19.9649	18.7641	16.6631	14.8981	13.4062	11.0511	9.3066	6.5335	4.9697	3.9923
29	26.9330	25.0658	23.3761	21.8444	20.4535	19.1885	16.9837	15.1411	13.5907	11.1584	9.3696	6.5509	4.9747	3.9938
30	27.7941	25.8077	24.0158	22.3965	20.9303	19.6004	17.2920	15.3725	13.7648	11.2578	9.4269	6.5660	4.9789	3.9950
35	32.0354	29.4086	27.0756	24.9986	23.1452	21.4872	18.6646	16.3742	14.4982	11.6546	9.6442	6.6166	4.9915	3.9984
40	36.1722	32.8347	29.9158	27.3555	25.1028	23.1148	19.7928	17.1591	15.0463	11.9246	9.7791	6.6418	4.9966	3.9995
45	40.2072	36.0945	32.5523	29.4902	26.8330	24.5187	20.7200	17.7741	15.4558	12.1084	9.8628	6.6543	4.9986	3.9998
50	44.1428	39.1961	34.9997	31.4236	28.3623	25.7298	21.4822	18.2559	15.7619	12.2335	9.9148	6.6605	4.9995	3.9999

Index

A

B

J

L

M

Q

R

S

T

U

V

W